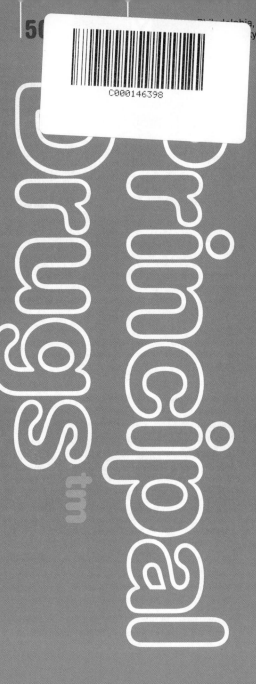

# Principal™

# Drugs

An Alphabetical Guide to
Modern Therapeutic Agents
and Their Use in Some
Common Disorders

## Eleventh Edition

## S.J. Hopkins

Honorary Consultant Pharmacist
Addenbrooke's Hospital
Cambridge

Philadelphia,
Tokyo

C000146398

| | |
|---|---|
| Publisher | **Jill Northcott** |
| Development Editor | **Gillian Harris** |
| Project Manager | **Louise Patchett** |
| Design | **Greg Smith** |
| Layout | **Gisli Thor** |
| Cover Design | **Greg Smith** |
| Production | **Hamish Adamson** |

Published by Mosby, an imprint of Mosby International Limited, Lynton House, 7–12 Tavistock Square, London WC1H 9LB, UK

ISBN 0 7234 3007 1

Printed by GraphyCems, Navarra, Spain

For full details of all Mosby titles, please write to Mosby International Publishers Limited, Lynton House, 7–12 Tavistock Square, London WC1H 9LB, UK.

A CIP catalogue record for this book is available from the British Library.

**Library of Congress Cataloging-in-Publication Data has been applied for.**

# Contents

# Preface

This book, primarily intended for nurses, has now reached its eleventh edition. The Dictionary section has been extensively revised and extended, and is an up-to-date guide to the wide range of drugs in current use, reflecting the advances that have been made in therapeutics in recent years. The section on some common illnesses has also been revised and now includes notes on angina, gout, prostatic hyperplasia and tuberculosis, and may extend the usefulness of the book to all those interested in modern drug therapy.

Most drugs are available under a proprietary or brand name and under an official approved or generic name. The British National Formulary (BNF) recommends that the latter should be used on prescription, so drugs are described under approved names in this book with brand names in brackets. An extensive list of both approved and proprietary names is given on pages 176–247. As this list includes some drugs not mentioned in the text, an indication is given of the nature or mode of action of the drug, so a reference back to a similar drug described in the Dictionary section may give helpful information. As a rule, no reference is given in the book to the numerous mixed products now available, the exceptions being those mixed products officially recognized by the BNF, exemplified by co-proxamol.

The doses given in this book are for guidance only, and although care has been taken to supply accurate information, the author does not assume any liability for errors or omissions. Before giving a drug, and for further information, reference should be made to official publications such as the **British National Formulary** or **Martindale's Extra Pharmacopoeia** or to Data Sheets and other literature issued by the manufacturer of the drug concerned.

It should be noted that three main groups of drugs are recognized:
(a) those generally available such as antacids and aspirin
(b) those available only from a pharmacy and
(c) those supplied only on the prescription of a medical practitioner.

There is a tendency to transfer some more commonly prescribed drugs to group (b), so no attempt has been made in this book to indicate any grouping.

As the side-effects and reactions of certain new drugs are not fully known, the Committee of Safety of Medicines keeps such new drugs under close surveillance, and requires any reactions to be reported on a 'Yellow Card'. Such drugs are distinguished by a blue inverted triangle. Controlled drugs (CDs), to which strict prescribing rules apply, are indicated by a dagger.

The publisher, in this edition, has used the international standard in abbreviating micrograms to μg. Readers should be aware that it is recommended that micrograms should be written out in full in all prescriptions.

Thanks are due to those readers who have commented on the book or suggested alterations, and a note of any errors or omissions will be appreciated. **S.J.H. 1998**

# Notes on dosage

In this dictionary of drugs, the doses, unless otherwise stated, are average daily doses for adults, and are normally given as divided doses at suitable intervals. An indication is given of those few drugs that are taken as a single daily dose, or where the dose is based on the surface area of the body expressed as square metres ($m^2$). When a dose range is indicated, a small initial dose is often followed by gradually increasing doses according to need and response, but with long-acting drugs care must be taken to avoid excessive dosage, as such drugs may then accumulate in the body and have toxic side-effects. It should be noted that the side-effects of a drug may prevent the administration of an optimum therapeutic dose, and a recommended dose is often a compromise between activity and toxicity. The gap is sometimes referred to as the 'therapeutic window', and the wider the gap the safer the drug.

Dosage is also influenced by the route of administration, as oral doses are normally larger than those given by intramuscular injection, and the latter are in turn larger than those given intravenously. The weight, age and sex of a patient may also have to be taken into account when assessing dosage. Renal and hepatic impairment may require an adjustment of dose, whereas if tolerance to a drug develops, a larger dose may be required to evoke an adequate response. Dosage also requires particular care during pregnancy if toxic effects on the fetus are to be avoided and, ideally, no drug should be given in pregnancy unless the need outweighs the risks.

Doses for infants also present problems. Their drug-detoxifying enzyme systems and renal excretory capabilities are not fully developed although, paradoxically, they have higher metabolic rates than adults, and so may sometimes require an apparently relatively high dose of a drug. Many schemes for basing children's doses on body weight, or body weight plus age, have been described, but doses based on surface area of the body are now considered more reliable. Taking the body surface of an average adult to be 1.8 $m^2$, the approximate dose of a drug for a child can be expressed as a percentage of the adult dose:

$$\frac{\text{surface area of patient as } m^2}{1.8} \times 100 = \text{per cent of adult dose}$$

(See Table 1)

Doses for the elderly also frequently require modification, as their reduced renal efficiency may cause accumulation of the drug and increase susceptibility to toxic effects, unless reduced doses are given. Elderly patients are, in any case, more susceptible to nephrotic drugs generally. Hepatic disease may also increase drug toxicity as liver enzymes play a major part in drug metabolism, and severe liver disease may give rise to a drug toxicity that might not otherwise occur. Hyperlipidaemic drugs, fusidic acid and some antifungal agents of the ketoconazole type are examples of drugs best avoided in hepatic disease. Multiple therapy may also lead to an increased and not always appreciated incidence of drug toxicity. For further information on these important aspects of drug dosage, a book for nurses on drugs and pharmacology should be consulted.

| Age | Body surface (m$^2$) | % of adult dose |
|---|---|---|
| *2 months | 0.28 | 15 |
| *4 months | 0.36 | 20 |
| 6 months | 0.4 | 22 |
| 12 months | 0.47 | 25 |
| 3 years | 0.62 | 33 |
| 7 years | 0.88 | 50 |
| 12 years | 1.25 | 75 |

* pre-term infants require reduced dose

Table 1 Estimating children's doses.

# Drug administration and responsibility

Nurses should remember that the responsibility for drug administration is delegated to them by doctors, and that they act under medical direction. There is a trend to extend nurses' responsibilities to certain aspects of drug administration that are normally dealt with by medical staff, and nurses should be clearly aware of what they are accountable for, and where their responsibility ends.

Before any drug is administered, the name of the drug and the dose should be checked with the prescription and the product. The golden rule is **READ THE LABEL**. If there is any doubt whatsoever, confirmation with a senior officer should be sought. **Belief** that the correct drug in the correct dose has been given is no substitute for certainty. Nurses are responsible for any errors that they may make, and must be prepared to accept the full consequences.

Recently the responsibilities of nurses have been extended by the publication of the Nurse Prescribers' Formulary, by which nurses are now allowed to prescribe a limited range of some commonly used drugs. This Formulary is a long overdue recognition of the part nurses play in medication generally and there can be little doubt that the limited range of prescribing now permitted will be extended as nurses rise to the new challenge of increased responsibility.

# Controlled drugs

Drugs likely to cause dependence and misuse are referred to as 'controlled drugs' (CDs), as they are subject to the strict prescription requirements of the Misuse of Drugs Act, 1971, and are distinguished in this book by a dagger †. They include opium, morphine, heroin (diamorphine), pethidine and other synthetic, potent analgesics/narcotics, dihydrocodeine injection, barbiturates (except intravenous anaesthetics) and amphetamines. Controlled drugs can be supplied only on receipt of a hand-written prescription from the prescriber, giving full details of the patient, the drug, the form and strength of the prescription to be dispensed, and the total amount to be supplied expressed in both words and figures. Certain weak preparations of some controlled drugs, such as Kaolin and Morphine Mixture for diarrhoea, with which misuse is unlikely, are exempt from control, and can be obtained without prescription.

# Drug compliance

An increasing problem of current therapy is patient compliance with prescribed treatment. It is easy for a doctor to prescribe, but to ensure that the patient takes the prescribed drugs in the right dose is a very different matter. The magnitude of the problem has increased with the rise in multiple therapy, and the reluctance on the part of some doctors to prescribe mixed products so that the number of different tablets or capsules to be taken daily can be reduced. It must be admitted that relatively few patients leave the consulting room with a clear idea of the nature and dose of the prescribed medication, partly as a result of fear of the doctor, and partly because of the difficulties of understanding complex therapy. Here, nurses can play a valuable part in reducing difficulties and misunderstandings, particularly when dealing with the elderly and/or confused patient, and it is often helpful to ask patients to repeat the directions that they believe they have been given. Misunderstandings and errors can then be cleared up at an early stage. The containers of the dispensed medicines should bear not only the name of the drug, but also useful additional information such as 'The Heart Tablets' or 'The Water Tablets'. Vague directions should be avoided: whenever possible definite times for administration of drugs should be arranged. Such timing can be linked with some regular activity, such as a meal time, or a favourite TV programme may be used as a memory aid for regular dosing. With multiple therapy, patients should be encouraged to set each day's dose aside, so that a double dose of a drug will not be taken by forgetfulness. Patients should be advised that the occasional missed dose is not always important, and a missed dose should *not* be made up by taking a double dose later on.

Although regular dosing is important in securing patient compliance, many modern drugs have relatively long half-lives so the regular administration of full doses for long periods may lead to overdose. The ideal dose depends on many factors, including absorption, metabolism, transport and excretion, but in many cases the margin of safety is fairly wide. In the elderly, however, reduced renal efficiency may lead to the gradual accumulation of a drug with insidious toxic effects. Many elderly patients, for example, on digoxin, may become over-digitalized because of poor metabolism and excretion of the drug. It is by no means unknown for elderly and confused patients, once admitted to hospital for observation, to make an apparently surprising recovery from an illness that was basically due to over-medication, often as a result of following blindly a misunderstood drug regimen. It is here that the community nurse has an exceptionally valuable part to play in ensuring regular and accurate medication, and reporting any incipient signs of overdose or side-effects.

# Dictionary of drugs

# A

**abciximab** A monoclonal antibody that inhibits platelet aggregation and thrombus formation. Used as an adjunct to heparin in percutaneous transluminal coronary angioplasty under expert supervision. (ReoPro).

**acamprosate** An analogue of GABA used in alcoholism. It assists in the maintenance of abstinence in alcohol-dependence, but prolonged treatment for a year may be required. **Dose:** 666 mg 3 times a day. (Campral).

**acarbose** An inhibitor of alpha-glucosidase, the enzyme that converts dietary carbohydrates to soluble sugars. Used in non-insulin-dependent-diabetes to reduce hyperglycaemic peaks after food.
**Dose:** 50 mg daily initially, rising to 150 mg daily if required. Side-effects are flatulence and diarrhoea; a hypoglycaemic reaction can be treated with oral glucose. (Glucobay). See page 131 and Table 13.

**ACE inhibitors** See angiotensin-converting enzyme inhibitors.

**acebutolol** A beta-adrenergic blocking agent with the actions, uses and side-effects of propranolol, but with a more cardioselective effect and less likely to cause bronchospasm.
**Dose:** in hypertension, 400–800 mg daily; in severe angina, up to 1.2 g daily. It is contraindicated in cardiogenic shock, atrioventricular-block and heart failure. Care is necessary in obstructive airway disease and renal failure (Sectral). See page 148 and Table 21.

**aceclofenac** A non-steroidal anti-inflammatory drug (NSAID) used for the relief of pain in arthritic and rheumatoid conditions. **Dose:** 200 mg daily. (Preservex). See page 131 and Table 29.

**acemetacin** A derivative of indomethacin with similar actions and uses, but said to be better tolerated.
**Dose:** 120–180 mg daily. (Emflex). See page 165 and Table 29.

**acetazolamide** An inhibitor of the enzyme carbonic anhydrase that has been given as a mild diuretic, as it increases the excretion of bicarbonate. Now used mainly in mild glaucoma, as it decreases intraocular pressure by reducing formation of aqueous humour. It has also been used in epilepsy.
**Dose:** 250 mg–1 g daily. In severe conditions it may be given in similar doses by i.v. injection. Side-effects are drowsiness, gastrointestinal disturbances and paraesthesia. (Diamox). See page 138 and Table 16.

**acetomenaphthone** A synthetic form of vitamin K, formerly used in prothrombin deficiency. Menadiol and phytomenadione are now preferred. Acetomenaphthone is present in some chilblain preparations.

**acetylcholine** The neurotransmitter of the parasympathetic nervous system. A 1% solution is sometimes used as a miotic to obtain rapid contraction of the pupil after cataract surgery. (Miochol).

**acetylcysteine** A mucolytic agent used as eye drops 5% in tear deficiency. Of value in the *early* treatment (10–15 hours) of paracetamol poisoning.
**Dose:** initially 150 mg/kg by slow i.v. injection, followed by smaller doses up to a total dose of 300 mg/kg over 20 hours. It is ineffective, and possibly harmful, if given at a later stage. (Parvolex). See methionine.

**acetylsalicylic acid** See aspirin.

**aciclovir** See acyclovir.

**acipimox** A derivative of nicotinic acid used in hypercholesterolaemia.
**Dose:** 500–750 mg daily. Side-effects are flushing, erythema, nausea and malaise. (Olbetam). See page 146 and Table 20.

**acitretin** A vitamin A derivative (retinol) used in severe psoriasis resistant to other treatment.
**Dose:** 20–30 mg daily. Teratogenic – see specialist literature. (Neotigason).

**aclarubicin** An anthracene cytotoxic agent of the doxorubicin type used in resistant acute non-lymphatic leukaemia. (Aclacin). See specialist literature.

**acrivastine** One of the newer antihistamines. It is less likely to cause drowsiness, as it does not cross the blood-brain barrier to any great extent, but is correspondingly less effective in non-allergic pruritus.
**Dose:** 24 mg daily. (Semprex). See page 110 and Table 2.

**ACTH** See corticotrophin.

**actinomycin D** A cytotoxic antibiotic, also known as dactinomycin, that inhibits cell division by forming a stable complex with DNA. It is used mainly in Wilm's tumour, and tumours of the uterus and testes.
**Dose:** 500 µg daily for 5 days by i.v. infusion, but other dosage schemes are in use. It is highly irritant to soft tissues, and great care must be taken to avoid extravasation. Close haematological control is necessary. Skin eruptions, alopecia and gastrointestinal disturbances are frequent side-effects. (Cosmogen). See page 122 and Table 8.

**acyclovir (aciclovir)** An antiviral agent highly active against herpes simplex and zoster viruses. It acts indirectly by inhibiting the DNA polymerase essential for viral replication.
**Dose:** 200 mg 5 times a day for 5 days in herpes simplex infections of the skin and mucous membranes, and in genital herpes; in shingles (herpes zoster), 800 mg orally 5 times a day for 7 days is given, but treatment should be started as soon as possible to obtain the maximum relief of pain. A 5% cream is used for superficial infections, and for herpes simplex keratitis a 3% ophthalmic ointment is available. Acyclovir is also of great value in herpes simplex infections in immunocompromised patients. Dose: 200 mg 4 times a day; 800 mg 5 times a day in zoster infections. In severe conditions, 5 mg/kg or more 8-hourly by i.v. infusion. It is also given orally for long-term prophylaxis in such patients. Reduced doses are necessary in renal impairment and in the elderly. Side-effects include gastrointestinal disturbances, rash and neurological reactions. (Zovirax). See page 144 and Table 19.

**adapalene∇** A new retinoid used like tretinoin in the treatment of acne. Applied as a 0.1% gel, once a day, taking care to avoid all mucous surfaces. Irritation may require temporary withdrawal. (Differin gel).

**adenosine** A cardiac drug that slows conduction through the AV node. It is used to restore normal sinus rhythm in paroxysmal tachycardia.
**Dose:** given by rapid i.v. injection as an initial dose of 3 mg. A second dose of 6 mg may be necessary after 1–2 minutes, and a third dose of 12 mg if the tachycardia

remains uncontrolled. For use only with close cardiac monitoring. (Adenocor).

**adrenaline (epinephrine)** Adrenaline is one of the principal hormones of the medulla of the adrenal gland, but is now made synthetically. It acts on both the alpha and beta receptors of the sympathetic nervous system. The effects of the alpha receptors result in vasoconstriction with a rise in blood pressure; stimulation of the beta receptors increases cardiac rate and output, and relaxes bronchial muscles.
**Dose:** in cardiac arrest, 0.2–0.5 ml of 1–1000 solution by s.c. or i.m. injection. In anaphylactic shock and allergic emergencies, 0.5–1 mg (0.5–1 ml of 1:1000 solution) is given by i.m. injection and repeated every 15 minutes as required. An i.v. injection of an antihistamine is sometimes given as supportive therapy. Doses of 100–200 µg (1–2 ml of 1:10 000 solution) have been given by intracardiac injection in cardiac arrest and syncope. In hypotensive crises, noradrenaline or metaraminol are preferred. Adrenaline is added to local anaesthetic solutions (1:50 000–1:200 000) to prolong the anaesthetic effect by reducing diffusion of the anaesthetic solution. Occasionally the solution is applied locally to stop capillary bleeding and epistaxis. It is also used as eye drops (1%) in chronic open angle glaucoma, but may cause redness and smarting of the eye. Solutions of adrenaline may darken on storage and lose activity.

**albendazole** An anthelmintic used in hydatid disease with larval cysts of the dog tapeworm. The cysts do not develop into worms, but increase in size to simulate liver abscess.
**Dose:** given as an adjunct to surgery in doses of 800 mg daily for 28 days, repeated after a 2-week rest period for 3 cycles, with liver tests and blood counts. (Eskazole).

**albumin (human)** Human albumin, obtained from pooled human plasma. Given by i.v. infusion as a 5–20% solution in the treatment of shock and other conditions where restoration of blood volume is urgent; in severe burns to prevent haemoconcentration, and in some conditions of hypoalbumaemia, and in acute oedema.

**alclometasone** A highly potent topical corticosteroid. It is used as a 0.05% cream or ointment in inflammatory and pruritic dermatoses likely to respond to such therapy. Contraindicated in infected skin lesions, and prolonged therapy should be avoided. (Modrasone).

**alcohol (ethanol)** Used occasionally by injection to destroy nerve tissue in the treatment of intractable trigeminal neuralgia. Industrial alcohol or methylated spirit contains 5% of wood naphtha; surgical spirit is industrial alcohol with the addition of methyl salicylate and other substances and is used for skin preparation and the prevention of pressure sores. Ordinary, coloured, methylated spirit contains pyridine, and is not suitable for medical purposes.

**aldesleukin** A recombinant form of interleukin-2, a lymphokinine that stimulates the production of interferon and T-lymphocytes. Used in metastatic renal cell carcinoma; severe toxicity is common. (Proleukin).

**aldosterone** The main mineralocorticoid hormone of the adrenal cortex. An excessive secretion of aldosterone may occur in some oedematous states and reduce the action of thiazide diuretics. See spironolactone and canrenoate.

**alendronate** A bisphosphonate used in postmenopausal osteoporosis. It inhibits osteoclast activity and increases bone strength, but continuous treatment is necessary.
**Dose:** 10 mg daily in the morning with water on an empty stomach, 30 minutes before food. Side-effects include severe oesophageal reactions. (Fosomax).

**alfacalcidol** A derivative of calciferol, with a more powerful and rapid action. It is used to treat hypocalcaemia in hypoparathyroidism, neonatal hypocalcaemia and other hypocalcaemic states, and in vitamin D-resistant conditions. Regular blood calcium determinations are essential as a drug-induced hypercalcaemia may take weeks to subside after withdrawal.
**Dose:** 1 mg orally or i.v. daily initially, according to response. (Alpha D; One-Alpha).

**alfentanil** A potent, rapidly acting narcotic analgesic, useful in short surgical procedures, or for longer operations in ventilated patients. The peak effect occurs

about 90 seconds after i.v. injection, with recovery after 5–10 minutes.
**Dose:** initially, 500 μg i.v., followed by 250 μg as required. (Rapiten).

**alfuzosin**∇ A selective alpha-adrenoceptor blocking agent for the symptomatic treatment of benign prostatic hypertrophy (BPH).
**Dose:** a first dose of 2.5 mg should be given in bed to avoid a marked first-dose hypotensive response, then 7.5 mg daily. Side-effects are dizziness, hypotension and tachycardia. (Xatral). See page 164 and Table 28.

**alglucerase**∇ An enzyme product used i.v. by specialists in Gaucher's disease. (Ceredase).

**alkylating agents** Cytotoxic drugs which act by damaging DNA, and so interfere with cell replication. Chlorambucil and cyclophosphamide are examples.

**allantonin** A natural substance said to promote wound healing. Present in some locally applied products for skin disorders.

**allergen vaccines** Weak allergen vaccines prepared from allergens such as grass pollens, house dust mites and bee stings are used to desensitize hypersensitive individuals but such treatment carries the risk of severe anaphylactic reactions, which may prove fatal in asthmatics, and it is now recommended that desensitization therapy should be carried out only when full cardiorespiratory resuscitation measures are immediately available.

**allopurinol** An enzyme inhibitor that blocks the formation of uric acid, and so is useful in the treatment of chronic gout. It also reduces the formation of uric acid calculi. It is useful in the hyperuricaemia of leukaemia but it should be given before cytotoxic therapy is commenced.
**Dose:** 100 mg daily as a single dose with food, slowly increased to 300 mg daily or more as required, reduced in cases of renal impairment. It may cause gouty arthritis initially, requiring colchicine or non-steroidal anti-inflammatory agent (NSAID) treatment for at least 1 month. Side-effects include nausea, headache and gastrointestinal disturbances, but skin reactions indicate withdrawal of the drug. (Zyloric). See page 140 and Table 17.

**alprazolam** A benzodiazepine used in the short-term treatment of anxiety and anxiety with depression.
**Dose:** 0.75–3 mg daily. Side-effects include dizziness and ataxia. Care is necessary in pulmonary insufficiency. (Xanax). See page 117 and Table 5.

**alprostadil** A preparation of prostaglandin E, for i.v. use in maintaining the patency of the ductus arteriosus in neonates with congenital heart lesions requiring surgical correction. The improvement in circulation so obtained permits diagnosis while surgery is being considered.
**Dose:** 50–100 ng/kg/min i.v. under strict control. Apnoea may occur, usually within an hour of the injection, requiring immediate ventilatory assistance. Bradycardia and hypotension may also occur. (Prostin VR).

**alteplase** A form of human plasminogen activator with a selective fibrinolytic action on blood-clot-bound plasminogen. It is of value in the *early* treatment (6 hours) of acute thrombosis, myocardial infarction and pulmonary embolism.
**Dose:** 10 mg initially by slow i.v. injection; then 90 mg over 3 hours by i.v. infusion. Side-effects are nausea, vomiting and local bleeding. (Actilyse). See streptokinase.

**aluminium** The powdered metal is used as a skin protective in ileostomy, as Baltimore paste, also known as Compound Aluminium Paste.

**aluminium acetate** An astringent used as an 8% solution for ear drops in otitis externa. A weak solution (0.65%) is used as a lotion in exudative eczematous states and in suppurative conditions.

**aluminium chloride** An antiperspirant used in the treatment of axillary hyperhydrosis by the local application of a 20% alcoholic solution. Over-use may cause skin irritation. (Anhydrol; Driclor).

**aluminium hydroxide** An antacid with a prolonged action.
**Dose:** as a gel, 7.5–15 ml, or as 500 mg tablets, to be chewed or crushed before swallowing. Best given between meals and at night. May interfere with the absorption of some other drugs. (Aludrox).

**alverine** An antispasmodic with a local action on intestinal smooth muscle.

**Dose:** used in irritable bowel syndrome in doses of 60–360 mg daily. (Spasmonal). See page 134 and Table 14.

**amantadine** An antiviral drug thought to act by inhibiting the penetration of the virus into the host cell, and used for the prophylaxis and treatment of influenza. It is also used with levodopa in the treatment of parkinsonism, but it may relieve the rigidity more than the tremor.
**Dose:** 200 mg daily. Many side-effects are dose-related. (Symmetrel). See page 160 and Table 26.

**amethocaine** Powerful local anaesthetic, used for anaesthetia of mucous membranes 1–2% solution, eye drops 0.25–1%. As spray for throat before endoscopy, etc, a 0.5% solution may be used. Hypersensitivity and allergic reactions may occur as with other local anaesthetics. Also used as 1% cream for pruritus and other skin conditions.

**amifostine**∇ An organic thiophosphoric acid used to reduce neutropenia-associated risks of infection after cyclophosphamide and platinum treatment of ovarian cancer.
**Dose:** by i.v. infusion 910 mg/m$^2$ daily 30 minutes before chemotherapy. Hypotension is a side-effect that may limit treatment. (Ethyol).

**amikacin** A semi-synthetic antibiotic similar in actions and uses to gentamicin, but more resistant to enzyme inactivation. Mainly used in the short-term treatment of serious infections due to Gram-negative, gentamicin-resistant organisms.
**Dose:** 15 mg/kg daily by i.m. injection or i.v. infusion, up to a total treatment dose of 15 g. Side-effects include ototoxicity, drug fever, rash and nausea. Dose should be reduced in renal impairment. (Amikin).

**amiloride** A potasssium-conserving diuretic with an action on the distal tubule similar to that of spironolactone, although it is not an inhibitor of aldosterone. It is used in hypertension and heart failure, often with a thiazide diuretic to obtain a more balanced response.
**Dose:** 5–20 mg daily. Rash is an occasional side-effect. See page 148 and Table 21.

**amino acids** Certain amino acids are essential for the formation of protein. When oral nutrition is not possible, amino acid preparations may be given by i.v. infusion, and such therapy can be extended if necessary to provide total parenteral nutrition by the addition of glucose, electrolytes, fats and vitamins as specially prepared solutions. In hospitals, a 24-hour supply for total parenteral nutrition can be provided in a single large container and patients may be taught to administer total parenteral nutrition at home. Representative amino-acid products for i.v. infusion are Aminoplex, Perfusin, Synthamin and Vamin.

**aminobenzoic acid** An absorbent of some of the erythema-producing ultra-violet light waves of sunlight. It is present in some sun screen preparations.

**aminoglutethimide** An inhibitor of adrenal steroid and oestrogen biosynthesis. It is used in the control of post-menopausal oestrogen-dependent mammary carcinoma and in the treatment of advanced prostatic carcinoma.
**Dose:** 250 mg daily, increased, if necessary, to 1 g daily. Supplementary corticosteroid therapy is essential. Side-effects include drowsiness, rash and drug fever. (Orimeten). See page 122 and Table 8.

**aminoglycosides** A group of antibiotics that includes amikacin, gentamicin, netilmicin, tobramycin, kanamycin, streptomycin, neomycin and framycetin. They act mainly against Gram-negative bacilli, although they are also active against some Gram-positive organisms. Kanamycin and streptomycin are also active against *Mycobacterium tuberculosis*. The aminoglycosides are not absorbed orally and when injected they are more toxic than most other antibiotics, and in renal impairment care is necessary, as the plasma concentration of the antibiotic may rise to an ototoxic or nephrotoxic level. The toxicity may also be increased by diuretics of the frusemide type. Measurement of plasma levels is essential in high dosage or continued therapy. Gentamicin is the most widely used aminoglycoside for systemic infections, and neomycin and framycetin, being too toxic for systemic use, are of value in skin infections.

**aminophylline** A derivative of theophylline with a similar bronchodilater action. It is used chiefly in asthma, cardiac oedema and congestive heart failure.
**Dose:** 300 mg–1.2 g orally daily; 5 mg/kg

may be given by slow i.v. injection. It is not suitable for i.m. administration. Sustained release oral products available cause less gastric disturbance. (Pecram; Phyllocontin). See page 118 and Table 6.

**amiodarone** An iodine-containing antiarrhythmic agent of value in all types of paroxysmal tachycardia, especially when the condition is resistant to other drugs.
**Dose:** 600 mg daily for 1 week; maintenance dose: 200 mg or less daily. When a rapid response is required, 5 mg/kg may be given by i.v. infusion under cardiac monitoring. It is contraindicated in bradycardia, pregnancy and thyroid disorders, and care is necessary in hepatic impairment. Pulmonary alveolitis, corneal microdeposits and photosensitivity have been reported as side-effects. (Cordarone).

**amitriptyline** A tricyclic antidepressant similar in action to imipramine, but it also has anxiolytic and sedative properties.
**Dose:** in depression complicated by anxiety, 30–150 mg daily initially; maintenance dose: 20–100 mg daily; sometimes as a single nightly dose to reduce daytime sedation. Lower doses are often adequate in elderly patients. Dose by injection, 40–80 mg daily. Full benefit may not be achieved for some weeks and prolonged therapy may be necessary to avoid relapse. Withdrawal of the drug should be gradual. Amitriptyline is also used in nocturnal eneuresis in children. Dose: 25–50 mg daily. Side-effects include dryness of the mouth, sedation and cardiac arrhythmias. It is contraindicated in glaucoma, prostatic hypertrophy and after recent myocardial infarction. (Lentizol; Tryptizol). See page 128 and Table 11.

**amlodipine** A calcium channel blocking agent used in hypertension and myocardial ischaemia associated with angina.
**Dose:** 5–10 mg as a single daily dose. Side-effects are headache, dizziness, flushing and oedema. Care is necessary in renal impairment. (Istin). See page 148 and Table 21.

**ammonium chloride** A mild expectorant present in Ammonia and Ipecacuanha Mixture.

**amorolfine** An antimycotic used in the treatment of fungal infections of the nails. It is applied to the nails as a lacquer (5%), but prolonged treatment at weekly intervals for some months is required until the nails are regenerated. Also cream 5% for skin infections. (Loceryl).

**amoxapine** A tricyclic antidepressant with the actions, uses and side-effects of imipramine, but giving a more rapid initial response.
**Dose:** 100–250 mg daily, with half dose for elderly patients. The side-effects of drowsiness may be reduced by giving a single daily dose at night. (Asendis). See page 128 and Table 11.

**amoxycillin** An orally active penicillin very similar to ampicillin, but absorption is less influenced by food. It is active against a wide range of organisms and is used in the treatment of respiratory, urinary and soft-tissue infections, and also in typhoid fever.
**Dose:** 750 mg–1.5 g daily. In severe infections doses up to 4 g daily by i.v. infusion. In simple, acute, urinary infections 2 oral doses of 3 g with 12 hours between doses. In the prophylaxis of bacterial endocarditis 1 or 2 doses of 3 g. The activity against penicillinase-producing organisms is increased by the combined use of clavulanic acid. (Amoxil).

**† amphetamine sulphate** A powerful central nervous system stimulant. It is now rarely prescribed because of the high risk of dependence. See dexamphetamine.

**amphotericin** An antifungal antibiotic, effective in systemic as well as superficial infections.
**Dose:** for systemic use, 250 µg/kg daily in 5% glucose solution by i.v. infusion, and increased if tolerated to a maximum of 1 mg/kg daily. Side-effects, often severe, are numerous and include vomiting, fever, cardio- and nephrotoxicity. (Abelcet and Ambisone are modified products with reduced toxicity.) For intestinal candidiasis, doses of 400–800 mg daily are given orally. For superficial infections 3% ointment is applied locally. (AmBisone; Fungicillin).

**ampicillin** An acid-stable and orally active penicillin. It is inactivated by penicillinase-producing organisms and most staphylococci are now resistant to ampicillin. It is used in chronic bronchitis, ear infections, and infections of the biliary and urinary tracts.
**Dose:** 1–2 g orally or by i.m. injection; in severe infections, up to 4 g daily by i.v.

infusion. In urinary infections, doses of 1.5 g daily are given, but in gonorrhoea, a single dose of 2 g with 1 g of probenecid is often effective. Skin reactions are relatively common but the urticarial type is indicative of penicillin allergy, and requires a change of treatment. A macro-papular rash is frequent with patients with infective mono-nucleosis and treatment with ampicillin should be discontinued. (Amfipen; Penbritin).

**ampiclox** A mixed product containing ampicillin 250 mg and cloxacillin 250 mg.

**amsacrine** A synthetic cytotoxic agent similar in action to doxorubicin but less cardiotoxic.
**Dose:** in refractory myeloid leukaemia 90 mg/m$^2$ daily for 5 days by i.v. infusion. Subsequent doses at intervals of 2–4 weeks according to response. Strict control is essential as hypokalaemia with fatal arrhythmia has occurred. Side-effects include nausea, stomatitis, alopecia, myelo-suppression and epileptiform seizures. (Amsidine). See page 112 and Table 8.

**amylobarbitone** A barbiturate of medium intensity.
**Dose:** 100–200 mg. Sodium derivative is more rapid in action, but the effect less prolonged; it has been given i.v. for the control of convulsions and in epilepsy. (Amytal). See page 152.

**anabolic steroids** Compounds related to testosterone with similar protein-building properties but reduced virilizing effects. They have been used to stimulate protein synthesis after major surgery and in wasting disease, but the response is often disappointing. They are sometimes used to relieve the itching of chronic biliary obstruction, but may exacerbate the associated jaundice. Some anabolic steroids have been used in high doses in aplastic anaemia, and as palliatives in breast cancer. Side-effects are oedema and jaundice, and hepatic impairment is a contraindication. They should not be given to children as they may cause premature closing of the epiphyses. See nandrolone; stanozolol.

**anastrozole** An inhibitor of aromatase, the enzyme involved in the conversion of androgens to oestrogens by the adrenal gland. Used in post-menopausal oestrogen-dependent breast cancer as it reduces the plasma level of oestrogens.

**Dose:** 1 mg as a single daily dose. Supplementary steroid therapy is unnecessary. Side-effects are hot flushes, vaginal dryness and hair thinning. (Arimidex). See page 122 and Table 8.

**aneurine hydrochloride** See thiamine.

**angiotensin converting enzyme inhibitors (ACE)** Drugs which inhibit the conversion of angiotensin I (secreted by the kidney) to angiotensin II (a powerful hypertensive) and thus, indirectly, lower blood pressure. ACE inhibitors are used in the treatment of hypertension, especially in severe conditions that have not responded to other therapy, and also in congestive heart failure. Initial therapy requires care, as a marked first-dose fall in blood pressure may occur. The first dose is best given at night, with the patient in bed, and if possible any diuretic treatment should have been suspended for a few days. Renal function should be monitored during ACE inhibitor therapy, as these drugs may cause a progressive and sometimes severe renal impairment. See page 148 and Table 21.

**anistreplase** A complex of streptokinase with human plasminogen, used to restore blood flow after myocardial infarction. It binds with the fibrin of blood clots, and is slowly metabolized to release the active fibrinolytic agent plasmin. It is given by i.v. infusion as a single dose of 30 units, within 6 hours of infarction up to a total dose of 100 mg over 3 hours. Side-effects include transient hypotension, nausea, flushing and allergic reactions. (Eminase).

**antazoline** A mild antihistamine, used with the vasoconstrictor naphazoline as a nasal spray to reduce local congestion in sinusitis and rhinitis, and as eye drops in allergic conjunctivitis. (Otrivine).

**antibiotics** Antibacterial substances which occur as by-products of the growth of certain moulds. The term now includes some synthetic derivatives. The first to be discovered was penicillin, but some penicillin derivatives (amoxycillin, ampicillin and pivampicillin) have a wider range of activity; others (cloxacillin and flucloxacillin) are effective against resistant staphylococci. Azlocillin, carfecillin, piperacillin and ticarcillin are more effective against *Pseudomonas aeruginosa*. Antibiotics with a more extensive range of

action are represented by aureomycin, chloramphenicol, the tetracyclines, and the cephalosporins. The aminoglycoside antibiotics represented by gentamicin are used mainly in infections due to Gram-negative organisms, but are more toxic than the penicillins or related drugs. Rifampicin is an antibiotic used mainly in tuberculosis. Broad-spectrum antibiotics should not be given for more than 5–10 days, to prevent disturbance of normal bacterial flora in the gut leading to overgrowth of other organisms such as candida. Certain antibiotics, including neomycin and bacitracin, are too toxic for systemic use but may be useful in the treatment of infected skin conditions.
A few antibiotics such as actinomycin, bleomycin, doxorubicin, mitomycin and aclarubicin have cytotoxic properties. Others, such as griseofulvin, have only an antifungal action.

**anticholinergic agents (antimuscarinics)** Drugs like atropine that inhibit the activity of the neurotransmitter acetylcholine. They are used as smooth muscle relaxants, as inhibitors of gastric secretion, and to reduce the excessive cholinergic activity associated with Parkinson's disease. By their nature, they have side-effects such as dryness of the mouth and blurred vision, and are contraindicated in glaucoma. See page 160 and Table 26.

**anticoagulants** Blood clots consisting mainly of fibrin may form in the venous circulation, and heparin and warfarin are used as anti-coagulants in deep vein thrombosis. Heparin is also used prophylactically against postoperative thrombosis and during renal dialysis, and in low doses to reduce the risks of pulmonary embolism.

**anticonvulsants** Also known as anti-epileptics, these are used to control the convulsions of epilepsy. The main types of convulsions or seizures are *grand mal* and *petit mal* (absence seizures) but atypical and myoclonic seizures may also occur. Some drugs are effective in most types of seizure, others are more selective in action, but in all cases dosage must be adjusted to need and response. Any change of treatment requires care with overlapping doses to avoid loss of control. Paradoxically, young children may require relatively high doses. See page 136 and Table 15.

**antidepressants** The drugs used in the treatment of depression fall into two main groups, the so-called tricyclic anti-depressants and the monoamine oxidase inhibitors (MAOIs). (Unrelated drugs include lithium carbonate, used only for the prophylaxis and treatment of manic depressive illness.) The tricyclic group, which also includes some other com-pounds with a similar action, appear to act by blocking the neuronal uptake of central transmitters such as noradrenaline and serotonin. They are more widely used than the MAOIs because they are more generally effective, and interact less exten-sively with other drugs and certain foods. The tricyclic drugs are widely used in endogenous depression, particularly when sleep disturbances are present, but the onset of action is slow, and improvement may not commence until after 2–4 weeks of treatment. Extended therapy is usually required to avoid the risk of a relapse, and patients should be advised accord-ingly. Some tricyclic antidepressants, such as amitriptyline, have a sedative action of value when anxiety is a complicating factor, whereas a less sedating drug such as imipramine may be useful in patients exhibiting apathy and withdrawal. Some of the side-effects, such as dryness of the mouth, are linked with their anti-cholinergic activity, but tolerance may develop with continued treatment. They also influence the cardio-vascular system and may cause arrhythmias, tachycardia and hypotension, and may interfere with the action of some antihypertensive drugs, although the response to beta-blocking agents is unaffected. Care is necessary in cardiac disease, and with the elderly initial doses should be low. The use of tricyclic antidepressants in epileptic patients may result in a lowering of the convulsive threshold. See page 128 and Table 11.

**antidiabetic agents** *Diabetes mellitus* is a deficiency disease due to a lack of insulin, and is characterized by an excessive level of glucose in the blood and urine. Treatment is either replacement therapy with daily injection of insulin, or orally by hypogly-caemic agents such as chlorpropamide. Such agents act by stimulating insulin secretion and release by the beta-cells of the pancreas, and are ineffective in the absence of such cells. See page 132 and Tables 12 & 13.

**anti-D(Rh$_o$) immunoglobulin** An immunoglobulin that is given to a rhesus-negative mother to prevent her forming anti-bodies against fetal rhesus-positive cells which may pass into the maternal circulation during childbirth or abortion and which, in a later pregnancy, could cause haemolytic disease.
**Dose:** 500 units i.m. within 60–72 hours of delivery or abortion. Doses of 1250 units are given prophylactically. It is of no value if given after anti-D antibodies have been formed. The immunoglobulin has also been given after the transfusion of rhesus-incompatible blood. (Partobulin).

**antiemetics** Nausea and vomiting may be due to several causes, including stimula-tion of the chemoreceptor trigger zone in the reticular formation of the brain. Many antiemetics have some degree of central activity, and in some cases their action may be mediated by blocking the effects of dopamine on the trigger zone. Effective drugs include some antihistamines and some phenothiazine-based tranquillizers such as prochlorperazine. The alkaloid hyoscine is widely used in travel sickness. More powerful drugs such as domperi-done, metoclopramide, nabilone and ondansetron, are of value in the control of the severe nausea and vomiting induced by cytotoxic drugs. The use of antiemetics in early pregnancy requires great care, and is seldom essential.

**antiepileptics** See anticonvulsants, page 136 and Table 15.

**antihistamines** Drugs such as prometh-azine are of value in conditions associated with the release of histamine from mast cells, such as hayfever, rhinitis, urticaria, pruritus, insect bites and stings. They are also useful in drug allergies. Some antihist-amines also have antiemetic properties, and are useful in travel sickness. Although all antihistamines have the same basic action, the degree and duration of response and the severity of side-effects may vary. Some antihistamines pass easily into the central nervous system and are more likely to cause drowsiness. Others may have reduced anticholinergic proper-ties, and cause less dryness of the mouth and blurring of vision. Care is necessary in epilepsy, glaucoma, hepatic disease or prostatic enlargement. See page 110 and Table 2.

**antihypertensive agents** See page 148 and Table 21.

**anti-inflammatory agents** See non-steroidal anti-inflammatory drugs (NSAIDS) and page 165 and Table 29.

**antimetabolites** Cytotoxic drugs that appear to act by combining irreversibly with cell enzymes, and so prevent cell division. Methotrexate and mercaptopurine are examples. See page 122 and Table 8.

**antimuscarinic agents** See anticholinergic agents, page 160 and Table 26.

**antineoplastic agents** Anti-cancer drugs. See page 122 and Table 8.

**antipsychotic agents** See pages 117 & 168, and Tables 5 & 30.

**antitetanus immunoglobulin** Human antitetanus immunoglobulin obtained from plasma is used in injured patients who have not previously been immunized, and when tetanus is a definite risk.
**Dose:** 250 units i.m. A course of tetanus vaccine should also be commenced.

**antitubercular agents** See rifampicin, page 170 and Table 31.

**antiviral agents** See page 144 and Table 19.

**anxiolytics** See page 117 and Table 5.

**apomorphine** A morphine derivative formerly used as a powerful emetic, but now considered to be too toxic. Occasionally used in the hospital treatment of parkinsonism. (Britaject).

**apraclonidine** A clonidine derivative used as eye drops 1% to control intraocular pressure during ophthalmic surgery. Some absorption may occur, so care is necessary in severe cardiovascular disease. (Iopidine).

**aprotinin** An inhibitor of the proteolytic enzyme plasmin, obtained from bovine lung tissue. It is used in the severe haemorrhage due to hyperplasminaemia.
**Dose:** 500 000–1 000 000 units by i.v. infusion. (Trasylol).

**arachis oil** Groundnut or peanut oil. It has emollient properties, and is used in dermatology and pruritus as oily calamine lotion. Arachis oil enema is used to soften impacted faeces.

**argipressin** A synthetic form of vasopressin.

**artificial tears** Some chronic sore eye conditions may occur in rheumatoid arthritis, and may be due to tear deficiency. Solutions of hypromellose or polyvinylalcohol, sometimes referred to as 'artificial tears', are useful as a bland lubricant to replace the tear deficiency. (Isopto; Hypotears).

**ascorbic acid (vitamin C)** Present in many citrus fruits. Deficiency is not uncommon in the elderly receiving inadequate diets. Severe deficiency causes scurvy, once the bane of seafarers.
**Dose:** for prophylaxis 25–75 mg daily; therapeutic dose 200–500 mg daily. Doses of 4 g daily are given for acidification of the urine. Claims that vitamin C prevents colds are unproven.

**asparaginase** Crisantaspase. See page 122 and Table 8.

**aspirin (acetylsalicylic acid)** Widely used as a mild analgesic and anti-inflammatory agent, often in association with other drugs such as paracetamol and codeine.
**Dose:** 1.2–4 g daily, but in acute rheumatoid conditions doses of 4–8 g daily have been given. Long-term treatment with doses of 75 mg daily are given for the prophylaxis of cardiovascular disease. Side-effects include gastric irritation with some blood loss, hyperventilation, and tinnitus, with the risk of deafness, may occur with high doses. Aspirin may cause rash and bronchospasm in asthmatic and other sensitive patients. As aspirin is now thought to be associated with Reye's syndrome, the drug should not be given to children under 12 years of age unless specifically indicated. Aspirin may increase the effects of certain hypoglycaemic and anticoagulant drugs.

**astemizole** An antihistamine with an extended action and reduced sedative effects.
**Dose:** 10 mg once daily before food, and must not be exceeded. Higher doses may cause cardiotoxic side-effects such as ventricular tachycardia. Arrhythmias may follow combined treatment with many other drugs. (Hismanol; Pollen-ese). See page 110 and Table 2.

**atenolol** A long-acting beta-adrenoceptor blocking agent of the propranolol type, but with a more cardioselective action. Used mainly in hypertension and angina.
**Dose:** 50–100 mg daily. Also given by slow i.v. injection in arrhythmias in doses up to 10 mg. The side-effects are similar to propranolol, although atenolol may cause fewer sleep disturbances. (Tenormin). See pages 114 & 148, and Tables 4 & 21.

**atorvastatin**∇ A lipid-lowering agent with an enzyme-inhibitory action on cholesterol synthesis used in hyperlipidaemia.
**Dose:** 10 mg daily initially, up to a maximum of 80 mg daily. Liver function tests are necessary before and during treatment. (Lipitor). See page 146 and Table 20.

**atovaquone** An antibacterial agent used in *Pneumocystis carinii* pneumonia resistant to co-trimoxazole.
**Dose:** 750 mg daily with food for 21 days. Side-effects are rash, nausea and diarrhoea. (Wellvone).

**atracurium** A non-depolarizing muscle relaxant of the gallamine type, but causing less histamine release.
**Dose:** 300–600 µg/kg i.v. initially followed by doses of 100–200 µg/kg at intervals as required. Its action can be reversed, if necessary, with neostigmine. Aminoglycoside antibiotics may increase the response and require an adjustment of dose. (Tracrium).

**atropine** An alkaloid with anticholinergic properties obtained from belladonna, hyoscymus and other plants. It is often given in doses of 300–600 µg by injection with morphine for preoperative sedation and to reduce bronchial secretion. Is also of value in gastrointestinal smooth muscle spasm.
**Dose:** 0.25–2 mg daily. It is used as eye drops (1%) to dilate the pupil, but such use in the elderly requires care, as the long action may precipitate glaucoma. It is also used with neostigmine in doses of 600 µg–1.2 mg to reverse the action of the vecuronium-type muscle-relaxants. Side-effects include dryness of the mouth, disturbed vision, and bradycardia followed by tachycardia. Care is necessary in prostatic enlargement and urinary disturbances, and glaucoma is a contraindication.

**augmentin** See co-amoxiclav.

**auranofin** An orally active gold compound used in the treatment of active rheumatoid arthritis not relieved by non-steroidal anti-inflammatory drugs (NSAIDs).
**Dose:** 6 mg daily, increased if necessary after 6 months to 9 mg daily. It should be withdrawn if the response is inadequate after 9 months. Side-effects are nausea and diarrhoea. See sodium aurothiomalate for the systemic side-effects of gold therapy. (Ridaura). See page 165 and Table 29.

**avomine** Derivative of promethazine used in travel sickness, nausea and vomiting.
**Dose:** 25–150 mg daily.

**azapropazone** A non-steroidal anti-inflammatory agent (NSAID) with actions and uses similar to those of naproxen and used when other NSAIDs are unsuitable.
**Dose:** 1.2 g daily, but in acute gout an initial, divided, dose of 1.8 g is given. Side-effects include rash and occasional photosensitivity, and care is necessary in peptic ulcer. Azapropazone may potentiate the action of warfarin and phenytoin, and require an adjustment of dose. (Rheumox). See page 165 and Table 29.

**azatadine** An antihistamine with the actions and uses of promethazine.
Dose: 1–2 mg twice daily. (Optimine). See page 110 and Table 2.

**azathioprine** An immunosuppressive agent mainly used to inhibit rejection after organ transplant surgery. It has also been used in some auto-immune conditions and in resistant ulcerative colitis.
**Dose:** 1–5 mg/kg daily, but dose and duration vary according to need and response. Side-effects include depression of bone marrow function, gastrointestinal disturbances, hepatotoxicity and rash. Severe secondary infections may occur as a result of the immunosuppression, and the use of the drug requires close control. (Azamine).

**azeolic acid** An organic acid with some antibacterial properties. Used as 20% cream for acne vulgaris. (Skinoren).

**azelastine** An antihistamine used as a nasal spray 0.1% in allergic rhinitis. (Rhinolast).

**azidothymidine** See zidovudine.

**azithromycin** A macrolide antibiotic with a longer action than erythromycin or clarithromycin, used chiefly in respiratory tract infections.
**Dose:** 500 mg daily for 3 days, 1 hour before or 2 hours after food or antacids. Side-effects include nausea, abdominal discomfort and diarrhoea. Not to be given with astemizole or terfenadine (risk of arrhythmias). (Zithromax).

**azlocillin** A broad-spectrum antibiotic with exceptional activity against *Pseudomonas*. Of value in respiratory and urinary infections, and in septicaemia.
**Dose:** in life-threatening infections, 5 g by i.v. infusion 8-hourly. Doses of 2 g 8-hourly may be given in less severe infections. In patients with impaired renal function, doses should be given 12-hourly. Allergy to penicillins or cephalosporins is a contraindication. (Securopen).

**AZT** See zidovudine.

**aztreonam** An antibiotic that is exceptional in being resistant to breakdown by beta-lactamases. It has a selective action against Gram-negative aerobes, and it is given in urinary, respiratory, bone and other infections caused by susceptible bacteria. When given in association with an aminoglycoside, the activity of aztreonam against *Pseudomonas aeruginosa* may be increased.
**Dose:** 4 g daily by i.m. injection and up to 8 g daily i.v. in severe infections. Reduced doses are indicated in renal impairment. Side-effects are skin reactions, nausea, jaundice, blood disorders, and malaise. (Azactam).

**B**

**baclofen** A muscle relaxant that acts on the spinal end of some motor neurones. Useful in multiple sclerosis and muscle spasms caused by spinal lesions.
**Dose:** 15 mg daily initially gradually increased, as required, up to a maximum of 100 mg daily. Side-effects include nausea, fatigue and hypotension. Care is necessary in epilepsy and psychiatric disorders. Withdrawal of treatment is slow over 1–2 weeks to avoid serioius side-effects. In severe spasticity and spinal injury, baclofen

is given by intrathecal injection in small doses via an implantable pump, but treatment requires specialist supervision. (Lioresal).

**BAL** See dimercaprol.

**balsalazide** A melsalazine complex used in ulcerative colitis. It reaches the colon unchanged, where it is broken down to release active melsalazine.
**Dose:** 9 g daily until remission or for 12 weeks. Side-effects are those of melsalazine. See page 172 and Table 32.

**bambuterol** A prodrug of terbutaline, with a similar but more prolonged bronchodilator action.
**Dose:** 10–20 mg at night. (Bambec). See page 118 and Table 6.

**† barbiturates** A group of hypnotic drugs exemplified by butobarbitone. Once widely used, but their value has declined sharply and safer drugs such as nitrazepam are now preferred.

**barium sulphate** A very insoluble powder, given orally or rectally as an aqueous suspension as contrast agent for X-ray examination of the alimentary system.

**BCG vaccine** A preparation of the Calmette–Guérin strain of *Mycobacterium tuberculosis*. It is used for active immunization against tuberculosis. particularly for individuals likely to be exposed to infection.
**Dose:** 0.1 mL by intradermal injection. A product obtained from an isoniazid-resistant strain of the organism is also used for the immunization of individuals receiving prophylactic treatment with isoniazid.

**beclomethasone** A potent corticosteroid used in the control of asthma and bronchospasm not responding to other drugs.
**Dose:** by oral aerosol inhalation, 100 µg (two puffs) repeated up to 4 times a day according to need and response. Dose: by powder inhalation 800 µg daily. Hoarseness may develop as a side-effect, and oral candidiasis may occur with high doses. Beclomethasone is also used as a cream or ointment (0.025%) in severe inflammatory skin conditions not responding to less potent corticosteroids. (Becotide; Propaderm).

**bendrofluazide** A widely used diuretic of the thiazide group, with a powerful and prolonged action. It is used in congestive heart failure, oedema and mild hypertension. In more severe hypertension it is given together with other drugs to increase the overall response.
**Dose:** 2.5–10 mg daily. It causes some loss of potassium, so potassium supplements are required if treatment is prolonged. Side-effects include rash and thrombocytopenia. Renal failure is a contraindication. (Aprinox; Neo-Naclex). See page 148 and Table 21.

**benorylate** A compound of aspirin and paracetamol, with the general properties of both drugs, but generally better tolerated than aspirin. Used in arthritic conditions and for the relief of painful musculoskeletal disorders.
**Dose:** 3–6 g daily. Like aspirin, it may cause gastrointestinal disturbances and increase the action of oral anticoagulants. (Benoral).

**benperidol** A tranquillizer of the haloperidol type with similar side-effects, but used to control antisocial sexual behaviour in adults.
**Dose:** 0.25–1.5 mg daily. (Anquil).

**benserazide** An enzyme inhibitor used with levodopa in parkinsonism. It inhibits the breakdown of levodopa to dopamine, enabling large amounts to reach the brain, and so permits a reduction in dose and a smoother response. Some of the side-effects of levodopa, such as nausea and vomiting, may also be reduced, although the incidence of involuntary movements may increase.
**Dose:** 12.5 mg with 50 mg of levodopa. (Madopan). See page 160 and Table 26.

**benzalkonium chloride** A detergent with antiseptic properties present in various skin preparations. It is also used as a preservative in eye drops.

**benzhexol** A spasmolytic drug used mainly to relieve the tremor and rigidity of parkinsonism.
**Dose:** 1 mg initially, slowly increased to 5–15 mg daily according to need. Side-effects include mouth dryness, dizziness and blurred vision. Care is necessary with high doses as some psychiatric disturbances may occur and warrant withdrawal of the drug, but abrupt discontinuance of treatment should be avoided. Benzhexol should be used with care in cases of glaucoma, hepatic and cardiac disease or urinary disturbances. (Artane; Broflex). See page 160 and Table 26.

**benzocaine** A local anaesthetic for topical application. Used as lozenges (100 mg) for painful oral conditions; ointment (5–10%); suppositories 200 mg.

**benzodiazepines** A widely used group of drugs with a powerful action on the central nervous system. They appear to have a selective action on certain serotonin receptors. The type of action varies within the group, and they may be used as sedatives, hypnotics, anxiolytics, anticonvulsants or muscle relaxants. As hypnotics they have virtually replaced the barbiturates, as they have a wide margin of safety and are less dangerous in overdose. Prolonged use should be avoided as dependence remains a possibility. The withdrawal of treatment with benzodiazepines should be gradual, as otherwise confusion, convulsions and toxic psychoses may occur. Nitrazepam has a relatively long action as a hypnotic, whereas flunitrazepam has a shorter action. Diazepam is the preferred drug for controlling the spasms of tetanus. Hypnotic benzodiazepines include flunitrazepam, flurazepam, loprazolam, lormetazepam, nitrazepam and temazepam. Those used as anxiolytics are alprazolam, bromazepam, chlordiazepoxide, clobazam, clorazepate, diazepam, ketazolam, lorazepam, medazepam and oxazepam. Most of these diazepines are referred to briefly under the above names. See page 117 and Table 5.

**benzoic acid** It has fungistatic properties similar to salicylic acid, and has been used as Whitfield's ointment (Compound Benzoic Acid Ointment) for the treatment of ringworm.

**benzoin** A balsamic resin used mainly as Compound Tincture of Benzoin for pressure sores and stoma care.

**benzoyl peroxide** An antifungal agent used locally for superficial fungal infections. It is also used, together with sulphur, as a cream or gel for acne.

**benzthiazide** A thiazide diuretic present with triamterene in Dytide.

**benztropine** An anticholinergic drug, used to relieve the rigidity, tremor and salivation of Parkinson's disease. It also has some sedative action, and in some cases may be preferred to benzhexol. Like benzhexol, it is sometimes useful in the control of drug-induced extrapyramidal symptoms.
**Dose:** 0.5–6 mg daily. In severe conditions, it may be given by injection of 1–2 mg, repeated according to response. The side-effects are those of the anticholinergic drugs generally. (Cogentin). See page 160 and Table 26.

**benzydamine** A mild analgesic used as a mouthwash (0.15%) for painful conditions of the mouth and throat, and as a cream (3%) for musculoskeletal pain.

**benzyl benzoate** A clear liquid with an aromatic odour. It is used as an emulsion in the treatment of scabies by two applications to the whole of the body except the head.

**benzyl penicillin** See penicillin.

**beractant** A pulmonary surfactant used in the respiratory distress syndrome of premature infants, by endotracheal tubing within 8 hours of birth. Monitor heart rate and arterial oxygenation. (Survanta). See also colfosceril, poractant and pumactant.

**beta-adrenoceptor blocking agents**
Adrenaline and related catecholamines are released into the circulation during exercise and stress, and stimulate cardiac output by acting on the beta-adrenoceptor sites in the heart. When such stimulation is excessive the increased oxygen demand of the heart may cause myocardial insufficiency and angina. Drugs such as propranolol block these receptor sites and so indirectly reduce cardiac stimulation, and are of value in the control of angina, cardiac arrhythmias and hypertension. Some blocking agents also act on other receptor sites and may cause bronchospasm by releasing histamine. Newer drugs, represented by acebutolol and meroprolol, are more cardioselective, and others such as sotalol are of more value in hypertension. Some of these blocking agents, such as atenolol, are less likely to reach the central nervous system and so may cause fewer sleep disturbances. By their nature and depressant action on the myocardium, care is necessary when giving beta-blockers in cardiac failure, heart block and bradycardia. See pages 114 & 148, and Tables 4 & 21.

**betahistine** A vasodilator with some of the properties of histamine. Used to reduce the vertigo of Ménière's disease. Should be used with care in asthmatics and in peptic ulcer.
**Dose:** 16–48 mg daily. (Serc).

**betamethasone** A corticosteroid characterized by its low dose, increased anti-inflammatory action, and reduced side-effects. It has virtually no salt-retaining properties, and causes little increase in the urinary excretion of potassium. It is indicated in all inflammatory, allergic and other conditions requiring corticosteroid therapy – with the exception of Addison's disease and after adrenalectomy when a salt-retaining steroid is required.
**Dose:** 0.5–5 mg daily; in cerebral oedema, 5–20 mg by i.m. or i.v. injection. In asthmatic states, oral aerosol inhalation of 800 μg (eight puffs) daily; for inflammatory conditions of the eye, ear and nose, a 0.1% solution is used locally. (Betnesol).

**betaxolol** A beta-adrenoceptor blocking agent of the propranolol type, with similar properties and side-effects, but with a more cardioselective action. It is used mainly in the treatment of hypertension.
**Dose:** 20 mg once daily. Betaxolol is also used as eye drops (0.5%) in ocular hypertension and glaucoma. (Betoptic; Kerlone). See page 148 and Table 21.

**bethanechol** A parasympathomimetic agent used in reflux oesophagitis, paralytic ileus and postoperative urinary retention.
**Dose:** 30–120 mg daily before food. Side-effects are nausea, bradycardia and colic. Care is necessary in asthma and cardiovascular disease. (Myotonine).

**bethanidine** A blocking agent that has an antihypertensive action by inhibiting the release of noradrenaline from post-ganglionic adrenergic nerve endings. It is useful in resistant hypertension, and when other agents are not well tolerated, and is usually given in association with a thiazide diuretic or a beta-blocker.
**Dose:** 20–200 mg daily. Postural hypotension, nasal congestion and diarrhoea are side-effects. (Bendogen). See page 148 and Table 21.

**bezafibrate** A plasma-lipid regulating agent with an action similar to clofibrate, and used in the treatment of hyperlipidaemia not responding to diet.
**Dose:** 600 mg daily with food. Contraindicated in renal or hepatic dysfunction. May potentiate oral anticoagulants. Side-effects are nausea, pruritus and urticaria. (Bezalip). See page 146 and Table 20.

**bicalutamide**∇ A nonsteroidal anti-androgen that binds selectively with androgen receptors. It is used with an LH–RH analogue such as goserelin in advanced prostatic cancer in doses of 50 mg daily. (Casodex). See page 122 and Table 8.

**biperiden** An antispasmodic and parasympatholytic drug used chiefly to control the rigidity and excessive salivation of parkinsonism. It has less effect on tremor.
**Dose:** 2 mg daily initially, increased, as required, up to 6 mg or more daily. If necessary it may be given by i.m. or slow i.v. injection in doses of 5–20 mg daily. Side-effects include dizziness, blurred vision and drowsiness. (Akineton). See page 160 and Table 26.

**BIPP** A mixture of bismuth subnitrate, iodoform and liquid paraffin, used occasionally as an antiseptic dressing.

**bisacodyl** A synthetic laxative that exerts its action by a direct stimulating effect on the nerve endings of the colon.
**Dose:** 10 mg orally, or as a suppository. Abdominal cramp is an occasional side-effect. It should not be used in intestinal obstruction.

**bismuth chelate** A potassium-bismuth-citrate complex used to promote the healing of peptic ulcers, mainly by a protective action.
**Dose:** 480 mg daily for 28 days, repeated if necessary at monthly intervals. Not to be given with food. It may blacken the faeces. (De-Noltab).

**bismuth subgallate** A yellow insoluble powder with astringent properties. Used as dusting powder, and as suppositories for rectal conditions.

**bisoprolol** A beta-blocking agent with the actions, uses and side-effects of propranolol.

**Dose:** It is given in hypertension and angina in doses of 5–20 mg daily. (Emcor; Monocor). See pages 114 & 148, and Tables 4 & 21.

**bisphosphonates** Substances used in Paget's disease of bone and hypercalcaemia of malignancy. See alendronate, disodium etidronate, disodium pamidronate and sodium clodronate.

**bleomycin** A cytotoxic antibiotic, exceptional in causing little or any disturbance of bone marrow activity. Used mainly in skin tumours, lymphomas and mycosis fungoides.
**Dose:** 15–30 mg twice-weekly by i.m. or i.v. injection up to a total dose of 500 mg. The onset of stomatitis is an indication of the maximum tolerated dose. Pigmentation of the skin may occur, but a severe dose-related, delayed reaction is pulmonary fibrosis, requiring immediate withdrawal of the drug. There is a risk of respiratory failure during general anaesthesia associated with a high oxygen intake. See page 122 and Table 8.

**botulinum toxin complex** Botulinum toxin causes severe respiratory muscle paralysis, but a modified form has a local action. The complex is used in severe blepharospasm and given by injection into the ocular muscle. Response is slow (1–2 weeks) and treatment may need to be repeated at intervals of 8 weeks. (Botox; Dysport).

**bretylium** An antihypertensive agent, now used only in the control of resistant ventricular arrhythmias.
**Dose:** 5 mg/kg, i.m., 6–8-hourly. It may also be given by slow i.v. injection in doses of 5–10 mg/kg, repeated as required. Side-effects include nausea, vomiting and severe hypotension. (Bretylate).

**brimonidine** A selective alpha$_2$-andrenergic receptor agonist. It is used in the treatment of glaucoma when beta-blockers are not suitable or not tolerated.
**Dose:** one drop of a 0.2% solution in the eye or eyes twice daily. Some initial burning and stinging may occur, and an ocular allergic reaction may occur with prolonged therapy. (Alphagan). See page 138 and Table 16.

**bromazepam** A benzodiazepine used mainly in the short-term treatment of anxiety.

**Dose:** 9–18 mg daily. Contraindicated in respiratory depression and phobic states. (Lexotan). See page 117 and Table 5.

**bromocriptine** An inhibitor of the release of prolactin from the pituitary gland. It is used to prevent or suppress lactation when other measures have failed.
**Dose:** 1–1.5 mg daily initially for a few days, then twice daily for 14 days. It also stimulates dopamine receptors in the brain and is used in parkinsonism, mainly in patients unable to tolerate levodopa, to stimulate any surviving dopamine receptors. Dose: 1.25 mg at night initially, with food, slowly increased according to response up to 40 mg. The use of the drug requires care, as it has many side-effects, including early hypotensive reactions. Bromocriptine is also used in some conditions of pituitary dysfunction such as acromegaly. (Pardolel). See page 160 and Table 26.

**brompheniramine** An antihistamine similar to promethazine, but with shorter action and reduced side-effects. It also has some antitussive properties.
**Dose:** 12–32 mg daily. (Dimotane). See page 110 and Table 2.

**budesonide** A steroid similar to beclomethasone, and used by oral aerosol inhalation in chronic airway obstruction and other asthmatic conditions.
**Dose:** 200–800 µg/kg (1–4 puffs) according to need. A long-acting form (Entocort) is used in the treatment of Crohn's disease. Dose: 9 mg daily before breakfast for up to 8 weeks. Also used locally as a cream (0.025%) in eczema, psoriasis and dermatitis. (Pulmocort; Preferid).

**bumetanide** A rapidly acting loop diuretic similar to frusemide, with comparable actions, uses and side-effects.
**Dose:** 1–5 mg daily. Much larger doses may be needed when renal function is impaired. In acute pulmonary and cardiac oedema, 1–2 mg may be given i.v. (Burinex). See page 148 and Table 21.

**bupivacaine** A local anaesthetic related to lignocaine but characterized by its increased potency and long duration of action which may be up to 8 hours when used for nerve blocks. It is also of value in continuous epidural analgesia. It is used as a 0.25% to 0.5% solution in doses

according to requirements with or without adrenaline. The side-effects are those of lignocaine, but it may cause more severe myocardial depression. (Marcain).

**buprenorphine** A powerful analgesic, related to morphine, but less likely to cause dependence. Valuable in pain of terminal cancer, after operation or myocardial infarction.
**Dose:** 200–400 µg 6–8-hourly as sublingual tablets, or 300–600 µg by i.m. or slow i.v. injection at intervals of 6–8 hours according to need. Side-effects include drowsiness, nausea and dizziness. Naxolone is only a partial antagonist. (Temgesic).

**buserelin** A synthetic gonadotrophin-releasing hormone that indirectly depresses androgen and oestrogen synthesis. It is used in the treatment of testosterone-sensitive prostatic carcinoma.
**Dose:** 500 µg by s.c. injection 8-hourly for 7 days, followed by intranasal maintenance doses of 100 µg 6 times a day. Patients should be warned that an increase in pain may occur initially. Side-effects are hot flushes and loss of libido. (Suprefact). It is also used as a nasal spray in the long-term treatment of endometriosis in doses of 900 µg daily. Side-effects are menstrual-like bleeding and mood changes. (Suprecur). See goserelin, leuprorelin and nafarelin.

**buspirone** A drug for the treatment of anxiety. It acts more selectively than the benzodiazepines on serotonin receptors in the brain, but the full response may take 1–2 weeks.
**Dose:** 10–15 mg daily initially, slowly increased as required up to a maximum of 45 mg daily. Side-effects are nausea, dizziness and drowsiness. Benzodiazepines must be withdrawn slowly before transfer to buspirone. (Buspar). See page 117 and Table 5.

**busulphan** A cytotoxic compound used in the palliative treatment of chronic myeloid leukaemia. Close haematological control is essential during treatment as remission of symptoms may not be complete for some weeks and overdose may cause irreversible myelodepression.
**Dose:** 0.5–4 mg daily. Side-effects include pigmentation of the skin. (Myleran). See page 122 and Table 8.

† **butobarbitone** A barbiturate of medium intensity and rapidity of onset.
**Dose:** 60–200 mg. (Soneryl).

# C

**cabergoline**∇ A dopamine agonist similar to bromocriptine, but with a longer action.
**Dose:** for suppression of lactation 1 mg, followed by doses of 0.25 mg for 2 days. Nausea, dizziness and breast pain are side-effects. (Cabaser; Dostinex).

**cadexomer iodine** A modified starch powder containing 0.9% of iodine in a slow release form. It is used as an antiseptic application for venous ulcers and pressure sores. It should not be used during prenancy or lactation, during thyroid investigations or in patients sensitive to iodine. (Iodosorb).

**caffeine** The central nervous system stimulant present in tea and coffee. It is used with paracetamol and other mild analgesics.

**calamine** Zinc carbonate. It has a mild astringent and soothing action and is widely used as Calamine Lotion for skin irritation and as Oily Calamine Lotion in eczema.

**calciferol (vitamin D₂)** The form of vitamin D used in the prophylaxis and treatment of deficiency states such as rickets in children and osteomalacia in adults, and in other bone disorders.
**Dose:** prophylactic 800 units daily; therapeutic 5000–50 000 units daily. In resistant rickets and parathyroid deficiency, higher doses may be required, but such therapy requires care, as hypercalcaemia and irreversible renal damage may occur. See also alfacalcidol and calcitriol.

**calcipotriol** An analogue of vitamin D with a selective inhibitory action on the proliferation of keratinocytes. Used in the treatment of psoriasis as a 0.005% cream or ointment twice a day. Not more than 100 g/week. (Dovonex).

**calcitonin** Pork-derived calcitonin is a hormone that has an action similar to that of the parathyroid gland in regulating blood calcium levels. It is used in the hypercalcaemia associated with malignancy, and in osteoporosis. It is also of value in Paget's disease of bone, in which it relieves bone pain and reduces the neurological symptoms.
**Dose:** 10–160 units daily by s.c. or i.m. injection according to need and response. In Paget's disease, prolonged treatment for some months may be required. Side-effects are nausea, flushing and paraesthesia, and local reactions may also occur. (Calcynar; Calcitare; Miacalcic). See salcatonin.

**calcitrol** The metabolite formed in the kidney from calciferol. It is the most powerful and rapidly acting metabolite with vitamin D activity. It is of value in chronic renal deficiency states when the normal metabolism of calcium and phosphorus is impaired, as in renal osteodystrophy.
**Dose:** 1–2 μg daily under biochemical control. Side-effects, such as hypercalcaemia and hypercalciuria, are usually reversible on withdrawing the drug. (Rocaltrol).

**calcium channel blocking agents** The movement of calcium ions through the calcium channels of the myocardium plays an essential role in cardiac activity. The inhibition of such movement by channel blocking agents reduces myocardial contractility and lowers the tone of the cardiovascular system. Such a reduction is of value in angina, hypertension and cardiac arrhythmias, and can be obtained by the use of calcium channel blocking agents such as diltiazem, felodipine, isradipine, nicardipine, nifedipine, nimidopine and verapamil. These compounds exhibit certain differences in action and in therapeutic applications, and their use requires care. Nifedipine and verapamil have been used in the prophylactic treatment of migraine. Their side-effects include nausea, oedema, rash and bradycardia. See pages 114 & 148, and Tables 4 & 21.

**calcium carbonate** A time honoured antacid now used less frequently. It also acts as a phosphate binder, and is used in hyperphosphataemia.

**calcium chloride** The calcium salt present in various intravenous electrolyte solutions.

**calcium folinate** See folinic acid.

**calcium gluconate** A soluble and well-tolerated calcium salt used in many conditions associated with calcium deficiency such as rickets, coeliac disease and parathyroid deficiency; also during pregnancy and lactation often in association with vitamin D. Calcium gluconate is also given in chilblains, urticaria and allergic reactions.
**Dose:** usually given in doses of 0.5–2 g, but in hypocalcaemic tetany it is given by slow i.v. injection in doses of 10 ml of a 10% solution, with laboratory control of the blood calcium levels. Calcium gluconate is also given i.v. in the early treatment of toxic hyperkalaemia.

**calcium lactate** The calcium salt most commonly given orally in mild deficiency states.
**Dose:** 1–5 g.

**Calcium Resonium** An ion-exchange resin that takes up potassium in exchange for calcium. Used in hyperkalaemia associated with anuria and haemodialysis. Should be used only when potassium and calcium serum levels are under biochemical control.
**Dose:** 15–30 g 3 or 4 times a day. In children, 0.5–1 g/kg daily. It is sometimes given as a retention enema.

**canrenoate** A steroid-derived aldosterone antagonist with the actions and uses of spironolactone.
**Dose:** given in oedema by slow i.v. injection or infusion in doses of 200–400 mg daily. Nausea and vomiting are high-dose side-effects. (Spiroctan–M).

**capreomycin** An antibiotic of value in resistant tuberculosis or when other drugs are not tolerated.
**Dose:** 1 g daily by i.m. injection. It may cause tinnitus, deafness, renal damage and allergic reactions. (Capastat).

**captopril** An inhibitor of the angiotensin converting enzyme. It is used in the treatment of hypertension, including that resistant to other therapy, but care is necessary as the initial dose may cause marked hypotension, and so is best taken in bed. It is often given with a thiazide diuretic to improve the response, and with a beta-blocker to maintain the effect.
**Dose:** 25 mg initially, slowly increased, as required, up to 450 mg daily. Similar doses are given in heart failure. Side-effects include proteinuria, neutropenia, agranulocytosis, rash and loss of taste. (Acepril; Capotin). See ACE inhibitors, page 148 and Table 21.

**carbachol** A parasympathomimetic agent used orally and by injection in the treatment of postoperative atony and retention of urine, and occasionally as eye drops (3%) in the treatment of glaucoma.
**Dose:** 2–4 mg orally, 250 μg by s.c. injection. Side-effects include nausea, bradycardia and colic.

**carbamazepine** An anticonvulsant effective in all types of epilepsy except petit mal (absence seizures). It is also of value in trigeminal neuralgia and is given prophylactically in manic-depressive states.
**Dose:** 200–400 mg daily initially, slowly increased up to 1.8 g daily if required. Suppositories of 125–250 mg are available. Carbamazepine has some antidiuretic properties, and has been used in diabetes insipidus in doses of 100–200 mg daily. Side-effects include dizziness, gastrointestinal disturbances and an erythematous rash. (Tegretol). See page 136 and Table 15.

**carbaryl** An insecticide used as a lotion and shampoo in pediculosis.

**carbenoxolone** A cytoprotectant derived from liquorice, used for mouth ulcers. (Bioplex; Bioral). See Table 27.

**carbidopa** An enzyme inhibitor used with levodopa in parkinsonism. It prevents the breakdown of levodopa, thus permitting a larger amount to reach the brain. See page 160.

**carbimazole** An antithyroid drug. It inhibits the formation of thyroxine and is valuable in the treatment of thyrotoxicosis and in preparation for thyroidectomy.
**Dose:** 30–60 mg daily initially; maintenance dose, 5–20 mg daily. It is sometimes given together with thyroxine in the 'blockage replacement' treatment of hyperthyroidism. Side-effects are nausea, rash and pruritus; alopecia and agranulcytosis have been reported. (Neo-Mercazole).

**carbocisteine** A mucolytic agent used to reduce the production and viscosity of sputum in respiratory disorders.
**Dose:** 1.5 g daily. (Mucodyne).

**carbon dioxide** A colourless, non-inflammable gas. It has a stimulating effect on the respiratory centre, and a mixture of 5% of carbon dioxide in oxygen is used for respiratory depression. Solid carbon dioxide is used to destroy warts, naevi, etc.

**carbonic anhydrase inhibitors** These drugs, represented by acetazolamide and dichlorphenamide, have been used as diuretics as they inhibit the reabsorption of sodium and bicarbonate in the kidneys. Their use has declined as more effective diuretics have become available. They also reduce the formation of the aqueous humour and so bring about a reduction in the intraocular pressure, and are used in the treatment of glaucoma. See page 138 and Table 16.

**carboplatin** An analogue of cisplatin but with generally reduced side-effects, although the myelodepression may be more severe. It is used mainly in ovarian and small-cell lung cancer.
**Dose:** 40 mg/m$^2$ i.v. as a single dose, repeated after 4 weeks. Blood tests during treatments are essential. Severe renal impairment is a contraindication. (Paraplatin). See page 122 and Table 8.

**carboprost** A prostaglandin with a selective action on the myometrium, and used in post-partum haemorrhage not responding to ergometrine.
**Dose:** 250 µg initially by deep i.m. injection, with subsequent doses according to need up to a total of 2 mg (not for i.v. injection). Care in asthma, epilepsy and hypertension. Nausea and vomiting are side-effects. (Hemabate).

**carisoprodol** A muscle relaxant used in musculoskeletal disorders and muscle spasm.
**Dose:** 1 g daily. (Carisoma).

**carmustine** A cytoxic agent similar to lomustine. It is used mainly in brain tumours, multiple myeloma and Hodgkin's disease, often in association with other drugs.
**Dose:** 200 mg/m$^2$ by slow i.v. injection, repeated at intervals of 6 weeks. Side-effects are nausea, vomiting and burning at the injection site. A delayed bone-marrow depression is often a dose-limiting factor. (BICNU). See page 122 and Table 8.

**carteolol** A beta-adrenaergic blocking agent used as eye drops (0.1–0.2%) in glaucoma. Some systemic absorption may occur from eye drops, and care is necessary in asthma and bradycardia. (Teoptic). See page 138.

**carvedilol**▽ A non-cardiac selective beta-blocker with the actions and uses of propanolol.
**Dose:** in hypertension 12.5 mg initially, rising to 25–50 mg as a single daily dose. (Eucardic). See page 148 and Table 21.

**cascara** A mild purgative.
**Dose:** dry extract 100–250 mg, liquid extract and elixir 2–5 ml.

**castor oil** A mild purgative.
**Dose:** 5–20 ml. The oil has emollient properties and is used together with zinc ointment for pressure sores and napkin rash.

**catecholamines** A term applied to the sympathomimetic drugs adrenaline, dopamine, noradrenaline, and related compounds, indicating that they are derivatives of catechol.

**CCNU** See lomustine.

**cefaclor** An orally active cephalosporin antibiotic used mainly in urinary and respiratory infections.
**Dose:** 750 mg or more, up to 4 g daily, with reduced doses in renal impairment. Nausea and diarrhoea are side-effects, but an allergic reaction indicating sensitivity may require withdrawal of the drug. (Distaclor). See Table 34.

**cefadroxil** An analogue of cephalexin. It is well absorbed orally and gives high blood levels.
**Dose:** 1–2 g daily. (Baxan). See page 248 and Table 34.

**cefamandole** See cephamandole.

**cefixime** A cephalosporin with the actions, uses and side-effects of the cephalosporins generally, but effective in single daily doses of 200–400 mg. (Suprax). See page 248 and Table 34.

**cefodizine** A cephalosporin used in lower respiratory tract infections and in urinary tract infections.
**Dose:** 2 g daily by i.m. injection or i.v.

injection/infusion. (Timecef). See page 248 and Table 34.

**cefotaxime** A cephalosporin with an increased activity against many Gram-negative organisms.
**Dose:** 2 g daily by injection, increased in severe infections up to 12 g daily. A single dose of 1 g is given in gonorrhoea. The side-effects are those of the cephalosporins generally. (Claforan). See page 248 and Table 34.

**cefoxitin** A cephamycin with a wide range of activity and an increased potency against Gram-negative bacteria. It is of value in many infections, and is also used in surgical prophylaxis.
**Dose:** 3–12 g daily by i.m. or i.v. injection. (Mefoxin). See page 248 and Table 34.

**cefpirome** A beta-lactamase-stable cephalosporin with a wide range of activity.
**Dose:** 2 g daily i.v. (Cefrom). See page 248 and Table 34.

**cefpodoxime** An oral cephalosporin for respiratory tract infections.
**Dose:** 200–400 mg daily with food. (Orelox). See page 248 and Table 34.

**ceftazidime** A cephalosporin resistant to most beta-lactamases, and active against a wide range of Gram-positive and Gram-negative organisms, including *Pseudomonas aeruginosa*, although it is less active against *Staphylococcus aureus*. Valuable in both single and mixed infections.
**Dose:** 1–6 g daily by injection, reduced in cases of renal impairment. In pseudomonal lung infections associated with cystic fibrosis, 100–150 mg/kg daily. Side-effects include abdominal disturbance and local reactions at the injection site. (Fortum; Kefadim). See page 248 and Table 34.

**ceftibuten** An oral cephalosporin similar to cefaclor, but with a longer action.
**Dose:** 400 mg as a single daily dose. (Cedax). See page 248 and Table 34.

**ceftriaxone** A cephalosporin of the cefaclor type given as a single daily dose of 1 g by deep i.m. or slow i.v. injection, doubled in severe infections. With high doses vary injection site. (Rocephin). See page 248 and Table 34.

**cefuroxime** A cephalosporin often effective against some organisms resistant to penicillin, and with increased activity against *Haemophilus influenzae*.
**Dose:** 3–6 g daily by injection. For surgical prophylaxis and in gonorrhoea a single dose of 1.5 g. Side-effects include nausea, diarrhoea, urticaria, rash and hypersensitivity reactions. (Zinacef). Cefuroxime-axetil is an orally active form. Dose: 500 mg–1 g daily. (Zinnat). See page 248 and Table 34.

**celiprolol** A selective $\beta_1$ receptor blocking agent, with some stimulating action on $\beta_2$ receptors. The former occur mainly in the heart, the latter in the bronchi and peripheral vessels. It is used in mild hypertension, as it has a vasodilatory and cardioselective action with reduced side-effects.
**Dose:** 200 mg daily, at breakfast. Occasional side-effects are nausea, headache and dizziness. (Celectol). See page 148 and Table 21.

**cephalexin** An orally active cephalosporin of value in infections of the respiratory and urinary tracts, and in naso-oral and soft-tissue infections.
**Dose:** 1–2 g daily, but lower doses are indicated in renal impairment. Cephalexin is usually well tolerated, but some gastrointestinal disturbances may occur. (Ceporex; Keflex). See page 248 and Table 34.

**cephalosporins** A group of antibiotics with properties similar to those of the penicillins, but having a wider range of activity. Some are active orally, others may have to be given by injection. Cefotaxime, ceftazidime and ceftizoxime have an increased activity against Gram-negative bacteria, but are less potent against *Staphylococcus aureus* and Gram-positive organisms generally. Cefotoxin is active against bowel organisms. An indication of the range and dose is given in the table on page 248. The higher doses are given in severe infections; reduced doses should be given in renal impairment. The main side-effect of the cephalosporins is hypersensitivity, and cross-sensitivity to the penicillins is not uncommon. Sensitivity to one is likely to extend to all members of the group. The cephalosporins can affect blood-clotting mechanisms. See page 248 and Table 34.

**27**

**C**

**cephamandole** A cephalosporin more resistant to inactivation by penicillinases. It is of value in serious infections resistant to other antibiotics.
**Dose:** 2–12 g daily by i.m. or i.v. injection. (Kefadol). See page 248 and Table 34.

**cephamycins** A small group of antibiotics closely related to the cephalosporins and having similar actions and uses. See cefoxitin. See page 248 and Table 34.

**cephazolin** A cephalosporin with the general properties of the group.
**Dose:** 1–12 g daily by injection. (Kefzol). See page 248 and Table 34.

**cephradine** A cephalosporin active orally as well as by injection.
**Dose:** 1–2 g orally daily; in severe infections 2–8 g daily by injection. (Velosef). See page 248 and Table 34.

**certoparin** A low molecular weight form of heparin. Used in prophylaxis of venous thromboembolism.
**Dose:** 3000 units once a day by s.c. injection (1–2 hours before surgery) for 7–10 days. (Alphaparin). See enoxaparin.

**cetirizine** A slower-acting antihistamine with reduced sedative effects, as it does not pass the blood-brain barrier to any extent. The anti-cholinergic side-effects are also reduced.
**Dose:** 10 mg at night. (Zirtek). See page 110 and Table 2.

**cetrimide** A detergent with some antiseptic properties. It is used chiefly in association with chlorhexidine.

**charcoal** Activated charcoal is a powerful adsorbent, and is used in the treatment of overdose or poisoning by many toxic drugs by preventing further absorption.
**Dose:** 50 g orally. It is also used in the charcoal-haemoperfusion system to promote elimination from the circulation of some already absorbed poisons. Charcoal has also been used as impregnated dressings to deodorize foul smelling wounds and ulcers.

**chenodeoxycholic acid** A bile acid derivative that has a solvent action on cholesterol-containing gallstones, and it is useful when surgical removal of the stones is contraindicated.

**Dose:** 1 g once daily, but prolonged treatment is necessary. Side-effects are diarrhoea and pruritus, and ursodeoxy-cholic acid, which has fewer side-effects, is often preferred. Chenodeoxycholic acid is not suitable for the dissolution of radio-opaque gallstones. (Chendol; Chenofalk).

**chloral hydrate** A water-soluble hypnotic with a rapid action that is useful in the treatment of insomnia in children and the elderly.
**Dose:** 0.3–2 g. It must be given well-diluted to reduce the gastric irritant side-effects, and is contraindicated in gastritis, and severe renal, hepatic and cardiac disease. (Notec). Chloral betaine (Welldorm) is a less irritant alternative. See page 152 and Table 22.

**chlorambucil** An orally active cytotoxic drug used mainly in the treatment of lymphomas and chronic lymphocytic leukaemia.
**Dose:** 100–200 µg/kg daily for 4–8 weeks. It is sometimes used as an immunosuppressant in the treatment of rheumatoid arthritis in doses of 2.5–7.5 mg daily. Chlorambucil is generally well tolerated, but bone marrow depression may occur, and haematological control during treatment is essential. (Leukeran). See page 122 and Table 8.

**chloramphenicol** A wide-range, orally active antibiotic but now used only in life-threatening infections where other drugs are unsuitable.
**Dose:** 2 g daily orally, but in severe infections, 50 mg/kg daily by i.v. injection. Care is necessary when giving chloramphenicol to infants as it may cause so-called 'grey syndrome'. Side-effects include nausea, neuritis and aplastic anaemia. Chloromycetin is also used locally in skin, eye and ear infections. (Chloromycetin; Kemicetine).

**chlordiazepoxide** A benzodiazepine used mainly in the short-term treatment of anxiety and alcoholism.
**Dose:** 30 mg daily, increased in severe anxiety up to 100 mg daily, with half doses for elderly patients. Withdrawal of treatment should be gradual to avoid rebound effects. Side-effects include dizziness, drowsiness and ataxia. Prolonged use carries the risk of dependence. (Librium). See page 117 and Table 5.

**chlorhexidine** An antiseptic of high potency and a wide range of activity, although it is ineffective against spores and viruses. For preoperative skin preparation, a 0.5% solution in alcohol is often used; an aqueous solution (0.05%) is for general topical application. Chlorhexidine is also used as a 1/10 000 (0.01%) solution for bladder irrigation. A general purpose cream and an obstetric cream are also available. Solutions of chlorhexidine may become contaminated with *Pseudomonas*, and all aqueous solutions should be sterilized. (Hibitane).

**chlormethiazole** A sedative with anticonvulsant properties.
**Dose:** in severe insomnia in the elderly, 200–400 mg orally; in alcohol withdrawal conditions, 400–800 mg initially, reduced and withdrawn over a 9-day period. It may also be given by i.v. infusion as a 0.8% solution. Chlormethiazole has also been given by injection in status epilepticus and the toxaemia of pregnancy in doses according to need and response. Side-effects are sneezing, gastrointestinal disturbances and headache. (Heminevrin). See page 136 and Table 15.

**chloroform** Once widely used as a general anaesthetic, but now obsolete. Used as chloroform-water in mixtures as a preservative and flavouring agent, and for its carminative effects.

**chloroquine** An antimalarial drug used for both prophylaxis and treatment of benign and malignant tertian malaria. It should be noted that chloroquine-resistant strains of *Plasmodium falciparum* are becoming increasingly common, and a return to treatment with quinine may be necessary.
**Dose:** adult prophylaxis, 300 mg once a week; for treatment of an attack of malaria, 600 mg initially followed by 300 mg daily for 2–3 days. Seriously ill or vomiting patients should be given 200–300 mg by i.m. or slow i.v. injection, repeated once if necessary before oral treatment can be tolerated. Other dosage schemes are also in use, and for details reference should be made to standard works on the treatment of malaria. It has also been used in hepatic amoebiasis, but metronidazole is now often preferred. Chloroquine also has an action in rheumatoid inflammatory conditions similar to that of penicillamine, dose: 150 mg daily after food. Such use requires care, as extended therapy is necessary, and the drug may cause corneal opacity and irreversible retinal damage. Other side-effects are gastrointestinal disturbances, rash and pruritus. (Avloclor; Nivaquine). See page 165.

**chlorothiazide** The first of the thiazide diuretics, now largely replaced by bendrofluazide and similar drugs.
**Dose:** 1–2 g daily in oedematous states; 0.5–1 g daily in hypertension. Potassium supplements may be necessary with extended treatment. (Saluric). See page 148 and Table 21.

**chloroxylenol** A general purpose antiseptic present in some popular products. Of no value against *Pseudomonas. aeruginosa* or *Proteus*.

**chlorpheniramine** An antihistamine with the action, uses and side-effects of the group, including drowsiness.
**Dose:** 16–24 mg daily: 10–20 mg by i.m. or s.c. injection as required. (Piriton). See page 110 and Table 2.

**chlorpromazine** A powerful tranquillizer or antipsychotic agent with a wide range of activity on the central nervous system. It is widely used in the treatment of schizophrenia and other psychoses, in agitation and tension, and the management of refractory patients. It is also effective as an antiemetic in terminal illness; in the short-term treatment of severe anxiety; and for the control of intractable hiccup.
**Dose:** initially 75 mg orally daily, slowly increased as required. In psychotic states, up to 1 g daily. Single doses of 25–50 mg may be given by *deep* i.m. injection in acute conditions. Suppositories of 100 mg are also available. Side-effects include extrapyramidal and anticholinergic symptoms, drowsiness, hypotension, weight gain, rash, jaundice and haemolytic anaemia. Prolonged use may cause pigmentation of the skin and eyes. Care is necessary in hepatic and renal dysfunction. Skin sensitization may occur after contact with solutions of chlorpromazine. (Largactil). See page 168 and Table 30.

**chlorpropamide** A long-acting hypoglycaemic agent of the sulphonylurea type. It is effective only if some insulin-secreting cells are still functional. It is used mainly in mild diabetes mellitus occurring in middle-aged patients not responding to dietary control. Its long action makes it unsuitable for elderly diabetics.

**Dose:** 250–500 mg daily as a single morning dose. Side-effects are rash, jaundice, blood dyscrasia and hypoglycaemia, but are uncommon with low doses. Flushing may occur if alcohol is taken. Chlorpropamide (but not other sulphonylureas) is sometimes used to check the polyuria of diabetes insipidus. It acts by sensitizing the renal tubules to endogenous vasopressin, but great care is necessary to avoid hypoglycaemic reactions. Dose: up to 350 mg daily in adults, or 200 mg daily in children. (Diabinese). See page 131 and Table 13.

**chlortetracycline** An orally effective antibiotic with the actions, uses and side-effects of the tetracyclines.
**Dose:** 1–2 g daily. (Aureomycin).

**chlorthalidone** A diuretic similar in action and uses to bendrofluazide, but with a longer duration of activity that permits a single morning dose. It is also useful in diabetes insipidus.
**Dose:** as diuretic 50–100 mg daily or on alternate days; in hypertension 25–50 mg; up to 350 mg daily in diabetes insipidus. (Hygroton). See page 148 and Table 21.

**cholecalciferol** See vitamin D.

**cholestyramine** An exchange resin that binds with bile acids in the intestines and prevents their absorption. Such acids are essential for cholesterol synthesis, and resin-binding leads indirectly to a lowering of plasma cholesterol levels.
**Dose:** in hyperlipidaemia: 12–24 g daily, with water; similar doses in the diarrhoea of Crohn's disease. It is also used in doses of 4–8 g daily to relieve the pruritus associated with biliary obstruction. Side-effects are rash and gastrointestinal disturbances. Cholestyramine and related agents may interfere with the absorption of anticoagulants and other drugs. (Questran). See page 146 and Table 20.

**choline theophyllinate** A bronchodilator with the actions, uses and side-effects of aminophylline.
**Dose:** 400–1600 mg daily, after food. (Choledyl). See page 118 and Table 6.

**chorionic gonadotrophin** A gonad-stimulating hormone prepared from the urine of pregnancy. It has been used in anovulatory sterility, metropathia haemorrhagica, habitual abortion and undescended testis.

**Dose:** 500–1000 units by i.m. injection. Nausea, vomiting and oedema are side-effects. (Pregnyl; Profasi).

**chymotrypsin** A proteolytic enzyme of the pancreas used in ophthalmology to facilitate intracapsular lens extraction. (Zonulysin).

**cidofovir** An antiviral agent used in cytomegalovirus retinitis resistant to ganciclivir.
**Dose:** 5 mg/kg by i.v. infusion every 2 weeks. (Vistide). See page 144 and Table 19.

**cilastatin** See imipenem.

**cilazapril** A long-acting ACE inhibitor with the actions, uses and side-effects of that group of drugs.
**Dose:** in essential hypertension 1 mg daily initially, increased up to 5 mg daily according to need. In renovascular hypertension 0.25–0.5 mg daily. (Vascace). See page 148 and Table 21.

**cimitidine** A selective histamine $H_2$ receptor antagonist. Unlike ordinary antihistamines, it inhibits gastric secretion, and is used in the treatment of peptic ulcer and other conditions of gastric hyperacidity.
**Dose:** 800 mg daily for at least 4 weeks, doubled in severe conditions. Dose by i.m. or slow i.v. injection 200 mg 4–6-hourly. The dose should be reduced in renal impairment. The drug may increase the effects of oral anticoagulants and phenytoin. Side-effects include diarrhoea, rash and dizziness. It has some anti-androgen activity, and gynaecomastia is an occasional side-effect with high doses. (Dyspamet; Tagamet; Zita). See page 162 and Table 27.

**cinchocaine** A local anaesthetic used as ointment 1% in haemorrhoids and pruritus. (Nupercainal).

**cinnarizine** An antihistamine, chiefly of value in Ménière's disease, although it is also used in travel sickness and in peripheral vascular disorders.
**Dose:** 45–90 mg daily. Drowsiness and gastrointestinal disturbances are side-effects. (Stugeron).

**cinoxacin** A quinolone derivative with actions, uses and side-effects similar to those of nalidixic acid.

**Dose:** in urinary tract infections, 1 g daily; prophylaxis 500 mg daily. Contraindicated in severe renal impairment. (Cinobac).

**ciprofibrate** A blood-lipid lowering agent used in diet-resistant hyperlipidaemia as a single daily dose of 100–200 mg. (Modalim). See page 146 and Table 20.

**ciprofloxacin** A quinolone with a wide range of activity against both Gram-positive and Gram-negative bacteria, including *Pseudomonas* and *Proteus*. It is effective in many systemic infections, as well as in bone, joint and urinary infections, and in gonorrhoea, but is indicated mainly in infections resistant to other antibacterial agents.
**Dose:** 500 mg –1.5 g daily for 5–7 days; in gonorrhoea, a single dose of 250 mg is given. In severe infections 200–400 mg daily by i.v. infusion for 5–7 days. Side-effects include nausea, dizziness, headache, rash and pruritus. Plasma levels of theophylline may be increased and should be closely controlled. Care is necessary in convulsive disorders. (Ciproxin).

**cisapride** A gastrointestinal stimulant given to relieve gastro-oesophageal reflux and delayed gastric emptying.
**Dose:** 30–40 mg daily before meals, and at night, for some weeks. Side-effects are abdominal pain and diarrhoea. Drugs that delay the excretion of cisapride and may cause arrhythmias are erythromycin and clarithromycin–antifungal agents of the ketoconazole type should also be avoided. Unlike metoclopramide, it has no central antiemetic properties. (Alimix; Prepulsin).

**cisatracurium** A non-depolarizing neuromuscular blocking agent with an intermediate duration of activity. It is used as a muscle-relaxing adjunct in general anaesthesia, and to facilitate tracheal intubation. (Nimbex).

**cisplatin** A cytotoxic agent containing platinum bound in an organic complex. The action is linked with drug-induced changes in DNA structure that inhibit cell development. It is used in ovarian, testicular and other solid tumours, and in resistant malignant conditions, sometimes in association with other antineoplastic agents.
**Dose:** by i.v. injection 15–20 mg/m$^2$ daily for 5 days a month, or 15–120 mg/m$^2$ monthly. Blood tests are essential

throughout treatment. Side-effects, which may be severe, include nausea, vomiting, and oto-, nephro- and myelotoxicity. See page 122 and Table 8.

**citalopram**▽ A selective serotonin-reuptake inhibitor (SSRI).
**Dose:** used in depression in single daily doses of 20 mg, increased up to 40 mg daily. Treatment for at least 6 months necessary to avoid relapse. (Cipramil). See page 128 and Table 11.

**cladribine**▽ A new agent used by specialists in hairy cell leukaemia. (Leustat).

**clarithromycin** A macrolide antibiotic similar to erythromycin, but with better absorption and reduced gastrointestinal side-effects.
**Dose:** 250 mg twice a day for 7 days, doubled in severe infections. Care in hepatic and renal impairment. It may potentiate the effects of warfarin and digoxin. Should not be given with astemizole or terfenadine (risk of arrhythmias). (Klaricid).

**clavulanic acid** An inhibitor of beta-lactamase. Many penicillin-resistant organisms contain that enzyme in the cell wall, which inactivates the penicillin before it can enter the cell and exert its bacterial action. Clavulanic acid inhibits such enzyme activity, and so facilitates the penetration of the antibiotic into the bacterial cell. It is used in association with amoxycillin as co-amoxiclav (Augmentin) and with ticarcillin as Timentin, in the treatment of infections due to amoxycillin-resistant bacteria.

**clemastine** An antihistamine used in allergic rhinitis, urticaria and allergic dermatoses.
**Dose:** 1 mg twice a day. In common with other antihistamines, it may cause drowsiness, and anticholinergic side-effects such as dryness of the mouth. (Tavegil). See page 110 and Table 2.

**clindamycin** An antibiotic used mainly in staphylococcal bone and joint infections not responding to other drugs. It is also useful in anaerobic abdominal infections.
**Dose:** 600–800 mg daily. A serious side-effect is a potentially fatal pseudomembranous colitis, and the drug should be withdrawn immediately if diarrhoea occurs. See vancomycin and metronidazole. It is used locally as a 1% solution in acne. (Dalacin).

**clobazam** A benzodiazepine tranquillizer with the actions and uses of diazepam, but with reduced sedative effects. It is used mainly in the short-term treatment of anxiety.
**Dose:** 20–30 mg as a single nightly dose. In severe anxiety larger but divided doses may be given under medical control. It is also useful in the auxiliary treatment of epilepsy. (Frisium). See page 117 and Table 5.

**clobetasol** A potent corticosteroid used as a cream or ointment (0.05%) in the short-term treatment of severe inflammatory skin conditions not responding to less powerful drugs. The application should be used sparingly as absorption with systematic and local side-effects may occur with excessive or prolonged treatment. (Dermovate).

**clobetasone** A locally acting corticosteroid, used as a cream or ointment (0.05%) in eczema and inflammatory skin conditions not responding to less potent drugs. (Eumovate).

**clodronate sodium** A bisphosphonate used like etidronate and pamidronate in the hypercalcaemia of malignancy.
**Dose:** 1.6–3.2 g daily as a single dose 1 hour before or after food. May also be given i.v. by infusion as a single daily dose of 300 mg for 7–10 days. Long oral treatment is necessary, and serum calcium and phosphate levels should be checked. Side-effects are nausea and diarrhoea. (Bonefos; Loron).

**clofazimine** An antileprotic agent given in association with dapsone and rifampicin to prevent the incidence of resistance.
**Dose:** 300 mg monthly; in lepra reactions, 300 mg daily for 3 months. It may cause discoloration of the urine, skin and lesions. (Lamprene).

**clofibrate** A plasma lipid-regulating agent used in hyperlipidaemia in conjunction with dietary measures, to reduce excessive plasma levels of cholesterol and triglycerides.
**Dose:** 2 g daily, with regular checks on plasma lipid levels. Side-effects are transient nausea and abdominal discomfort. It increases the biliary excretion of cholesterol, and gall stones are a contraindication. A myositis-like reaction may occur in renal impairment, and the drug should

be withdrawn. Clofibrate may potentiate the action of oral anticoagulants, the dose of which may require adjustment. (Atromid–S). See page 146 and Table 20.

**clomiphene** An anti-oestrogen used to stimulate ovulation in some types of anovulatory sterility.
**Dose:** 50 mg daily for 5 days a month, repeated if ovulation does not occur. Its use has resulted in occasional multiple births. If pregnancy does not follow up to 6 courses, further treatment is of little use. Side-effects are hot flushes, and abdominal discomfort; visual disturbances indicate that treatment should be withdrawn. Contraindicated in hepatic disease and ovarian neoplasm. (Clomid; Serophene).

**clomipramine** A tricyclic antidepressant with the actions, uses and side-effects of imipramine and related drugs, but with reduced sedative properties.
**Dose:** 30–150 mg daily orally; up to 150 mg daily by i.m. injection. (Anafranil). See page 128 and Table 11.

**clonazepam** A benzodiazepine with a marked anticonvulsant action of value in all types of epilepsy.
**Dose:** 1 mg daily initially, increased up to 8 mg daily according to need. In status epilepticus, 1 mg by slow i.v. injection, but apnoea and hypotension, requiring prompt treatment, may occur. Side-effects include drowsiness, dizziness and irritability and occasionally, paradoxical aggression. (Rivotril). See page 136 and Table 15.

**clonidine** A centrally acting antihypertensive agent, now used less frequently.
**Dose:** 150–300 µg daily initially, increased if required up to 1.2 mg daily. Doses of 150–300 µg have been given by slow i.v. injection. Sudden withdrawal of the drug may provoke a hypertensive crisis. (Catapres). Clonidine is also used in doses of 100 µg daily in the prophylaxis of migraine. (Dixarit). The side-effects include sedation, dry mouth, fluid retention and bradycardia. See pages 154 and Table 21.

**clorazepate** A benzodiazepine tranquillizer with the actions, uses and side-effects of diazepam. Used mainly in the short-term treatment of anxiety.
**Dose:** 7.5–22.5 mg daily, or a single dose of 15 mg at night. (Tranxene). See page 117 and Table 5.

**clotrimazole** An antifungal agent used locally in vaginal candidiasis.
**Dose:** 100–200 mg as vaginal tablets or pessaries for nightly insertion. Also used as a 1% cream, lotion or dusting powder for fungal infections of the skin and ears. Side-effects are local irritation and erythema. (Canestan).

**cloxacillin** An acid-stable, semi-synthetic penicillin that is not broken down by the enzyme penicillinase, and so is effective in infections due to penicillin-resistant staphylococci.
**Dose:** 2 g daily before food. In severe infections 250–500 mg by injection 6-hourly. Now largely replaced by flucloxacillin. The side-effects are those of the penicillins generally. (Orbenin).

**clozapine** A potent but potentially toxic dopamine-receptor blocking agent used in schizophrenia resistant to other drugs.
**Dose:** 12.5–50 mg daily initially (with care – risk of hypotension), slowly increased to 300 mg daily according to need. A serious side-effect is neutropenia that may lead to agranulocytosis, and treatment must be under hospital supervision with regular blood monitoring. Patient, doctor and hospital pharmacist must be registered with the Clozaril (clozapine) Patient Monitoring Service to maintain the necessary strict control of treatment. (Clozaril). See page 168 and Table 30.

**coal tar** The black viscous liquid obtained from the distillation of coal. It is used mainly as Zinc and Tar Paste in psoriasis and atophic eczema.

**co-amilofruse** Tablets of the diuretics amiloride and frusemide. (Frumil; Lasoride).

**co-amilozide** Tablets of the diuretics amiloride and hydrochlorothiazide. (Moduretic).

**co-amoxiclav** A mixture of clavulinic acid and amoxycillin. The resistance to penicillin by staphylococci and other organisms is due to penicillinases such as beta-lactamase in the bacterial cell wall. Those enzymes inactivate penicillin before it can enter the cell and exert its antibacterial action. Such inactivation can be prevented by inhibitors of beta-lactamase such as clavulanic acid. That acid has no antibacterial action, but when given with a penicillin the antibiotic is able to penetrate into the cell without loss of activity. The combination is of value in infections due to penicillin-resistant penicillinase-producing bacteria, including most staphylococci.
**Dose:** as amoxycillin 750 mg daily, doubled in severe infections, or 3–4 g daily by slow i.v. injection. The side-effects are similar to those of ampicillin, but a post-treatment reaction is cholestatic jaundice. (Augmentin).

**co-beneldopa** Tablets of levodopa and benzerazide. (Madopar). See levodopa.

**†cocaine** A local anaesthetic. Still used occasionally in ophthalmology as a 2% solution, often with homatropine.

**co-careldopa** Tablets of levodopa and carbidopa. (Sinemet). See levodopa.

**co-codamol** Tablets of codeine and paracetamol.

**co-codaprin** Tablets of codeine and aspirin.

**co-danthramer** Tablets of danthron and poloxamer.

**cod-liver oil** A rich source of vitamins A and D. It is used as a dietary supplement to improve general nutrition, promote calcification and prevent rickets.
**Dose:** 2–10 ml daily.

**codeine** One of the alkaloids of opium. It depresses the cough centre and is used in the treatment of useless cough. It also reduces intestinal motility, and is useful in the symptomatic treatment of diarrhoea. It also has mild analgesic properties, and is present with aspirin in co-codaprin and similar preparations. In large doses the constipating action may be a disadvantage.
**Dose:** 10–60 mg.

**co-dergocrine** A cerebral vasodilator, sometimes used in the treatment of senile dementia.
**Dose:** 4.5 mg daily, but the response is unreliable. Side-effects include nausea, rash and bradycardia. (Hydergine).

**co-dydramol** Tablets of dihydrocodeine and paracetamol.

**co-fluampicil** Tablets of flucloxacillin and ampicillin.

**co-flumactone** Tablets of spironolactone and hydrochlorothiazide.

**colchicine** The alkaloid obtained from meadow saffron. It is used in acute gout.
**Dose:** 500 µg every 2 hours until relief is obtained. A total dose of 10 mg should not be exceeded, but relief of pain or the onset of vomiting or diarrhoea usually renders full doses unnecessary. It is also used prophylactically in doses of 500 µg 2 or 3 times a day during early treatment with allopurinol, probenecid and sulphinpyrazone. Care is necessary in the elderly, and in renal impairment. See page 140 and Table 17.

**colestipol** An exchange resin used in hyperlipidaemia that acts by binding with bile salts in the gut and preventing their reabsorption, and so indirectly lowers the plasma level of cholesterol.
**Dose:** 10–30 g daily. May interfere with the absorption of many drugs. (Colestid). See page 146 and Table 20.

**colfosceril** A pulmonary surfactant used in the respiratory distress syndrome of the new-born. (Exosurf). See beractant.

**colistin** An antibiotic used mainly for bowel sterilization.
**Dose:** 4.5–9 mega-units daily. In systemic gram-negative infections 2 mega-units 8-hourly by injection have been used, but less toxic antibiotics are now preferred. (Colomycin).

**collodion** When applied to the skin, it dries to form a flexible film, and is used as a vehicle for the extended local application of drugs such as salicylic acid.

**co-phenotrope** Tablets of diphenoxylate and atropine. (Lomotil; Tropergen).

**co-prenozide** Tablets of oxprenolol and cyclopenthiazide. (Trasidex).

**co-proxamol** Tablets of dextropropoxyphene and paracetamol. (Distalgesic).

**corticosteroids** Hormones secreted by the cortex of the suprarenal gland. The principal hormone is hydrocortisone but more potent synthetic derivatives such as dexamethasone are also in use.

**corticotrophin** The adrenocorticotrophic hormone of the anterior pituitary gland. It stimulates the production of corticosteroid hormones by the adrenal cortex. It is now used mainly as a test of adrenocortical function. See tetracosactrin.

**cortisol** Hydrocortisone.

**cortisone** One of the corticosteroids secreted by the adrenal cortex. Although it is rapidly absorbed orally, it is inactive until converted in the liver to hydrocortisone. It therefore has the actions, uses and side-effects of hydrocortisone, which is often the preferred corticosteroid. It should be noted that cortisone is of no value for topical application. See hydrocortisone, page 250 and Table 36.

**co-tenidone** Tablets of atenolol and chlorthalidone. (Tenoretic).

**co-triamterzide** Tablets of hydrochlorothiazide and triamterine. (Diazide).

**co-trimoxazole** A mixture of trimethoprim and sulphamethoxazole. Trimethoprim, like the sulphonamides, interferes with the folic acid cycle of bacterial metabolism, but at a different point, and the mixture has an increased antibacterial action. It was once widely used, but is now advised only for *Pneumocystis carinii* pneumonia. Occasionally given in acute bronchitis and urinary infections when no other drug is acceptable.
**Dose:** 120 mg/kg daily for 14 days; 960 mg 12-hourly by i.v. infusion. (Bactrim; Septrin).

**coumarins** Compounds that depress the formation in the liver of prothrombin and other blood coagulation factors. See warfarin and phenindione.

**counter-irritants** Substances, also referred to as rubifacients, that, when applied to the skin, produce a mild, local irritation and inflammation, and give symptomatic relief in painful conditions of the muscles and joints. Creams and liniments containing methyl salicylate, turpentine, capsicum resin and menthol are examples of rubifacients.

**crisantaspase** Asparagine is an aminoacid essential for the development of some malignant cells. Crisantaspase is an enzyme, also known as asparaginase, that

breaks down asparagine, and so has an indirect cytotoxic action. It is used to induce remission in acute lymphoblastic leukaemia in children.
**Dose:** (after pre-treatment with other drugs): 1000 units/kg by slow i.v. injection daily for 10 days. Side-effects include anaphylactic reactions, and skin tests to detect hypersensitivity are essential before initial and re-treatment. (Erwinase). See page 122.

**crotamiton** An ascaricide and antipruritic. Used by local application as cream or lotion (10%) in the treatment of scabies and itching conditions. (Eurax).

**crystal violet** A dyestuff with a selective action against Gram-positive organisms and yeasts. Used as a 0.5% solution for infected skin conditions, and for skin preparation.

**cyanocobalamin** The anti-anaemic factor present in liver. It is specific in the treatment of pernicious anaemia and its neurological complications, and of value in some other anaemias due to nutritional deficiencies.
**Dose:** in pernicious anaemia, 1 mg by i.m. injection at monthly intervals. It has been largely replaced by hydroxocobalamin, which has a more prolonged action. (Cytamen). See page 112 and Table 3.

**cyclizine** An antihistamine, used mainly in travel sickness and nausea generally. Also useful in vertigo.
**Dose:** 100–150 mg daily. Side-effects include dryness of the mouth, headache and drowsiness. (Valoid).

**cyclopenthiazide** A thiazide diuretic with the actions, uses and side-effects of bendrofluazide.
**Dose:** 1 mg initially, 250–500 µg daily or on alternate days, in the morning, according to need. (Navidrex). See page 148 and Table 21.

**cyclopentolate** An anticholinergic agent used to produce cycloplegia and mydriasis. The action is more rapid and less prolonged than atropine, particularly in children. (Mydrilate).

**cyclophosphamide** A widely used alkylating cytotoxic agent, active orally and by injection. Used in Hodgkin's disease, chronic

lymphocytic leukaemia and lymphomas.
**Dose:** 100–300 mg daily, orally or i.v., or 500 mg–1 g weekly. A high fluid intake is necessary, as a metabolite may cause haemorrhagic cystitis, and it is sometimes used with mesna to reduce the risk of such cystitis. Nausea and vomiting are common side-effects, as is epilation with high doses. (Endoxana). See page 122 and Table 8.

**cyclopropane** An inhalation anaesthetic of high potency with which induction and recovery are rapid. It causes some respiratory depression and cardiac irregularities, and its administration requires care. It is used with closed-circuit apparatus as it forms an explosive mixture with air and oxygen. Supplied in orange-coloured cylinders.

**cycloserine** An antibiotic used in pulmonary tuberculosis when standard drugs are ineffective. Occasionally used in urinary infections.
**Dose:** 250–750 mg daily. Side-effects include drowsiness, vertigo and rash. See page 170 and Table 31.

**cyclosporin** An antibiotic with a powerful immunosuppressant action. It is used under expert control to prevent graft rejection in organ and bone marrow transplantation, and in the prevention of graft-versus-host disease (GVHD). Prolonged therapy over some months may be required. Side-effects may include tremor, gastrointestinal disturbance, hypertrichosis and nephrotoxicity. (Neoral; Sandimmun).

**cyproheptadine** A compound with antihistamine and antiserotonin properties. Some allergic reactions are due not only to histamine, but also to serotonin, and cyproheptadine is useful in conditions not responding completely to an antihistamine.
**Dose:** 4–20 mg daily. It has been used as an appetite stimulant in doses of 12 mg daily and in refractory migraine. (Periactin). See page 110 and Table 2.

**cyproterone** An anti-androgen used to reduce libido in sexual deviants. *Dose*: 50–100 mg daily. It is also used in the palliative treatment of prostatic carcinoma, particularly in advanced cases that have become resistant to other therapy.
**Dose:** 300 mg daily. For severe, refractory acne in females, 2 mg daily with ethinyloestradiol. Side-effects are fatigue and

lassitude, weight gain and gynaecomastia. Contraindicated in severe depression and acute hepatic disease. Care is necessary in diabetics. (Cyprostat).

**cytarabine** A cytotoxic agent that prevents cell development by inhibiting the formation of nucleic acid. It is used mainly in the control of acute myeloblastic leukaemia.
**Dose:** 0.5–3 mg/kg daily by i.v. or s.c. injection. Close haematological control is essential as the drug is a powerful myelodepressant. Other side-effects are those of the cytotoxic drugs, generally, but fever, myalgia and bone pain may also occur. (Alexan; Cytosar). See page 122 and Table 8.

**cytotoxic drugs** A term applied to drugs that can kill cancer cells. In practice, many factors influence their therapeutic value. They are rarely selective, and therapeutic doses usually have a toxic effect on some normal cells. They may attack cancer cells at different stages of development, as actively dividing cells are more susceptible than resting cells. They may not reach the cancer cells in adequate concentration, or resistance to the drug may develop. The dose may also depend to some extent on the patient's tolerance of the drug, and combined treatment with two or more drugs may have the advantages of increased potency with reduced toxicity. All cytotoxic drugs, with the exception of bleomycin and vincristine, bring about a depression of the bone marrow, which may be severe, and some degree of hair loss, which is usually reversible. Severe nausea and vomiting are also common, and early use of powerful antiemetics is essential. Many cytotoxic agents are tissue irritants, and with i.v. treatment great care must be taken to avoid extravasation, as severe local tissue damage can occur. See alkylating agents and antimetabolites. See page 122.

# D

**dacarbazine** A cytotoxic drug that appears to depress purine metabolism and the formation of DNA. It is used mainly in malignant melanoma, and in combination with other agents it is of value in other malignant conditions.

**Dose:** 2.5-4.5 mg/kg, daily for 10 days, repeated after 4 weeks. Side-effects are severe nausea, bone marrow depression and an influenza-like syndrome. The drug should be handled with care, as it is a tissue irritant. (DTIC). See page 122 and Table 8.

**dactinomycin** See actinomycin D.

**dalteparin** A low-molecular weight heparin given by s.c. injection for pre- and postoperative thrombo-embolic prophylaxis.
**Dose:** 2500 units daily for 5 days. (Fragmin). See enoxaprin and tinzaparin.

**danazol** A derivative of ethisterone that inhibits the release of pituitary gonadotrophins. Used in conditions such as endometriosis and gynaecomastia.
**Dose:** 200–800 mg daily, starting during menstruation. Side-effects are nausea, dizziness, rash, flushing and hair loss. Care is necessary in cardiac, renal or hepatic impairment, and in epilepsy and diabetes. (Danol).

**danthron** A synthetic anthraquinone laxative used mainly for constipation in the aged, and in drug-induced constipation in the terminally ill. Not suitable for routine use by other patients.
**Dose:** given in doses of 25–25 mg as co-danthramer, and acts within 6–12 hours. The urine may be coloured red.

**dantrolene** A skeletal muscle relaxant that acts on the muscle fibre, and not at the myoneural junction. The action may be linked with an interference with the movement of calcium ions. It is used in the severe and chronic spastic states that occur after stroke, spinal cord injury, and in multiple sclerosis.
**Dose:** 25 mg daily initially, increased at weekly intervals up to a maximum of 400 mg daily, as the response is slow and may be inadequate. The side-effects of weakness and fatigue are mild, and often transient, but liver function tests during treatment are essential. Dantrolene is also of value in malignant hyperthermia, a rare but serious complication of anaesthesia, and is given in doses of 1 mg/kg by i.v. injection as soon as the condition is diagnosed, and repeated up to a total of 10 mg/kg. (Dantrium).

**dapsone** A sulphone compound used in the treatment of leprosy.
**Dose:** 25–400 mg orally twice weekly and continued for some years. Resistance to dapsone may occur, and combined treatment with clofazimine and rifampicin may be necessary. Dapsone is sometimes given with pyrimethamine in chloroquine-resistant malaria. Side-effects are nausea, rash, neuropathy and myelodepression.

**daunorubicin** See doxorubicin.

**debrisoquine** An adrenergic neurone blocking agent with the actions, uses and side-effects of guanethidine, except that it is less likely to cause diarrhoea. It is used mainly in resistant hypertension, in association with other drugs. (Declinax). See page 148 and Table 21.

**deflazacort** A glucocorticoid with the actions and uses of related drugs, and comparable in activity with prednisolone.
**Dose:** initially in acute conditions up to 120 mg daily; maintenance dose 3–18 mg daily. (Calcort). See hydrocortisone, page 55 and Table 36.

**demeclocycline** An antibiotic with the actions, uses and side-effects of tetracycline, but more likely to cause photoallergic reactions.
**Dose:** 600 mg daily. Used occasionally in hyponatraemia due to overactivity of the antidiuretic hormone. (Ledermycin).

**desferrioxamine** A chelating agent that combines with iron salts to form a soluble non-toxic complex. Of great value in acute ferrous sulphate poisoning in children.
**Dose:** 2 g immediately by i.m. injection, together with gastric lavage (2 g of desferrioxamine/l) followed by a single oral dose of 10 g. It may also be given by continuous i.v. infusion, 15 mg/kg hourly up to a maximum of 80 mg/kg. It may cause hypotension if the infusion is given too rapidly. It is also useful in the treatment of iron-overload caused by repeated blood transfusions, and for aluminium overload in patients on dialysis. (Desferal).

**desflurane** An inhalation anaesthetic similar to enflurane. (Suprane).

**desmopressin** A derivative of vasopressin, with increased potency and longer duration of action. Used in the diagnosis and control of diabetes insipidus, and in the treatment of nocturnal enuresis.
**Dose:** 10–20 µg intranasally once or twice a day; 1–4 µg daily by injection. (DDAVP).

**desoxymethasone** A corticosteroid, for local application in acute inflammatory and allergic skin conditions. Used as oily cream 0.25%. (Stiedex).

**dexamethasone** A potent synthetic corticosteroid, with reduced salt-retaining properties. Useful in all conditions requiring systemic corticosteroid therapy (except Addison's disease), including inflammatory and allergic disorders, shock, cerebral oedema and adrenal hyperplasia.
**Dose:** 0.5–2 mg daily up to a maximum of 15 mg daily; in shock, 5–20 mg by slow i.v. injection or infusion; in cerebral oedema, 10 mg initially by i.v. injection, followed by 4 mg i.m. 6-hourly. Dexamethasone is also given by intra-articular injection for local inflammation of joints in doses of 0.4–4 mg. It is also used as eye drops (0.1%) in uveitis, but care is necessary with prolonged treatment as with some patients a 'steroid glaucoma' may be precipitated. (Decadron). See page 250 and Table 36.

**†dexamphetamine sulphate** A central nervous system stimulant. It is used in the treatment of narcolepsy and, paradoxically, it is sometimes useful in hyperkinesia in children.
**Dose:** in narcolepsy, 20–60 mg daily; in hyperkinesia 2.5 mg initially, slowly increased up to a maximum of 20 mg daily. Side-effects are insomnia, anorexia and agitation. Dependence and tolerance may occur early. (Dexedrine†).

**dextran** A blood-plasma substitute obtained from sucrose solutions by bacterial action, and used as solutions of varying molecular weight (dextran 40, 70). Dextran 70 is used as a blood volume expander by i.v. injection in some cases of shock; dextran 40 is used mainly to improve postoperative peripheral circulation, reduce blood viscosity, and to prevent thrombo-embolism. Care must be taken to adjust dose to avoid overloading the circulation. Any blood-matching should be carried out before giving dextran. (Gentran; Macrodex; Rheomacrodex).

37

D

**†dextromoramide** A powerful synthetic analgesic with a shorter and less sedating action than morphine. Of value in severe and intractable pain, and in terminal disease.
**Dose:** 5 mg or more either orally or by injection, according to need and response. Care is necessary in liver dysfunction and respiratory depression. (Palfium†).

**dextropropoxyphene** An orally effective analgesic. Of value in many painful conditions, and in malignant disease its use may delay the need to resort to the opiate analgesics.
**Dose:** 250 mg or more daily, but doses in excess of 700 mg daily may cause toxic psychoses and convulsions. (Doloxene). See co-proxamol.

**dextrose** See glucose.

**†diamorphine** A derivative of morphine with a more powerful analgesic and cough-suppressant action. It is also less liable to cause nausea. Valuable for the relief of severe pain and the suppression of useless cough. Addiction is a constant risk owing to the euphoric effects of the drug.
**Dose:** 5–10 mg orally or by injection, repeated as required. For severe pain in the terminally ill, addiction is of no consequence, and much larger doses are given according to need: if necessary, by continuous infusion or a syringe-pump device.

**diazepam** A benzodiazepine of value in anxiety states, insomnia, acute alcoholic withdrawal, and for premedication. It also has a muscle relaxant action, and is valuable when given by injection in status epilepticus and in the control of the spasm of tetanus.
**Doses:** 5–30 mg daily, 10–20 mg by slow i.v. injection as required, up to a maximum of 3 mg/kg in 24 hours. Absorption after i.m. injection is unreliable. It is sometimes given as suppositories of 5–10 mg. Side-effects are drowsiness, dizziness, respiratory depression and hypersensitivity reactions. Care is necessary in glaucoma and renal and hepatic impairment. Extended treatment may lead to dependence and addiction, and withdrawal should be slow to avoid the risks of precipitating toxic psychosis, confusion and convulsions. (Stesolid; Valium). See pages 177 & 136, and Tables 5 & 15.

**diazoxide** An inhibitor of insulin secretion.
**Dose:** given orally in doses of 5 mg/kg or more daily in severe hypoglycaemia. Also of value in severe hypertensive crisis, in doses up to 150 mg by rapid i.v. injection. Side-effects are nausea, tachycardia and oedema. (Eudemine).

**diclofenac** A non-steroidal anti-inflammatory drug (NSAID) of the naproxen type, and used in rheumatoid, arthritic and similar conditions.
**Dose:** 75–150 mg daily, after food. Suppositories of 100 mg are useful at night, but may cause local irritation. In acute conditions and in postoperative pain, doses of 75 mg once or twice a day by deep i.m. injection for not more than 2 days. (Diclomax; Voltarol). Like other NSAIDs, diclofenac may cause gastric disturbance and hypersensitivity reactions. See page 165 and Table 29.

**dicobalt edetate** A specific antidote in acute cyanide poisoning; toxic in other conditions.
**Dose:** 300 mg by slow i.v. injection, followed by 50 ml of glucose solution 50%, repeated if required. (Kelocyanor). See sodium nitrite.

**dicyclomine** An anticholinergic agent used to reduce gastric hyperacidity and the smooth muscle spasm of gastrointestinal disorders.
**Dose:** 30–60 mg daily. Side-effects include dryness of the mouth and blurred vision. (Merbentyl).

**didanosine** An antiviral agent used in HIV infections not responding to zidovudine.
**Dose:** 400 mg daily before food. Diarrhoea, vomiting and peripheral neuropathy are side-effects. (Videx contains didanosine with antacids). See page 144 and Table 19.

**dienoestrol** A synthetic oestrogen used as a 0.025% cream for senile or atrophic vaginitis.

**diethylcarbamazine** A synthetic drug used in filariasis but long-term treatment is necessary.
**Dose:** 1 mg/kg daily initially, slowly increased to 6 mg/kg daily, and continued for 21 days. Low initial doses are necessary to reduce allergic reactions due to proteins released from dead worms. Side-effects include headache, nausea, rash and conjunctivitis. (Hetrazan). See ivermectin.

**diflucortolone** A corticosteroid used topically as a 0.1% or 0.3% cream or ointment in steroid-responsive dermatoses. Of value in resistant conditions. (Nerisone).

**diflunisal** An anti-inflammatory and analgesic drug (NSAID), chemically related to aspirin, but with actions and uses similar to naproxen.
**Dose:** 500 mg–1 g daily. Care is necessary in aspirin-sensitive patients, and in peptic ulcer. (Dolobid). See page 165 and Table 29.

**Digibind** A highly purified preparation of sheep-derived digoxin-specific antibodies, given by i.v. infusion in digoxin overdose or poisoning. It mobilizes digoxin from cardiac receptor sites and binds it as an inert complex which is excreted into the urine, and symptoms of digoxin toxicity subside within an hour.
**Dose:** depends on the amount of digoxin absorbed; 40 mg can neutralize about 600 µg of digoxin.

**digitalis** The dried leaf of the foxglove. It has a powerful strengthening and regulatory action on the heart, but is now used as digoxin.

**digitoxin** The most powerful cardiac glycoside of digitalis and of value in heart failure and atrial fibrillation. Absorption is rapid but excretion, which depends on metabolism by the liver, is very slow, and cumulative effects may occur.
**Dose:** (maintanence) requires careful adjustment, varying from 50–200 µg daily.

**digoxin** The principal cardiac glycoside obtained from digitalis leaf. It is rapidly absorbed orally, and is widely used in cardiac failure, paroxysmal tachycardia and atrial fibrillation. The diuresis of digoxin therapy is a secondary effect following the improvement in the renal circulation.
**Dose:** for rapid digitalization, 1–1.5 mg initially over 24 hours; subsequent maintenance dose 62.5–500 µg daily. For slow digitalization, 250–500 µg may be given daily for about a week, with subsequent doses based on the response. Elderly patients and children respond adequately to smaller doses, and tablets of 62.5 µg (Lanoxin-PG) are available for such patients. In emergency, digoxin can be given by slow i.v. injection in doses of

250–500 µg initially according to need. Nausea and vomiting are often signs of overdose. If the heart rate falls below 60 beats per minute, dosage requires adjustment. See page 141 and Table 18.

**digoxin-specific antibody** See Digibind.

**dihydrocodeine** An analgesic derived from codeine, but with a more powerful action. Of value in many painful conditions where mild analgesics are inadequate.
**Dose:** 30 mg orally after food, or 50 mg by i.m. or deep s.c. injection at intervals of 4–6 hours according to need. Dizziness and constipation are side-effects. (DF118).

**dihydrotachysterol** A sterol related to calciferol, but with more rapid calcium-mobilizing properties. It is used mainly in hypocalcaemia and parathyroid tetany, but is sometimes effective in calciferol-resistant rickets.
**Dose:** 200 µg daily, adjusted to need according to plasma calcium levels as a solution in oil. (AT 10).

**diloxanide** A well-tolerated amoebicide used in chronic intestinal amoebiasis when only cysts are present in the faeces. It is also used in acute infections, 5 days after a course of metronidazole.
**Dose:** 1.5 g daily for 10 days. (Furamide).

**diltiazem** A calcium channel blocking agent, used in the prophylaxis and treatment of angina, and useful when beta-blocking agents are unsuitable or ineffective.
**Dose:** 180–360 mg daily, reduced in renal impairment. It may cause bradycardia, ankle oedema and hypotension. (Adizen; Tildiem). Some long-acting products with various brand names are used in hypertension. They should not be regarded as interchangeable, as the duration of action may vary. See page 114 and Table 4.

**dimenhydrinate** An antihistamine used mainly as an antiemetic in nausea, travel sickness and vertigo.
**Dose:** 100–300 mg daily. It may cause more drowsiness than some related drugs. (Dramamine).

**dimercaprol (BAL)** A specific drug for the treatment of poisoning by arsenic, mercury, gold and other heavy metals.

**Dose:** up to 3 mg/kg 4-hourly by i.m.
injection for 2 days, gradually reduced to
twice or once daily for 10 days. Side-
effects include malaise, sweating, tachycardia, lachrymation and muscle spasm.

**dimethicone** Activated dimethicone is an
antifoaming agent, said to reduce
flatulence and protect mucous
membranes. It is a constituent of many
antacid preparations. It is also present in
some water-repellent skin creams.

**dimethylsulphoxide (DMSO)** An organic
liquid, it has been used for the symptomatic relief of interstitial cystitis
(Hunner's ulcer) by the bladder instillation
of 50 ml of a 50% solution. (Rimso–50).

**dinoprost** Prostaglandin $F_{2\alpha}$. It has actions
and uses similar to dinoprostone.
(Prostin F2).

**dinoprostone** A synthetic form of
prostaglandin $E_2$. It has been used to initiate contractions of the pregnant uterus.
**Dose:** 500 µg orally to induce labour,
repeated if necessary at hourly intervals; as
vaginal tablets or gel, 3 mg. Side-effects are
nausea, diarrhoea, shivering and dizziness.
(Prostin E2; Prepidil).

**dioctyl sodium sulphosuccinate** See
docusate.

**diodone injection** A solution of a complex
organic iodine compound, used as a
contrast agent in X-ray examination of
kidneys and ureters.

**diphenhydramine** One of the early antihistamines, with a more sedative action, and
used in the temporary relief of insomnia.
**Dose:** 10–25 mg. (Medinex, Nytol). It is
also present in some cough preparations
and nasal decongestants.

**diphenoxylate** A derivative that resembles
codeine in reducing intestinal activity. It is
used for the symptomatic relief of diarrhoea, and is usually given with a small dose
of atropine to discourage excessive dosage
and to reduce the risk of dependence.
**Dose:** 10 mg initially, then 5 mg every 6
hours as required. (Lomotil; Tropergen).

**diphenylpyraline** An antihistamine used as
a decongestant in colds and sinusitis.
Present in Eskornade.

† **dipipanone** A rapidly acting morphine-
like analgesic of value in the severe pain of
terminal disease.
**Dose:** 30–360 mg daily, but it is usually
given in association with cyclizine as
†Diconal. The side-effects are similar to
those of morphine.

**dipivefrine** A pro-drug that is converted
into adrenaline after absorption. It is used
in chronic *open* angle glaucoma as eye
drops (0.1%). (Propine). See page 138 and
Table 16.

**dipyridamole** An inhibitor of thrombus
formation by reducing the adhesiveness of
blood platelets in the arterial circulation.
**Dose:** 300–600 mg daily before food.
Side-effects include nausea, diarrhoea and
headache. (Persantin).

**disodium cromoglycate** See sodium
cromoglycate.

**disodium etidronate** See etidronate.

**disodium pamidronate** See pamidronate.

**disopyramide** A quinidine-like drug used
in the treatment of cardiac arrhythmias
especially after myocardial infarction.
**Dose:** 300–800 mg daily; dose by slow i.v.
injection under ECG cover, 2 mg/kg up to
150 mg, followed by oral therapy as soon
as possible. By its anticholinergic action
care is necessary in glaucoma and prostatic enlargement. Contraindicated in heart
block. (Dirythmin; Rythmodan). See
page 156 and Table 24.

**distigmine** An inhibitor of cholinesterase
similar to neostigmine but with a longer
action.
**Dose:** in the control of myasthenia gravis
5–20 mg as a single morning dose before
breakfast; in urinary retention after
surgery, 5 mg daily. It is sometimes used
in neurogenic bladder disorders. Side-
effects are nausea, abdominal cramp,
diarrhoea and weakness. (Ubretid).

**disulfiram** When taken with even small
amounts of alcohol, disulfiram permits the
accumulation of acetaldehyde in the body,
with side-effects such as flushing, giddiness,
vomiting and headache that may be severe.
Disulfiram is used in chronic alcoholism,
but prolonged treatment and co-operation
of the patient are essential.

**Dose:** after at least 24 alcohol free hours: 800 mg on the first day, falling over 5 days to 100–200 mg daily. Acute confusion may occur if given at the same time as metronidazole. (Antabuse).

**dithranol** Synthetic compound used locally in the treatment of psoriasis. It is a powerful irritant, and treatment should be commenced with a simple ointment or zinc paste containing 0.1% of dithranol, gradually increased to 1% if well tolerated. Higher concentrations are sometimes used in 'short-contact-time' therapy.

**diuretics** The most widely used group of diuretics is the thiazides, represented by bendrofluazide (see page 141). They act mainly by increasing the excretion of sodium by inhibiting its re-absorption by the distal tubule of the kidney, and evoke a rapid response which may persist over 12–24 hours, although some, such as chlorthalidone, have a still longer action. They are given in mild cardiac failure, oedema and in hypertension, but in more severe conditions, and in pulmonary oedema, the more powerful 'loop' diuretics, such as frusemide, which act at a different point, are preferred. A side-effect of some thiazides is an increase in the excretion of potassium which may require the use of potassium supplements or a change to a potassium-sparing diuretic such as triamterene. Spironolactone, an aldosterone antagonist, is a more powerful diuretic, of value in resistant oedema. Osmotic diuretics such as mannitol are used mainly in cerebral oedema. Simple diuretics such as potassium citrate are mainly used to alkalize the urine and promote diuresis in cystitis and similar conditions. See page 141 and Table 18.

**dobutamine** A sympathomimetic agent similar to isoprenaline, but with a more selective stimulant action on the beta$_1$ receptors in the heart. It increases cardiac contractility but is less likely to cause tachycardia. Useful in acute heart failure and cardiogenic and septic shock.
**Dose:** 2.5–5 µg/kg/min by i.v. infusion, carefully adjusted to need. (Dobutrex; Posiject). See page 141 and Table 18.

**docetaxel** A potent cytotoxic agent derived from the Pacific Yew. Used in advanced breast cancer resistant to other therapy.

**Dose:** 100 mg/m$^2$ by i.v. infusion over 1 hour. Rapid and severe hypersensitivity reactions (hypotension, bronchospasm) may occur, and treatment must be immediately available. Reaction risks may be reduced by premedication with dexamethasone given the day before treatment and continued for 5 days. Rash, pruritus and neutropenia may occur, and blood counts and liver function tests are necessary. (Taxotere). See page 122 and Table 8.

**docusate** A surface-active agent used as a faeces-softening laxative.
**Dose:** up to 500 mg daily. (Dioctyl).

**domperidone** An antiemetic that functions as a dopamine antagonist, as it prevents dopamine from reaching the receptors in the chemoreceptor trigger zone (see antiemetics). It is mainly of value in the severe nausea and vomiting caused by cytotoxic drugs, and is also useful in functional dyspepsia. It is of little value in postoperative and travel sickness.
**Dose:** 10–20 mg 4–8-hourly; 30–60 mg by suppository. Sedative side-effects are infrequent, as domperidone does not cross the blood-brain barrier. (Motilium). See page 77.

**donepezil** A reversible inhibitor of anticholinesterase. Alzheimer's disease is linked with a deficiency of acetylcholine in the brain, and donepezil may relieve some of the symptoms of that disease by increasing brain acetylcholine.
**Dose:** 5–10 mg at night. Diarrhoea and muscle cramps are side-effects. (Aricept).

**dopamine** A sympathomimetic agent with actions and uses similar to dobutamine.
**Dose:** 2.5–10 µg/kg/min by slow i.v. infusion. Careful control of dose is essential, as dopamine may cause vasoconstriction with higher doses and increase the risk of heart failure. (Intropin). Dopamine is also a central neurotransmitter, and a deficiency is associated with parkinsonism. See levodopa, page 141 and Table 18.

**dopexamine** A short-acting drug of the dopamine type but with a more powerful action on the β$_2$-receptors. It is used in heart failure during cardiac surgery.
**Dose:** 500 ng/kg/min by i.v. infusion (caval catheter), slowly increased if required up to a maximum of

6 µg/kg/min. Side-effects include tachycardia and anginal pain that subside following withdrawal. (Dopacard). See page 141 and Table 18.

**dornase alfa** A recombinant form of human deoxyribonuclease (rhDNase) used in cystic fibrosis. The viscous purulent airways secretion of that disease is due to the presence of large amounts of extra-cellular DNA from degenerating leucocytes. Dornase alfa breaks down the DNA and reduces the sputum viscosity.
**Dose:** 2500 units daily by inhalation from a jet nebulizer. Daily treatment is necessary to maintain the response. (Pulmozyme).

**dorzolamide** An inhibitor of carbonic anhydrase that reduces the amount of sodium bicarbonate in the aqueous humour of the eye. It is used as eye drops (2%) 2 or 3 times a day as adjunctive therapy in ocular hypertension when beta-blockers are unsuitable or ineffective. (Trusopt). See page 138 and Table 16.

**dothiepin (dosulepin)** A tricyclic antidepressant with the uses and side-effects of amitriptyline. It is used in the treatment of depression when a sedative action is also indicated.
**Dose:** 75–150 mg daily. It may also be given as a single nightly dose to reduce daytime drowsiness. (Prothiaden). See page 128 and Table 11.

**doxapram** A respiratory stimulant useful in postoperative respiratory failure under expert control.
**Dose:** by i.v. injection 1–1.5 mg/kg according to need. It is also given by i.v. infusion in doses controlled by arterial blood gas studies. Side-effects include hypertension, bronchospasm and tachycardia. (Dopram).

**doxazocin** An alpha-adrenoceptor blocking agent of the prazosin type, but with a longer action that permits a single daily dose.
**Dose:** in hypertension 1 mg initially, slowly increased after 7–14 days to 2 mg daily, up to a daily maximum of 16 mg, usually in association with other antihypertensive drugs. It is also used in the symptomatic treatment of benign prostatic hyperplasia. Side-effects are

dizziness and postural hypotension, and initial therapy, as with prazosin, requires care. (Cardura). See pages 148 & 164, and Tables 21 & 28.

**doxepin** An antidepressant with the actions, uses and side-effects of dothiepin.
**Dose:** 30–300 mg daily; a single dose of 100 mg is sometimes given at night. (Sinequan). See page 128 and Table 11.

**doxorubicin** A cytotoxic antibiotic widely used in leukaemia, lymphosarcoma, breast and lung cancer.
**Dose:** by fast i.v. infusion 60–75 mg/m$^2$ at intervals of 3 weeks, or 20–25 mg/m$^2$ daily for 3 days. It is also used by bladder installation (50 mg in 50 ml of saline solution) for superficial bladder tumours. Side-effects include bone marrow depression, cardiac damage, alopecia, buccal ulceration and nausea. Doxorubicin is a skin irritant, and should be handled with care. See page 122 and Table 8.

**doxycycline** A long-acting tetracycline.
**Dose:** 200 mg initially, followed by 100 mg as a single daily dose. In acne, a dose of 50 mg daily is given for some weeks. It should be taken with adequate fluid, with the patient in a sitting or standing position. (Nordox; Vibramycin).

**droperidol** A tranquillizer with unusual properties. It is given in severe psychotic conditions such as mania, in drug-induced nausea and vomiting and for preoperative sedation. It is also given with fentanyl to produce a state of detachment (neuroleptanalgesia).
**Dose:** 20–120 mg daily; 5–10 mg by injection; in cancer therapy induced vomiting doses of 1–3 mg/hr have been given by continuous i.v. infusion. Side-effects are those of chlorpromazine and haloperidol. (Droleptan).

**dydrogesterone** An orally active progestogen that is virtually free from any oestrogenic or androgenic side-effects. It is used in amenorrhoea, endometriosis, functional uterine bleeding, and threatened abortion.
**Dose:** 10–30 mg daily. (Duphaston).

**econazole** An antifungal agent similar in actions and uses to clotrimazole. (Ecostatin; Pevaryl).

**ecothiopate** A potent and long-acting miotic that has been used in glaucoma as eye drops of 0.03–0.25%. It may cause cataract; its availability is strictly limited.

**edrophonium** A very short-acting drug of the neostigmine type. It is used in the diagnosis of myasthenia gravis.
**Dose:** 2–10 mg by i.v. injection, which causes a marked but transient increase in muscle power if myasthenia gravis is present.

**eformoterol**∇ A selective β₂ stimulant (agonist) with a rapid initial action, used as supplementary treatment in patients receiving other bronchodilator therapy for reversible airway obstruction.
**Dose:** by inhalation: 12 µg twice daily, doubled if necessary. Care is necessary in ischaemic heart disease and diabetes. Not to be used for acute attacks. (Foradil). See page 118 and Table 6.

**enalapril** An ACE inhibitor used in the treatment of all types of hypertension, and in congestive heart failure, often together with a diuretic.
**Dose:** 5 mg daily initially, increased as required up to 40 mg daily, and often given as a single dose. Dizziness, hypotension and loss of taste are some side-effects. (Innovac). See page 148 and Table 21.

**enflurane** An inhalation anaesthetic with the actions and uses of halothane, but less potent.

**enoxaparin** A low-molecular weight and longer acting form of heparin. It has the general properties of heparin, but with less effect on blood platelet activity. It is used in the prevention of venous thrombosis.
**Dose:** 20 mg by s.c. injection once daily (1 hour before surgery) for 7–10 days. (Clexane). See certoparin, dalteparin and tinzaparin.

**enoximone** An inhibitor of the enzyme phosphodiesterase. It has a digoxin-like action on the myocardium and is used in

congestive heart failure not responding to other drugs.
**Dose:** by i.v. infusion, 90 µg/kg/min initially; followed by supportive doses of 5–20 µg/kg as required up to a maximum of 24 mg/kg over 24 hours. Side-effects are hypotension, ectopic beats and gastro-intestinal disturbances. (Perfan). See milinone, page 141 and Table 18.

**ephedrine** A sympathomimetic agent once used in asthma and bronchospasm, but now largely replaced by drugs of the salbutamol type. It is still used to prevent spinal anaesthesia hypotension.
**Dose:** 15–30 mg by i.m. injection; and to reverse such hypotension with i.v. injections of 3–6 mg at intervals of 3–4 minutes according to need. It is also used as nose-drops (0.5%) to relieve nasal congestion.

**epirubicin** A cytotoxic agent with the actions, uses and side-effects of doxorubicin.
**Dose:** 75–90 mg/m² as free-flowing i.v. infusion repeated at intervals of 3 weeks. The side-effects and cardiotoxicity are less severe than those of doxorubicin. (Pharmarubicin). See page 122 and Table 8.

**epoetin alfa and beta** Recombinant forms of human erythropoietin. (Eprex; Recormon). See erythropoietin.

**epoprostenol** A prostaglandin present in the walls of blood vessels that inhibits platelet aggregation. It is used to prevent platelet aggregation during cardio-pulmonary bypass and charcoal haemo-perfusion, and as an alternative to heparin in renal dialysis.
**Dose:** 10–20 ng/kg/min by continuous i.v. infusion. Smaller doses in renal dialysis. It is also a vasodilator, and side-effects are flushing and hypotension. (Flolan).

**eptacog alfa** See Factor VIIa.

**ergocalciferol** See calciferol.

**ergometrine** The principal alkaloid of ergot. It promotes uterine contraction and is used for the rapid control of post-partum haemorrhage. Dangerous in the early stages of labour.
**Dose:** 0.5–1 mg orally; or 200–500 µg by injection. It is often used together with oxycytocin as Syntometrine. Side-effects are nausea and transient hypertension.

**ergot** A fungus that develops in rye and replaces the normal grain. The active principles include ergometrine and ergotamine. Chronic toxic effects characterized by gangrene of the extremities have followed the use of ergot-contaminated rye bread.

**ergotamine** An alkaloid of ergot that constricts the cranial arteries, and is used solely for the relief of migraine not responding to analgesic therapy. Early treatment evokes the best response.
**Dose:** 2 mg initially up to 6 mg during an attack, not to be repeated until after an interval of some days. Total dose in 1 week: 10–12 mg. It is also given by oral inhalation in doses of 360 µg (1 puff), repeated after 5 minutes, up to a maximum of 6 puffs daily. Side-effects include headache and nausea, and the drug should be withdrawn if tingling of the extremities occurs. Ergotamine is *not* suitable for prophylaxis because of the risks of toxicity. (Lingraine). See page 154 and Table 23.

**erythromycin** An antibiotic, resembling penicillin in its general range of activity, with the advantage of being active orally. It is useful in streptococcal and respiratory infections and in penicillin-resistant staphylococcal infections. Erythromycin is also of value in penicillin-sensitive patients. It is also given as a prophylactic before dental surgery.
**Dose:** up to 4 g daily; in severe infections it may be given by slow i.v. infusion in doses of 50 mg/kg daily. Side-effects include nausea and vomiting, and diarrhoea may occur after high doses. Care is necessary in hepatic impairment. Preparations of erythromycin *estolate* are contraindicated in liver disease. Erythromycin may potentiate the action of warfarin. It should not be given with astemizole or terfenadine.

**erythropoietin (epoetin)** A renal hormone that regulates blood cell production in the bone marrow. Patients with renal failure maintained by haemodialysis do not produce epoetin, and so become anaemic. A recombinant form of erythropoietin is available for replacement therapy.
**Dose:** 20–50 units/kg 3 times a week by s.c. or i.v. injection under haematological control. Side-effects include headache and hypertension, but a sudden migraine-like pain may indicate an impending hypertensive crisis. (Eprex; Recormon).

**eserine** See physotigmine.

**esmolol** A very short-acting beta-adrenoceptor blocker used in the emergency treatment of supra-ventricular arrhythmias, tachycardia and peri-operative hypertension.
**Dose:** by i.v. infusion 50–200 µg/kg/min under close control. (Brevibloc).

**estramustine** A compound of oestradiol and mustine, designed to release mustine at oestrogen-receptor sites. It has a more localized action and so causes less myelodepression. It is used mainly in prostatic carcinoma, especially when resistant to other therapy.
**Dose:** 0.56–1.4 g daily. It should not be taken with food or milk products. Side-effects include gastrointestinal disturbances, nausea and gynaecomastia. (Estracyt). See page 122 and Table 8.

**ethacrynic acid** A loop diuretic with a rapid and intense action used mainly in oliguria due to renal failure.
**Dose:** 50 mg daily initially, increased as required up to a maximum of 400 mg daily or on alternate days. Ethacrynic acid is also given by slow i.v. injection in doses of 50–100 mg in acute or refractory conditions. Side-effects include nausea, diarrhoea and deafness. Some hypotension may occur initially. (Edecrin).

**ethambutol** An antitubercular drug.
**Dose:** 15 mg/kg daily, together with rifampicin or isoniazid. Lower doses should be given in renal damage. It may cause visual disturbances with loss of acuity, but recovery is usually complete on withdrawal of the drug. (Myambutol). See page 170 and Table 31.

**ethamsylate** A haemostatic used in the prophylaxis and treatment of peri-ventricular haemorrhage in low birth-weight infants.
**Dose:** 12.5 mg/kg by injection 6-hourly within 2 hours of birth and continued for 4 days. It is also used orally in menorrhagia. Dose: 2 g daily. (Dicynene).

**ethanolamine oleate** A sclerosing agent used for varicose veins and bleeding oesophageal varices.
**Dose:** by local i.v. injection, 2–5 ml.

**ether** A colourless inflammable liquid, once widely used as a general anaesthetic but now replaced by halothane.

**ethinyloestradiol** A synthetic oestrogen formerly used to control menopausal symptoms and other conditions where oestrogen therapy is indicated.
**Dose:** 10–50 μg daily. It is present with a progestogen in many oral contraceptive products. See page 264 and Table 40.

**ethosuximide** An anticonvulsant for the treatment of petit mal epilepsy (absence seizures). May be used alone, or combined with other anticonvulsants, and it is often of value in patients not responding to other drugs.
**Dose:** 500 mg daily initially, gradually increased if required, to a maximum of 2 g daily. Care is necessary in renal or hepatic disease. Drowsiness, headache and gastro-intestinal disorders are some side-effects. (Emeside; Zarontin). See page 136 and Table 15.

**etidronate disodium** A bisphosphonate used in Paget's disease of bone, as it slows down the rapid turnover of bone and relieves the pain of that disease.
**Dose:** 5 mg/kg as a single daily dose between meals for 6 months or more. Side-effects are nausea and diarrhoea; high doses may increase bone pain and the risks of fracture. (Didronel). Didronel PMO also contains calcium carbonate, and is used in the extended treatment of vertebral osteoporosis. See clodronate and pamidronate.

**etodolac** A non-steroidal anti-inflamma-tory agent (NSAID) of the naproxen type, with similar actions, uses and side-effects.
**Dose:** in rheumatoid conditions, 400 mg daily. (Lodine). See page 169 and Table 29.

**etomidate** A short-acting i.v. hypnotic used for the induction of anaesthesia. It causes little cardiac disturbance or hypertension, but muscle movement and pain may occur during injection.
**Dose:** 300 μg/kg by i.v. injection. (Hypnomidate).

**etoposide** A cytotoxic agent used in small-cell lung cancer and resistant testicular cancers. It is given in daily doses based on skin area for 5 days, repeated after 21 days according to response.
**Dose:** 120–240 mg/m² daily orally; by i.v. infusion 60–120 mg/m², and care must be taken to avoid extravasation. Side-effects include nausea, alopecia and myelo-suppression. (Vespid). See page 122 and Table 8.

**eusol** A chlorine antiseptic solution used as lotion, or as compress. The solution should be freshly prepared. Now less popular, thought to be irritant.

**evening primrose oil** See gamolenic acid.

**eye drops** Weak solutions of drugs for the treatment of ocular conditions. They may be antibacterial, antifungal or antiviral in action, or may be used for non-infective conditions such as glaucoma, or for diag-nosis. For routine use they are supplied sterile in multiple-application containers, but are intended for individual use only. They contain preservatives, and for home use may be used for up to one month after the container has been opened. In eye surgery, single application products should be used. Occasionally, enough of a drug may be absorbed from eye drops to have systemic effects, and corticosteroids, if used as eye drops over a prolonged period, may cause 'steroid glaucoma'. Care should be taken with contact lenses, and ideally they should not be worn during eye drop treat-ment. Soft contact lenses can absorb the preservatives, which may cause irritation.

**F**

**Factor VIIa** A recombinant and active form of the blood coagulation Factor VII. The treatment of haemophilia with Factors VIII and IX is complicated by the development of antibodies to those factors. Factor VIIa acts as a late stage in the conversion of fibrinogen to fibrin, can function independently of Factors VIII and IX, and does not induce the formation of antibodies. It is used to control serious bleeding in haemophiliac patients and during surgery, under specialist supervision.
**Dose:** 60–120 μg initially by i.v. injection, followed by a second dose after 2–3 hours, then 4–12-hourly as required for 2–3 weeks or more. (NovoSeven).

**Factor VIII** Haemophilia A is caused by a deficiency of the blood clotting agent Fac-tor VIII, and highly purified preparations

45

**F**

of human Factor VIII as well as recombinant forms are used as replacement therapy in doses based on the degree of deficiency of that factor. (Kogenate; Monoclate P; Recombinate).

**Factor IX** Haemophilia B is due to a deficiency of Factor IX, and preparations of that factor, obtained by monoclonal antibody techniques, are given i.v. in doses based on the degree of efficiency of the factor. (Monomine; Replenine).

**famiclovir** An antiviral agent similar to acyclovir, and used in herpes zoster (shingles) and genital herpes infections.
**Dose:** 75 mg daily for 7 days. (Famvir). See page 144 and Table 19.

**famotidine** An $H_2$-receptor antagonist with the uses and side-effects of cimetidine, but a longer action.
**Dose:** in benign peptic ulcer, 40 mg at night for 4–8 weeks; 20 mg at night for the prevention of recurrence, also used in reflux oesophagitis. In Zollinger–Ellison syndrome, doses of 20 mg 6-hourly are given. (Pepcid). See page 162 and Table 27.

**Fansidar** Pyrimethamine, 25 mg with sulfadoxine 500 mg. Both these antimalarial drugs block the formation of folinic acid in the malarial parasite, but the combination is more effective. Mainly used with quinine in resistant falciparum malaria. (Fansidar is no longer recommended for prophylaxis, as fatalities have followed such use.)

**felodipine** A calcium antagonist used in the treatment of hypertension generally (see calcium channel blocking agents).
**Dose:** 5 mg daily initially, adjusted to maintenance doses up to 10 mg daily. Tablets should be taken in the morning, and swallowed whole with water. No adjustment of dose necessary for elderly patients, but care is required in marked hepatic impairment. Hypotension with tachycardia may occur with susceptible patients. (Plendil). See page 148 and Table 21.

**felypressin** A vasopressin derivative, used as a vasoconstrictor in local anaesthetic solutions for dental use, when sympathetic pressor drugs are contraindicated.

**fenbufen** A non-steroidal anti-inflammatory agent (NSAID) used for the relief of pain and inflammation in rheumatoid arthritis and similar conditions.
**Dose:** 600–900 mg daily. Like other NSAIDs, it may cause gastrointestinal disturbance and dizziness, but the incidence of rash requires withdrawal of the drug. (Lederfen). See page 165 and Table 29.

**fenofibrate** A plasma-lipid regulating agent of the clofibrate type, with similar uses and side-effects.
**Dose:** 300 mg initially, with food, later 200–400 mg daily according to need. (Lipantil). See page 146 and Table 20.

**fenoprofen** A non-steroidal anti-inflammatory and anti-rheumatic agent. It is also used as a mild analgesic in a variety of painful conditions.
**Dose:** 900 mg–3 g daily. Side-effects include nausea, dizziness, vertigo and rash. (Fenoprofen; Progesic). See page 165 and Table 29.

**fenoterol** A sympathomimetic agent with the actions, uses and side-effects of salbutamol.
**Dose:** by oral inhalation, 100–200 µg (1–2 puffs) up to 4 times a day. (Berotec). See page 118 and Table 6.

**†fentanyl** A narcotic analgesic, used mainly in thiopentone anaesthesia to increase the response and permit a reduction in dose of thiopentone, especially in poor-risk patients. It is also used with droperidol to produce a state of neuroleptanalgesia.
**Dose:** 50–200 µg by i.v. injection. (Sublimaze). Also used as a patch for the relief of chronic pain. (Durogesic).

**fenticonazole** An antifungal used in vaginal candidiasis as pessaries of 200 mg. (Lomexin).

**ferrous sulphate, fumarate, gluconate & succinate** These iron salts are used in the prophylaxis and treatment of iron-deficiency anaemias. Ferrous sulphate is the standard drug, given in doses of 600 mg daily, but it may cause gastric disturbance in some patients, and ferrous fumarate, gluconate and succinate are better tolerated alternatives. Some better tolerated slow-release products are available, but may be less well absorbed. Ferrous sulphate tablets are potentially dangerous for small children, and death has occurred after accidental administration. See desferrioxamine.

**fexofenadine**∇ An antihistamine with the general properties of that group of drugs. It is less likely to affect the ability to drive. **Dose:** 120 mg once daily. (Telfast). See page 110 and Table 2.

**fibrinolytic agents** Drugs used to break up blood clots, and so are of value in thrombosis. See alteplase, anistreplase, streptokinase and urokinase.

**filgrastim**∇ A recombinant form of human granulocyte colony stimulating factor (G–CSF), one of a group of natural growth factors concerned with bone marrow activity. It stimulates the development of neutrophils, the production of which is depressed during cytotoxic therapy. The neutropenia thus caused increases the risks of infection, but the neutrophil count can be restored by filgrastim. It is used mainly in the neutropenia associated with the cytotoxic treatment of non-myeloid malignancy. **Dose:** 500 000 units/kg daily by s.c. injection or i.v. infusion for 14 days, or until the neutrophil count returns to normal. Double doses are given after bone marrow transplantation. The first dose should be given within 24 hours of chemotherapy. The main side-effects are musculoskeletal pain and dysuria. (Neupogen). See lenograstim and molgrastim.

**finasteride** An inhibitor of the enzyme 5–alpha reductase, and so prevents the conversion of testosterone to dihydro-testosterone, the biologically active form of the male hormone. It is used for the symptomatic relief of benign prostatic hyperplasia, as prolonged therapy promotes a reduction in the size of the prostate gland. **Dose:** 5 mg daily for 6 months or more. Side-effects are reduced libido and impotence. (Proscar). See page 164 and Table 28.

**flavoxate** An antispasmodic of value in urinary disorders such as dysuria, frequency and related conditions. **Dose:** 600 mg daily. Side-effects include dry mouth and blurred vision. Contra-indicated in glaucoma and bladder obstruction. (Urispas).

**flecainide** An orally active anti-arrhythmic agent of the lignocaine type. It chiefly influences conduction in the bundle of

His, and is of value in serious ventricular tachycardia and extrasystoles. **Dose:** 200–400 mg daily. May be given by slow i.v. injection in doses of 2 mg/kg in acute conditions resistant to other therapy, and under hospital control. Care is necessary in patients with pace-makers, and in renal impairment. Dizziness and visual disturbances are side-effects. (Tambocor). See page 141 and Table 18.

**flucloxacillin** A derivative of cloxacillin, that is absorbed more readily when given orally. It is used mainly in infections due to penicillinase-producing penicillin-resistant staphylococci. **Dose:** 1 g daily before food; by injection 1–4 g daily, but larger doses are given in very severe infections. Side-effects are those of the penicillins generally. (Floxapen). See co-fluampicil.

**fluconazole** A systemically acting synthetic antifungal agent. **Dose:** in oral candidiasis, 50 mg daily for 7–14 days: in vaginal candidiasis, a single dose of 150 mg. Dose in systemic candidiasis and cryptococcosis, 200–400 mg daily orally or by i.v. infusion. Side-effects include nausea and abdominal discom-fort. Combined treatment with astemizole, cisapride or terfenadine should be avoided. (Diflucan).

**flucytosine** An antifungal agent used in systemic yeast infections such as candidiasis and cryptococcosis. **Dose:** 100–200 mg/kg daily i.v. It may cause some bone marrow depression, and sensitivity tests should be carried out before and during treatment, as resistance to the drug may limit its value. Care is necessary in renal and hepatic impair-ment. Side-effects include nausea, diarrhoea and rash. (Alcobon).

**fludarabine** A fluorinated cytotoxic agent used in chronic lymphocytic leukaemia (CLL) after other treatment has failed. **Dose** by i.v. infusion 25 mg/m$^2$ for 5 days a month. It is generally well tolerated, but myelosuppression may occur as with related drugs. (Fludara). See page 122 and Table 8.

**fludrocortisone** A synthetic steroid with a very powerful salt-retaining action. Valuable in adrenal deficiency states such

as Addison's disease to supplement hydro-cortisone treatment.
**Dose:** 50–300 µg daily. The side-effects are those common to the corticosteroids in general. (Florinef).

**flumazenil** A benzodiazepine antagonist used in anaesthesia to reverse the sedative effects of benzodiazepines.
**Dose:** 200 µg initially by i.v. injection, with subsequent doses of 100 µg at 1-minute intervals, up to a maximum of 1 mg. Further doses may be given by i.v. infusion if drowsiness returns, as the action of flumazenil is brief. (Anexate).

**flunisolide** A potent corticosteroid used locally in the more severe forms of hay fever and other nasal allergies.
**Dose:** by nasal inhalation, 50 µg (2 sprays), 2 or 3 times a day, continued for 2–3 weeks, or longer if required. (Syntaris).

**flunitrazepam** A benzodiazepine with a hypnotic action used for the short-term treatment of insomnia.
**Dose:** 0.5–2 mg. Side-effects include drowsiness, ataxia and visual disturbances. (Rohypnol). See page 152 and Table 22.

**fluocinolone** A topically active potent corticosteroid. Used as cream, ointment or gel (0.00625–0.025%) in severe, inflamed, corticosteroid-responsive skin disorders. Excessive application should be avoided. (Synalar).

**fluocinonide** A potent locally effective anti-inflammatory steroid similar to fluocinolone, used as cream, ointment or lotion (0.05%). (Metosyn).

**fluocortolone** A locally acting corticosteroid used as cream or ointment (0.25%) in severe, inflamed skin conditions. (Ultralanum).

**fluorescein** An orange-red dye; solutions have a strong green fluorescence. Used as eye drops (1–2%) for detecting corneal lesions, as areas of cornea denuded of epithelium stain green.

**fluorometholone** A corticosteroid used as eye drops (0.1%) for inflammatory conditions of the eye. (FML).

**fluorouracil** A cytotoxic agent used in the palliative treatment of carcinoma of the breast and gastrointestinal tract and other solid tumours.
**Dose:** 15 mg/kg orally or by i.v. infusion weekly, up to a total dose of 12–25 g. Side-effects include alopecia and dermatitis, but haematotoxicity, severe gastro-intestinal disturbance and haemorrhage may limit treatment. Fluorouracil is used locally as a 5% cream (Efudix) in malignant skin lesions.

**fluoxetine** An antidepressant that acts by selectively inhibiting the uptake of sero-tonin. Given in single daily doses of 20 mg.
**Dose:** 60 mg daily are given in bulimia nervosa. Side-effects are gastrointestinal disturbances, dizziness and anorexia; rash is an indication of withdrawal. It should not be used with other drugs that influence serotonin uptake. (Prozac). See page 128 and Table 11.

**flupenthixol** A tranquillizer similar to fluphenazine and used in the treatment of schizophrenia with apathy and withdrawal. It also has an antidepressant action.
**Dose:** 6–18 mg daily initially, with subsequent adjustment according to need. It may cause some restlessness and insomnia. Dose by deep i.m. injection, 20–40 mg every 2–4 weeks. Dose in depression: 500 µg–3 mg daily. The side-effects are similar to those of chlorpromazine. (Depixol; Fluanxol). See page 168 and Table 30.

**fluphenazine** An antipsychotic drug with the actions and uses of chlorpromazine, but with reduced sedative and anti-cholinergic side-effects, although extra-pyramidal symptoms may be increased.
**Dose:** 2–10 mg initially in schizophrenia adjusted up to 20 mg daily. In severe anxiety states 1–4 mg. For depot treatment, 12.5–100 mg of the decanoate by deep i.m. injection every 12–14 days according to response. (Modecate; Moditen). See page 168 and Table 30.

**flurandrenolone** A potent locally acting corticosteroid used as a cream or ointment (0.0125%) in severe skin disorders not responding to other therapy. (Haelan). An adhesive tape is used for small resistant dermatoses.

**flurazepam** A benzodiazepine hypnotic for the short-term treatment of insomnia.

**Dose:** 15–30 mg nightly. It may cause some daytime sedation. (Dalmane). See page 152 and Table 22.

**flurbiprofen** A non-steroid anti-inflammatory drug with the actions, uses and side-effects of naproxen. It is used in the relief of pain and inflammation in rheumatoid and arthritic conditions, and in other musculoskeletal disorders.
**Dose:** 150 mg daily, after food, increased up to 300 mg daily if necessary. Suppositories of 100 µg are available. Care is necessary in peptic ulcer and in aspirin-sensitive asthmatic patients. (Froben). See page 165 and Table 29.

**flutamide** An androgen blocking agent that inhibits the action of androgens on target organs. It is used in advanced prostatic cancer not responding to other drugs, usually in association with goserelin or related agents.
**Dose:** 750 mg daily. Side-effects include gynaecomastia, and liver function should be checked. (Drogenil). See page 122 and Table 8.

**fluticasone** A corticosteroid of increased potency. Used as a metered dose pump for the prophylaxis and treatment of seasonal allergic rhinitis and hay fever.
**Dose:** 100 µg (2 sprays) into each nostril once a day in the morning. Maximum relief may not be obtained for 3–4 days. Systemic absorption extremely low. (Flixonase).

**fluvastatin**∇ An inhibitor of the enzyme HMG-CoA-reductase used in the treatment of hyperlipidaemia.
**Dose:** 20–40 mg daily in the evening. (Lescol). See page 146, Table 20 and atorvastatin, provastatin and simvastatin.

**fluvoxamine** An antidepressant that acts by inhibiting the central re-uptake of serotonin. It is used mainly for maintenance treatment during depressive illness.
**Dose:** 100–300 mg daily in the evening; a steady plasma level is normally reached within 10–14 days. Side-effects after initial nausea may include somnolence, constipation and agitation. It should not be used with other drugs that increase serotonin uptake, or with aminophylline or theophylline. (Faverin). See page 128 and Table 11.

**folic acid** A constituent of the vitamin B group. It is essential for cell division and the growth and development of normal red blood cells. The main therapeutic use is in the treatment of megaloblastic anaemias due to folic acid deficiency.
**Dose:** 5 mg daily for 4 months initially; 5 mg weekly may be adequate after the haematological response has been obtained. Sometimes given with anti-epileptic drugs, as long-term therapy may cause a folic acid deficiency. Small doses are present in many iron preparations to prevent the megaloblastic anaemia that may occur in later stages of pregnancy. It must not be used alone in pernicious anaemia, as it cannot prevent the degeneration of the central nervous system associated with that disease.

**folinic acid** A methotrexate antidote. It is given at the end of a course of methotrexate to reduce the toxic effects on normal cells and in methotrexate-overdose.
**Dose:** up to 120 mg over 24 hours by i.m. injection (or i.v.), with 60 mg orally for another 48–72 hours.

**follitropin** A recombinant form of the follicle stimulating hormone used in some forms of infertility. It is given by injection in doses dependent on the degree of ovarian response. (Puregon).

**formaldehyde** A powerful but toxic germicide used mainly in the disinfection of rooms, and as 'formalsaline' (5% in normal saline) for the preservation of pathological specimens. Warts have been treated with a 3% solution.

**formestane** An inhibitor of aromatase, the enzyme that converts androgens to oestrogens. It is used in advanced post-menopausal breast cancer, as it has a cytotoxic action mediated by causing an oestrogen deficiency state.
**Dose:** 250 mg by deep intragluteal injection at intervals of 2 weeks, with variations of the injection site. Side-effect are rash, pruritus and occasional vaginal bleeding. (Lentaron). See page 122 and Table 8.

**foscarnet** An antiviral agent for the treatment of sight-damaging cytomegalovirus retinitis in AIDS patients as an alternative to ganciclovir.
**Dose:** 60 mg/kg daily by i.v. infusion for

2–3 weeks, with subsequent infusion at a rate dependent on renal function. (Foscavir). See page 144 and Table 19.

**fosfestrol** A water-soluble derivative of stilboestrol. It is metabolized by the enzyme acid phosphatase to liberate stilboestrol in tissues rich in that enzyme, and so it is of value in prostatic carcinoma.
**Dose:** by slow i.v. injection, 600–1200 mg daily for 5 days or more. Oral maintenance dose: 120–360 mg daily. Perineal pain is a side-effect. (Honvan). See page 122 and Table 8.

**fosfomycin** A phosphorus-containing antibiotic used mainly for infections of the lower urinary tract.
**Dose:** 3 g nightly after voiding the bladder. Also used prophylactically before prostatectomy. Rash, nausea and diarrhoea are side-effects. (Monuril).

**fosinopril** An ACE inhibitor indicated in hypertension when standard therapy is ineffective or unsuitable.
**Dose:** 10 mg daily initially, adjusted after 4 weeks up to 40 mg according to need. It is eliminated by the liver as well as the kidneys, and may have some advantages in renal impairment. (Staril). See ACE inhibitors, page 148 and Table 21.

**framycetin** An antibiotic resembling neomycin in general properties. Used in eye infections as drops or ointment 0.5%. (Soframycin).

**friar's balsam** Contains benzoin, storax, aloes, balsam of tolu. Official name Compound Tincture of Benzoin. See benzoin.

**frusemide** A loop diuretic with a powerful and intense action of short duration. Often effective in conditions no longer responding to thiazide diuretics.
**Dose:** 20–40 mg daily or on alternate days, or 20–50 mg i.m. or i.v. Much larger oral doses, varying from 250 mg up to a single maximum dose of 2 g may be required in renal failure and oliguria. Side-effects include nausea, diarrhoea and cramp. (Lasix). See page 141 and Table 18.

**fusafungine** An antibiotic with anti-inflammatory properties used for upper respiratory tract infections.
**Dose:** as aerosol spray 125 µg 5 times a day. (Locabiotal).

**fusidic acid** See sodium fusidate.

# G

**gabapentin** An anticonvulsant used in the control of the partial seizures of epilepsy, although the mode of action is not yet clear.
**Dose:** 300 mg initially, slowly increased to 1.2 g daily according to need. Drowsiness, tremor and weight gain are some side-effects. Withdrawal is with slowly reduced doses over 2–3 weeks. (Neurontin). See page 136 and Table 15.

**gallamine** A synthetic non-depolarizing (competitive) muscle relaxant.
**Dose:** 80–120 mg initially i.v. with small subsequent doses according to need and response. The action of the drug may be terminated by the injection of neostigmine, 2.5–5 mg, together with atropine, 0.5–1 mg. (Flaxedil). Now used less frequently as tachycardia is a side-effect.

**gamolinic acid** A derivative of linoleic acid present in evening primrose oil. It is said to be of value in atopic eczema.
**Dose:** 320–480 mg daily. It is also used in mastalgia (breast pain) in doses of 240–320 mg daily, but the response is slow (8–12 weeks). (Epogam; Efamast).

**gammaglobulin** See immunoglobulin.

**ganciclovir** An antiviral agent similar to aciclovir, but more toxic. It is used only in sight- and life-threatening infections with cytomegalovirus (CMV) in immuno-compromised patients.
**Dose:** by i.v. infusion, 5 mg/kg every 12 hours for 14–21 days, with maintenance dose of 5 mg/kg daily. Later oral dose 3 g daily. The solution is very alkaline, and injection requires care. Regular blood counts are essential. (Cymevene). See page 144 and Table 19.

**G–CSF** Human granulocyte colony stimulating factor. See filgrastim and lenograstim.

**Gee's linctus** A soothing cough linctus containing camphorated tincture of opium, oxymel of squill and syrup of tolu.
**Dose:** 2–4 ml.

**gelatin** A protein obtained by the hydrolysis of animal tissues. Used orally as nutrient jellies, and specially refined solutions have been used as blood volume expanders (see dextran). (Gelofusine; Haemaccel).

**gemcitabine**∇ A cytotoxic agent related to cytarabine, but with increased potency and a longer action. It blocks cancer cell replication by inhibiting DNA synthesis, and may enhance the action of other agents. It is used mainly in the palliative treatment of non-small cell lung cancer.
**Dose:** 1000 mg/m² by slow i.v. infusion over 30 minutes, once a week for 3 weeks, repeated after a rest period. It is generally well tolerated, but a common side-effect is a transient influenza-like reaction. Myelo-suppression is less severe than that of related cytotoxic agents. (Gemzar). See page 122 and Table 8.

**gemeprost** A synthetic prostaglandin used to dilate the cervix uteri in first trimester abortion.
**Dose:** 1 mg as a pessary 3 hours before surgery. Side-effects are mild uterine pain and vaginal bleeding initially, nausea and diarrhoea.

**gemfibrozil** A plasma lipid regulating agent, with the actions and uses of bezafibrate and clofibrate.
**Dose:** 900 mg–1.5 mg daily, with regular checks on plasma lipid levels. Treatment should be withdrawn after 3 months if the response is unsatisfactory. Gemfibrozil may potentiate the action of oral anti-coagulants, the dose of which should be adjusted. Side-effects include nausea, diarrhoea, abdominal pain, rash and dizziness. (Lopid). See page 146 and Table 20.

**gentamicin** An aminoglycoside antibiotic, active against a wide range of Gram-negative organisms, including *Pseudomonas aeruginiosa*, as well as against many Gram-positive bacteria, although it is not very active against anaerobic organisms. It is of great value in septicaemia and meningitis, as well as in bacterial endocarditis.
**Dose:** 2–5 mg/kg daily by i.m. injection or i.v. infusion. In serious or undiagnosed infections, supplementary treatment with a penicillin or metronidazole may be required. In common with other amino-glycosides, gentamicin has ototoxic and nephrotoxic side-effects, and dosage requires care when renal function is inadequate, and also in elderly patients. Gentamicin is also used locally as cream or ointment (0.3%) and as eye drops (0.3%). (Cidomicin; Genticin).

**gentian violet** See crystal violet.

**gestrinone** An antiprogestogen used in endometriosis that acts indirectly by suppressing gonadotrophin production.
**Dose:** 2.5 mg twice weekly on the same days each week for 6 months. Side-effects are fluid retention, acne and voice changes. (Dimetriose).

**gestronel** A synthetic progestogen used in the treatment of breast and endometrial carcinoma and benign prostatic hyper-trophy.
**Dose:** 200–400 mg i.m. once a week. (Depostat).

**glibenclamide** An orally active hypogly-caemic agent similar to chlorpropamide.
**Dose:** 5–15 mg daily, according to need and response. (Daonil; Euglucon). See page 131 and Table 13.

**gliclazide** A sulphonylurea with the actions and uses of chlorpropamide and related drugs.
**Dose:** 40–320 mg orally. (Diamicron). See page 131 and Table 13.

**glimepiride** A sulphonylurea used in non-insulin-dependent (Type II) diabetes mellitus.
**Dose:** 2 mg after breakfast, increased up to 4 mg daily. Side-effects include transient visual disturbances, rash and urticaria. (Amaryl). See page 131 and Table 13.

**glipizide** A sulphonylurea, used like chlor-propamide in diabetes, but effective in much lower doses.
**Dose:** 5 mg initially, maintenance dose 2.5–40 mg daily. (Glibenese; Minodiab). See page 131 and Table 13.

**gliquidone** An oral hypoglycaemic agent similar to chlorpropamide. Effective in maturity-onset diabetes.
**Dose:** 15 mg initially; maintenance dose 40–60 mg daily, but up to 180 mg daily have been given. (Glurenorm). See page 131 and Table 13.

51

**G**

**glucagon** A hormone of the alpha cells of the pancreas which raises the blood sugar level by mobilizing liver glycogen. Used in acute hypoglycaemia.
**Dose:** 0.5–1 mg by s.c., i.m. or i.v. injection. (GlucaGen). Give i.v. glucose if there is no response within 10 minutes.

**glucocorticoids** Those corticosteroids with an anti-inflammatory action similar to hydrocortisone, as distinct from the mineralocorticoids, such as fludro-cortisone, used in Addison's disease. They differ in anti-inflammatory potency, and 0.75 mg of dexamethasone is considered equivalent to 20 mg of hydrocortisone. See Table 36.

**glucose** Also known as dextrose. A readily absorbed carbohydrate present in many sweet fruits, but obtained commercially by the hydrolysis of starch. It is given orally as a dietary supplement; in acidosis; and to raise the glycogen reserves of the liver in hepatic damage. Given by i.v. infusion as a 5% solution, or as a glucose-saline infusion in dehydration and shock, and after surgery until fluids can be taken by mouth.

**glutaraldehyde** A disinfectant of the formaldehyde type, but with a more rapid and powerful action. Effective against a wide range of organisms, including viruses. Used mainly for instrument sterilization as a 2% solution. Usually activated before use by the addition of a corrosion inhibitor. Such activated solutions are stable for about 2 weeks. It is also used as a 10% solution for the removal of plantar warts.

**glycerin (glycerol)** A clear syrupy liquid used as a sweetening agent in mixtures and linctuses. It promotes drainage when applied to inflamed areas, and is used as a paste with magnesium sulphate for boils. It is also used as suppositories for constipation.
**Dose:** sometimes given orally in doses of 1–1.5 g/kg in glaucoma and before surgery to lower the intraocular pressure.

**glyceryl trinitrate** A powerful but short-acting vasodilator used in the control of angina pectoris. See page 114.
**Dose:** 300, 500 or 600 μg tablets which should be dissolved under the tongue for a rapid response. An aerosol spray (400 g per dose), as well as long-acting tablets are also available. Tolerance may occur with pro-longed therapy. Side-effects are a throbbing headache, flushing and tachycardia. It is also used locally for an extended action, particularly at night, as ointment and medi-cated patches. Also given by i.v. infusion to control hypertension and ischaemia during cardiovascular surgery and in left ventricu-lar failure. Dose: 10–200 μg/min in dextrose-saline. A new use of the drug is as an ointment (0.2%) to promote healing of anal fissure. See page 114 and Table 4.

**glycopyrronium** A synthetic atropine-like antispasmodic used for preoperative medication.
**Dose:** 200–400 μg by i.m. or i.v. injection. It has the side-effects of anticholinergic drugs such as dryness of the mouth and blurred vision. Contraindicated in glaucoma. (Robinul).

**GM–CSF** Granulocyte-macrophage colony stimulating factor. See molgramostim.

**gold therapy** See sodium aurothiomalate.

**gonadotrophins** The follicle-stimulating hormone (FSH) and the luteinizing hormone (LH) of the anterior pituitary gland. They stimulate ovarian develop-ment and the production of oestrogens; in the male LH controls the formation of androgens. See gonadorelin.

**gonadorelin** A synthetic form of the gonadotrophin-releasing hormone of the pituitary gland (LH–RH). It is used to assess pituitary function.
**Dose:** 100 μg by i.v. injection normally lead to a rapid rise in the plasma level of the luteinizing and follicle-stimulating hormones. In amenorrhoea and infertility due to gonadorelin insufficiency, it is given by pulsed s.c. infusion in doses of 1–20 μg every 90 minutes, day and night. Treatment for up to 6 months may be required. Side-effects are uncommon. (Fertilol; Relefact). Some analogues of gonadorelin are used in certain cancers. See page 122.

**goserelin** A synthetic analogue of the hypo-thalamic hormone (LH–RH). It suppresses the production of testosterone, and is used in the treatment of hormone-dependent carcinoma of the prostate. It is also used in endometriosis and post-menopausal breast cancer.

**Dose:** 3.6 mg by s.c. injection every 28 days or as an implant. Side-effects include impotence, hot flushes, rash, breast swelling and tenderness. (Zoladex). See page 122 and Table 8.

**gramicidin** A mixture of antibiotics effective against many Gram-positive organisms, but it is too toxic for systemic use. Used topically in infected skin conditions, usually in association with neomycin and hydrocortisone.

**granisetron** A serotonin (5–HT) antagonist with a highly selective and powerful antiemetic action mediated by its effects on the $5-HT_3$ receptors. It is used in the prevention and treatment of the severe nausea and vomiting induced by potent cytotoxic drugs such as cisplatin.
**Dose:** 1 mg 1 hour before treatment, then 1 mg twice daily, or by i.v. infusion in doses of 3 mg, repeated up to 3 times over 24 hours. For prophylaxis, a dose of 3 mg should be given before chemotherapy is commenced. Headache, rash and constipation are common side-effects. (Kytril). See page 158.

**griseofulvin** An orally effective but slow acting antifungal antibiotic that is deposited selectively in the skin, hair and nails. It is used in the systemic treatment of ringworm and other dermatophyte infections of the keratin-containing tissues, but only when local treatment has failed.
**Dose:** 0.5–1 g daily, but prolonged therapy is required. Side-effects are headache, nausea, dizziness, rash and photosensitivity. It may also reduce the effects of oral contraceptives. (Fulcin; Grisovin).

**growth hormone** See somatropin.

**guanethidine** An anti-hypertensive drug that brings about a reduction in blood pressure by blocking transmission in adrenergic nerves, and preventing the release of noradrenaline. It has been used in the treatment of hypertension, often with a thiazide diuretic, but its use has declined as it may cause postural hypotension. Still used as part of combined therapy in resistant hypertension.
**Dose:** 20 mg daily, increased by 10 mg at weekly intervals according to response, up to 50 mg daily, although sometimes larger doses are required. Dose by i.m. injection,

10–20 mg as required. Diarrhoea, weakness, nasal congestion and bradycardia are common side-effects. (Ismelin). See page 148 and Table 21. Guanethidine is occasionally used as eye drops (1–3%) in glaucoma. (Ganda). See page 138 and Table 16.

**guar gum** A vegetable gum that, when taken with food, appears to retard the absorption of carbohydrates. It is used in the supplementary treatment of diabetes mellitus.
**Dose:** up to 15 g daily, usually sprinkled on food. It is essential that a dose should be taken with an adequate fluid intake, and that the final dose is not taken at bedtime. Side-effects are flatulence and abdominal distension. (Guarem). See page 131 and Table 13.

# H

**halcinonide** A powerful corticosteroid used in severe inflammatory skin conditions not responding to other corticosteroids. It is applied sparingly as a 0.1% cream. (Halciderm).

**halibut-liver oil** A rich source of vitamins A and D.
**Dose:** 0.2–0.5 ml.

**halofantrine** An antimalarial, acting at the erythrocytic stage of the life cycle of *Plasmodium*, and useful in chloroquine or multi-drug resistant malaria.
**Dose:** 500 mg 6-hourly for 3 doses between meals. Side-effects are nausea, vomiting and diarrhoea. It must not be given with or after mefloquine (risks of fatal arrhythmias). Contraindicated in pregnancy. (Halfan).

**haloperidol** A powerful tranquillizer used in schizophrenia, mania and psychoses.
**Dose:** 5–20 mg daily, up to a maximum of 200 mg, reduced later according to response. Dose by i.m. injection for rapid control of hyperactive psychotic patients, 5–30 mg initially, followed by 5 mg or more as required. For depot treatment, it is given as haloperidol decanoate, 50–300 mg by deep i.m. injection every 4 weeks. It is also given orally in doses of 500 g twice daily in severe anxiety. Doses of 1.5 mg

have been given for intractable hiccup. Care is necessary in liver disease. It has reduced anticholinergic and sedative side-effects, but the incidence of extra-pyramidal symptoms may be a limiting factor. (Dozic; Haldol; Serenace). See page 168 and Table 30.

**halothane** A potent non-inflammable inhalation anaesthetic. It suppresses mucous and bronchial secretions, and reduces capillary bleeding. It has some muscle-relaxant properties, but in major surgery, supplementary treatment with a muscle relaxant is necessary. Halothane may cause some cardiac irregularities, but an occasional serious side-effect is severe hepatotoxicity, particularly after further exposure to the drug within periods of 4–6 weeks. Such susceptibility cannot yet be detected, so great care is necessary in any cases of liver dysfunction. (Fluothane).

**hamamelis** An extract of witch hazel leaves referred to as hamamelis or witch hazel water is used as a soothing application for bruises and sprains.

**Hartmann's solution** An electrolyte-replacement solution containing sodium lactate, sodium chloride, potassium chloride and calcium chloride.

**heparin** The natural anticoagulant obtained from lung and liver tissue. It is widely used in deep-vein thrombosis and pulmonary embolism.
**Dose:** by i.v. injection 5000 units initially, followed by 1000–2000 units hourly by i.v. infusion, or 15 000 units by s.c. injection 12-hourly under laboratory control. Pro-phylactic dose before surgery 5000 units, then 5000 units every 8–12 hours for 7 days. Overdosage can be controlled by the i.v. injection of protamine sulphate. Treatment with heparin may be combined with that of oral anticoagulants such as phenindione or warfarin to provide immediate action before the slow-acting oral drugs begin to take effect. Occasional side-effects include hypersensitivity reac-tions and alopecia. Heparin is a complex polysaccharide, but certain fragments of that large molecule retain some anti-coagulant activity, and are referred to as low molecular weight heparins. They are used mainly in the prophylaxis of venous thrombo-embolism, as they have a longer

action than standard heparin. They are given by once-daily s.c. injection, and laboratory control of the bleeding time is not necessary. The dose varies to some extent with the product used.

**hepatitis A & B vaccines** Inactivated hepatitis virus antigens for the protection of individuals highly exposed to the infections.
**Dose:** see data sheets. (Haverix A; Energix B; H–B–Vax).

**†heroin** See diamorphine.

**hetastarch** A soluble modified starch that is used as a 6% solution with 0.9% sodium chloride as a plasma volume expander.
**Dose:** 500–1500 ml daily by i.v. infusion, up to a maximum of 20 ml/kg daily. It is excreted by the kidneys, and care must be taken to avoid circulatory overload. Not for use in congestive heart failure or renal insufficiency. Side-effects are vomiting, chills, fever and urticaria. (eloHAES; Hespan).

**hexachlorophane** A slow-acting antiseptic used for skin sterilization, and present in some medicated soaps.

**hexamine (methenamine)** A formalde-hyde derivative of low toxicity, occasionally used as a urinary antiseptic.
**Dose:** 2 g daily. It is usually given as hexamine hippurate to ensure the neces-sary acidification of the urine. (Hiprex).

**histamine** A compound present in a bound form in all mammalian tissues; its release is probably the ultimate cause of many allergic conditions.

**histamine H$_1$-receptor antagonists** See antihistamines. See page 110 and Table 2.

**histamine H$_2$-receptor antagonists** Drugs that differ from conventional anti-histamines in having a selective blocking action on receptors in the gastric cells that secrete acid. They are widely used in the treatment of peptic ulcer and other condi-tions requiring a reduction in gastric acid secretion. See page 162 and Table 27.

**homatropine** An atropine derivative with a similar but more rapid mydriatic action (15–30 minutes), but a shorter duration of effect of about 24 hours. Eye drops (1–2%) sometimes with cocaine.

**hyaluronidase** A 'spreading' factor used to increase the absorption of large-volume s.c. injections. The injection of 1500 units of hyaluronidase, either into the injection site or mixed with the injection fluid, will promote the absorption of 500–1000 mL of electrolyte solution by s.c. drip infusion. (Hyalase).

**hydralazine** A vasodilator that is useful in the supplementary treatment of hypertension.
**Dose:** 50–100 mg daily, usually with a thiazide diuretic or a beta-blocking agent. Also given in hypertensive crisis by *slow* i.v. injection in doses of 5–10 mg; over-rapid injection may cause a marked fall in blood pressure. Side-effects are nausea, tachycardia and fluid retention (less likely with low doses), but a lupus erythematosus-like syndrome may occur with extended high-dose therapy. (Apresoline). See page 148 and Table 21.

**hydrochlorothiazide** A thiazide diuretic that brings about a marked increase in the excretion of salts and water, and is of value in congestive heart failure and other oedematous conditions. It is also of value in hypertension, as it reduces peripheral resistance, and potentiates the action of some other antihypertensive drugs.
**Dose:** 50–100 mg daily initially in oedema; maintenance dose 25–50 mg daily or on alternate days. In hypertension, 25–50 mg daily according to need. Hydrochlorothiazide, like other thiazides, increases the excretion of potassium as well as sodium, and in extended treatment supplementary treatment with potassium chloride or effervescent potassium tablets may be required. Side-effects include nausea, rash, dizziness and photosensitivity. (HydroSaluric). See page 148 and Table 21.

**hydrocortisone** The principal corticosteroid, also known as cortisol, that is secreted by the adrenal cortex. It plays a major role in the metabolism of glucose, protein and calcium, in maintaining the electrolyte balance, and in reducing inflammatory and allergic responses. It is used in all cases of adrenocortical insufficiency, including Addison's disease and after adrenalectomy. It is also used in anaphylactic shock, asthma, rheumatoid disease and allergic states. It is valuable in acute lymphoblastic leukaemia and some lymphomas. In common with some other corticosteroids, hydrocortisone inhibits organ-transplant rejection and in high doses it is given to control incipient rejection.
**Dose:** varies considerably according to need: for replacement therapy, 20–30 mg daily; in shock, 100–300 mg or more by slow i.v. injection, repeated as required. Side-effects are numerous and include hypertension, oedema, mental disturbances, re-activation of peptic ulcer, muscle weakness and diabetes. Cushing's syndrome may occur with high doses. Hydrocortisone, unlike cortisone, is active topically, and is used as eye drops 0.5% (usually with an antibiotic), ointment and cream (0.5% and 1%), often with an antibiotic to control any secondary infection.

**hydroflumethiazide** A thiazide diuretic with the actions, uses and side-effects of bendrofluazide.
**Dose:** 25–100 mg daily in the morning; 25–50 mg daily in hypertension. (Hydrenox). See page 148.

**hydrogen peroxide solution** It contains 5–7% of $H_2O_2$, equivalent to about 20 volumes of oxygen. It has antiseptic and deodorizing properties, and is used mainly for cleaning wounds. It is also used as a mouthwash (diluted 1:7), and as ear drops (1:4 in water or 50% alcohol).

**†hydromorphone** A potent opioid analgesic of the morphine type.
**Dose:** in severe pain 1.3–2.6 mg 4–6-hourly. (Palladone).

**hydrotalcite** Aluminium magnesium hydroxide carbonate. An antacid used in dyspepsia and related conditions.
**Dose:** 1 g as required.

**hydroxocobalamin** A derivative of cyanocobalamin, and now the preferred form of vitamin $B_{12}$ as it has a more prolonged action.
**Dose:** in pernicious anaemia and other vitamin $B_{12}$ deficiency states, 1 mg initially i.m. repeated 5 times at intervals of 2–3 days; maintenance dose 1 mg by injection every 3 months. It is also given prophylactically after total gastrectomy. (Cobalin–H; Neo-Cytamen). See page 112.

**hydroxyapatite** A natural substance with a mineral composition somewhat similar to that of bone. It is used as a source of calcium and phosphorus in osteoporosis and other deficiency states. Tablets of 830 mg are available. (Ossopan).

**hydroxychloroquine** An antimalarial with the actions, uses and side-effects of chloroquine. It is also useful in rheumatoid arthritis in doses of 200–400 mg daily, and in lupus erythematosus, but side-effects are numerous, and treatment requires expert supervision. (Plaquenil). See page 165.

**5–hydroxytryptamine** See serotonin.

**hydroxurea (hydrocarbamide)** A cytotoxic agent sometimes used in chronic myeloid leukaemia.
**Dose:** 20–30 mg/kg as a single dose daily or 80 mg/kg every third day. Side-effects are nausea, skin reactions and myelosuppression. (Hydrea). See page 122 and Table 8.

**hydroxyzine** A mild tranquillizer with some sedative and antihistaminic properties. It is given in the short-term treatment of anxiety, and in pruritus and dermatoses complicated by emotional tension.
**Dose:** 50–400 mg daily. It has the side-effects of the antihistamines, and is not recommended where some sedation is undesirable. (Atarax; Ucerax). See page 117 and Table 5.

**hyoscine (scopolamine)** An alkaloid obtained from plants of the belladonna group. It is a powerful hypnotic and is widely used together with papaveretum for premedication before anaesthesia in doses of 300–600 µg by s.c. or i.m. injection. It has some antiemetic properties, and is useful in travel sickness and vertigo.
**Dose:** 300 mg 30 minutes before starting the journey, followed by up to 3 doses 6-hourly. Scopoderm is a patch of 500 µg. The side-effects of mouth dryness and dizziness are those of the anticholinergic drugs generally. It is contraindicated in glaucoma. It is used occasionally in terminal care for bowel colic and excessive respiratory secretions. Dose: 600 µg–2.4 mg daily by s.c. infusion.

**hyoscine butylbromide** A derivative of hyoscine that differs in lacking any central action. It is given in spasm and

hypermotility of the gastrointestinal tract, and may be useful in spasmodic dysmenorrhoea.
**Dose:** 40–80 mg daily; in acute spasm, 20 mg by injection. (Buscopan).

**hypromellose** A cellulose-derivative that dissolves in water to form a viscid, colloidal solution. Such a solution is used as a base for eye drops to extend the action of a dissolved ophthalmic drug; to lubricate contact lenses; and to act as a lubricant in chronic, sore eye conditions.

# I

**ibuprofen** A non-steroidal anti-inflammatory agent (NSAID) widely used in rheumatoid and arthritic conditions. It is also given as an analgesic for mild to moderate pain, but not for acute gout.
**Dose:** 1.8 g daily initially; maintenance dose, 600 mg–1.2 g daily after food. A 5% cream is available for local use. The side-effects are those of the NSAIDs generally. (Brufen; Fenbid). See page 165.

**ichthammol** A thick, dark brown liquid with a characteristic odour, derived from certain bituminous oils. It is a mild antiseptic and is used mainly in chronic eczema as a 10% ointment or zinc paste. A solution (10% in glycerin) has been used on ulcers and inflamed areas.

**idarubicin** A potent cytotoxic agent similar in actions and uses to doxorubicin. It is given orally and i.v. in acute non-lymphocytic leukaemia, breast cancer, and as second-line therapy in acute lymphatic leukaemia. Dose is based on skin area. (Zavedos). See page 122 and Table 8.

**idoxuridine** An antiviral agent now virtually superseded by acyclovir and related drugs. Used occasionally in herpes zoster skin infection by local application of a 5% solution. See page 144 and Table 19.

**ifosfamide** A derivative of cyclophosphamide with similar actions and uses. It is effective in lung, ovary, breast and soft-tissue tumours, as well as some malignant lymphomas.
**Dose:** based on skin area, and is given by i.v. infusion over a 5-day course. As with

cyclophosphamide, ifosfamide must be given with mesna to reduce its urothelial toxicity. (Mitoxana). See page 122 and Table 8.

**imipenem** An antibiotic with a range of activity that includes Gram-positive and Gram-negative bacteria, as well as aerobes and anaerobes, and is indicated in infections due to such organisms. It is given by i.v. infusion in doses of 1–2 g daily. Also used in surgical prophylaxis. As it is inactivated to some extent by kidney enzymes, it is always given together with the specific enzyme inhibitor cilastatin. The side-effects are numerous and include those common to other antibiotics. Care is necessary in hypersensitivity to the penicillins, cephalosporins and related antibiotics, and in epilepsy. (Primaxin).

**imipramine** A tricyclic antidepressant with the general action, uses and side-effects of amitriptyline, but with a reduced sedative action. It has been widely used in acute endogenous depression, although the initial response may be slow, and long treatment may be required.
**Dose:** 75 mg daily, increased up to 200 mg. A single dose of 150 mg may be given at night. It is sometimes used in the treatment of enuresis in doses of 25–50 mg. Imipramine should not be given in association with or soon after monoamine oxidase inhibitors, as the effects of both drugs may be increased. Imipramine may also reduce the response to some anti-hypertensive drugs. (Tofranil). See page 128 and Table 11.

**immunoglobulin** The normal product obtained from plasma is given for protection against hepatitis, measles, rubella and hepatitis A in susceptible patients. More specific products are hepatitis B immunoglobulin, tetanus human immunoglobulin (HTIG) and varicella-zoster immunoglobulin (VZIG). Anti-D(Rh$_o$) immunoglobulin is used to prevent a rhesus-negative mother from forming antibodies to fetal rhesus-positive cells that may reach the maternal circulation, and so protect any further child from the risks of haemolytic disease.

**immunosuppressants** Drugs such as azathioprine that suppress the normal immune response are used in transplant surgery to prevent tissue rejection, but as their action includes depression of the immune defence system of the body, their use requires care. The systemically acting corticosteroids such as prednisolone also have valuable immunosuppressant properties. Cyclosporin has a powerful immunosuppressant action with little myelotoxicity, and is also used in the prophylaxis of graft-versus-host disease (GVHD). Tacrolinus is a new product with the actions and uses of cyclosporin.

**indapamide** A slow-acting thiazide-related drug used in hypertension.
**Dose:** 2.5 mg daily, continued for some months, until a maximum response has been obtained. Combined treatment with beta-blocking agents and other drugs may increase the response, but saluretic diuretics are not recommended as they may cause hypokalaemia. (Natrilix). See page 148 and Table 21.

**indigo carmine** A blue dye that has been used as a 0.4% solution by injection as a renal function test. Normally the urine is coloured blue in 10 minutes or so.

**indinavir**▽ An antiviral agent that functions as an inhibitor of HIV-protease. It prevents the development of immature virus particles into infective virus. It is best given in combination with another antiviral agent such as acyclovir which acts by a different mechanism.
**Dose:** 2.4 g daily, with ample fluid between meals. Care is necessary in hepatic impairment. (Crixivan). See page 144 and Table 19.

**indomethacin** A non-steroidal anti-inflammatory and analgesic agent (NSAID) of value in arthritic and rheumatoid conditions, and in acute gout.
**Dose:** 50–200 mg daily with food. Suppositories 100 mg are useful at night to reduce morning stiffness. Dose in dysmenorrhoea, up to 75 g daily. Side-effects are numerous and include gastrointestinal disturbances, which may be severe and cause bleeding, dizziness and confusion. Hypersensitivity reactions with blood disorders have been reported, and blurred vision with corneal deposits may occur with prolonged treatment. Indomethacin is also used by i.v. injection for the closure of the patent ductus arteriosus in premature babies, but the dose requires careful assessment under specialist supervision. (Iridocid; Imbrilon). See page 165 and Table 29.

**indoramin** An alpha-adrenoceptor blocking agent used in hypertension. It has a selective action on the alpha-receptors, and by preventing the release of noradrenaline it reduces peripheral resistance and lowers the blood pressure. The response may be increased by combined treatment with a thiazide diuretic or a beta-blocking agent.
**Dose:** 50 mg initially daily, increased, if required, up to 200 mg daily. Side-effects include drowsiness, dizziness and some anticholinergic reactions such as dryness of the mouth. (Baratol). It is also used for the symptomatic relief of benign prostatic hypertrophy in doses of 40–100 mg daily, although in elderly patients small doses of 20 mg at night may be effective. (Doralese). See page 148 and Table 21.

**inosine pranobex** A complex containing the purine metabolite inosine. The complex has antiviral properties, and may act more by stimulating the immune system than by a direct action on viral replication. Indicated in herpes simplex virus infections of the skin and mucous membranes.
**Dose:** 4 g daily for 1–2 weeks. Care is necessary in renal impairment, gout or hyperuricaemia. (Immunovir).

**inositol nicotinate** A vasodilator agent used mainly in peripheral vascular disorders such as Raynaud's disease, and acrocyanosis.
**Dose:** 1–4 g daily. (Hexopal).

**insulin** The antidiabetic principle of the pancreas, regulating the metabolism of carbohydrates and fats. It is widely used in the treatment of diabetes mellitus by s.c. injection in doses adjusted to individual need. Many modified insulin products are available, designed to extend the duration of action and reduce the frequency of injections, and so simulate the effects of the natural hormone more closely. Human insulins, obtained by the modification of pork insulin (emp) or by biosynthesis (crb) are also available, and are used routinely to an increasing extent. A transfer from animal to human insulin requires monitoring, and patients should be warned that the usual early symptoms of hypoglycaemia may be less marked. In diabetic emergency, soluble insulin remains the preparation of choice. See page 131 and Table 12.

**interferons** Protective proteins formed in mammalian cells in response to viral invasion. Interferon alfa, obtained by DNA technology, has cytotoxic properties, and is used in hairy cell leukaemia and renal cell carcinoma. Interferon gamma is used with antibiotics in chronic granulomatous disease.
**Dose:** see data sheets.

**interleukin** See aldesleukin.

**iodine** Powerful antiseptic used as povidone-iodine for skin preparation. Hypersensitivity to iodine skin applications is not unknown. Given orally in preoperative treatment of thyrotoxicosis.
**Dose:** as Aqueous Iodine Solution (Lugol's solution) 0.3–1 ml diluted with milk or water.

**iodized oil** Poppy-seed oil containing 40% iodine in combination. Used as a contrast agent in lymphangiography, hysterosalpingography, and other radiological examinations.

**iodoform** Yellow powder with strong odour. Mild antiseptic used occasionally as BIPP.

**iopanoic acid** A radio-opaque substance used as a contrast agent in cholecystography. It is largely excreted in the bile when given orally.
**Dose:** 2–6 g.

**iophendylate** An oily liquid containing 30% of combined iodine. It is mainly used as a contrast agent in myelography.
**Dose:** 6–9 ml by injection into the subarachnoid space. Before intrauterine blood transfusion, 9 ml have been injected into the amniotic sac to outline the fetus. Shock and violent coughing may occur if any iophendylate reaches the circulation.

**ipecacuanha** The dried root from which emetine is obtained. It has emetic properties, and is used mainly as Ipecacuanha Emetic Mixture in some forms of poisoning.
**Dose:** 30 ml in adults; 10–15 ml in children.

**ipratropium** An anticholinergic agent with bronchodilator properties. Of value in bronchoconstrictive states not responding to selective beta$_2$-receptor stimulants represented by salbutamol. It is relatively free from the side-effects associated with anticholinergic drugs.

**Dose:** by aerosol inhalation, 20–40 μg (1–2 puffs) 4 times a day. Similar doses are given by nasal spray in watery rhinorrhoea. (Atrovent). See page 118 and Table 3.

**irbisartan** An angiotensin II-receptor antagonist used in hypertension. It acts at a later stage than the ACE-inhibitors, and is less likely to cause drug-induced cough.
**Dose:** 150–300 mg once a day. (Aprovel). See page 148 and Table 21.

**irinotecan**∇ An inhibitor of topo-isomerase I, an enzyme involved in DNA replication. Used in colorectal cancer.
**Dose:** 150–350 mg/m$^2$ by i.v. infusion. Side-effects are neutropenia and diar-rhoea. (Campto). See page 122.

**iron-sorbitol** An injectable iron product for use when oral iron therapy is not possible or not effective. It is given by deep i.m. injection, taking care to prevent leakage back along the injection track to avoid staining the skin, in doses based on the degree of iron deficiency. (Jectofer). See page 112 and Table 3.

**iron salts** See ferrous sulphate.

**isocarboxazid** A monoamine oxidase inhibitor with the antidepressant action, uses and side-effects of phenelzine.
**Dose:** 30 mg initially daily, subsequently increased if necessary up to 60 mg daily, reduced later to 10–20 mg daily according to need. (Marplan). See page 128 and Table 11.

**isoconazole** An antifungal agent similar to miconazole. Used for the single-dose local treatment of candidal and trichomonal vaginal infections.
**Dose:** 600 mg as 2 vaginal pessaries. (Travogyn).

**isofluorane** An inhalation anaesthetic with the action and uses of halothane and enflurane. It is given as a 0.5–3% oxygen-nitrous oxide mixture from a calibrated vaporizer.

**isonlazid** A pyridine derivative with a spe-cific action against *Mycobacterium tuber-culosis*. Widely used in the treatment of tuberculosis, but as bacterial resistance soon develops combined treatment with other drugs such as rifampicin is essential.
**Dose:** 300 mg daily, or 1 g twice a week,

and often continued for some months. Side-effects include nausea and peripheral neuritis, rash and psychotic episodes. See page 170 and Table 31.

**isoprenaline** An old adrenaline-like beta-receptor agonist. It is used occasionally for the short-term treatment of severe heart block and bradycardia.
**Dose:** 5–10 μg/min by i.v. injection. Also used in airways obstructive conditions by aerosol inhalation in doses of 80–240 μg (1–3 puffs) as required. (Saventrine).

**isosorbide dinitrate** A vasodilator with the actions, uses and side-effects of glyceryl trinitrate, but with a more prolonged action.
**Dose:** in acute angina, 5–10 mg, sublin-gually; for extended treatment 30–120 mg orally daily; in left ventricular failure up to 240 mg daily; by i.v. infusion, 2–10 mg/hr. See page 114 and Table 4.

**isosorbide mononitrate** The active metabolite of the dinitrate. It escapes first-pass loss in the liver, and has a more rapid action. May cause peripheral vasodilata-tion and headache.
**Dose:** 40–120 mg daily. See page 114 and Table 4.

**isotretinoin** A potent, orally active deriva-tive of vitamin A. It is used for *severe* acne not responding to other treatment, and brings about a prolonged remission of symptoms.
**Dose:** 500 μg/kg daily for 4 weeks to assess response, followed by treatment for 8–10 weeks. An exacerbation of symptoms is common after 2–8 weeks which usually subsides later. Side-effects include dryness of mucous membranes, conjunctivitis, nausea and muscle pain. Isotretinoin is teratogenic so pregnancy must be avoided. Its use requires care under expert supervi-sion. (Roaccutane).

**ispaghula** The husk of ispaghula seed. It swells in water and is used as a bulk laxative It is also useful in irritable bowel syndrome and diverticulitis.
**Dose:** 3–5 g daily.

**isradipine** A calcium channel blocking agent used in hypertension.
**Dose:** 5 mg daily initially, increased after 3–4 weeks to 10 mg daily, with subsequent

adjustment to maintenance doses of 2.5–5 mg daily according to response. Side-effects include dizziness, headache, palpitations and local oedema. (Prescal). See page 148 and Table 21.

**itraconazole** An orally active antifungal agent used in the treatment of vulvovaginal candidiasis, pityriasis and tinea infections.
**Dose:** 200 mg twice a day for the 1-day treatment of vulvovaginal infections; 200 mg daily for 7 days in pityriasis, 100 mg daily for 15–30 days in tinea infections. Side-effects are nausea and abdominal pain. Liver disease is a contraindication. Combined treatment with astimazole or terfenadine should be avoided. (Sporonox).

**ivermectin** A fungal derivative effective against the microfilaria causing 'river blindness'. It does not kill either the adult worms or their larvae, but prevents the growth of the latter, and treatment must be continued until the adult worms die out.
**Dose:** 150 µg/kg as a single dose, repeated annually. (Mectizan).

# K

**kanamycin** An aminoglycoside antibiotic now used mainly in gentamicin-resistant infections.
**Dose:** 1 g daily by i.m. injection; 15–30 mg/ kg daily by i.v. infusion. (Kannasyn).

**kaolin** Aluminium silicate. Used as an absorbent in diarrhoea, colitis, food poisoning, etc., often as Kaolin and Morphine Mixture.
**Dose:** 10–20 ml as required. It is also used externally as Kaolin Poultice to relieve the pain of sprains, etc.

**kelocyanor** A specific antidote for cyanide poisoning. See dicobalt edetate.

**ketamine** A short-acting i.v. anaesthetic with analgesic properties.
**Dose:** 1–2 mg/kg i.v. over 1 minute, repeated as required; 4–10 mg/kg by deep i.m. injection. It is used mainly in paediatric anaesthesia, and its analgesic action is also of value in neurodiagnostic procedures, and other painful investigations. Hallucinations may occur during the recovery period. (Ketalar).

**ketoconazole** A broad-spectrum, orally active antifungal agent. It is of value in systemic and deep mycoses, and in severe and resistant mycoses of the gastrointestinal tract and the vagina. It is also effective in severe mycoses of the skin, but it should be used only for superficial fungal infections not responding to other treatment.
**Dose:** 200 mg daily with food, up to a maximum of 400 mg daily. Side-effects include nausea, rash and pruritus. It may cause hepatitis; liver function tests may be necessary if given for more than 14 days. (Nizoral).

**ketoprofen** A non-steroidal anti-inflammatory and analgesic agent of the ibuprofen type. It is of value in rheumatoid arthritis, gout, spondylitis and related conditions, and in dysmenorrhoea.
**Dose:** 100–200 mg daily with food; 100 mg by suppository at night, 50–100 mg by deep i.m. injection 4-hourly. Care is necessary in peptic ulcer and hepatic disease. May increase the action of anti-coagulants and other drugs bound to plasma protein. (Alrheumat; Orudis; Orivail). See page 165 and Table 29.

**ketorolac**∇ A potent analgesic used for the short-term relief of acute postoperative pain.
**Dose:** 10 mg 4–6-hourly up to 40 mg daily for not more than 7 days; dose by deep i.m. or slow i.v. injection. 10 mg initially, then 30 mg 4–6-hourly up to 90 mg daily for not more than 2 days. Side-effects are numerous; see data sheet. (Toradol). Also used as eye drops (0.5%) to reduce pain and inflammation after ocular surgery. (Acular).

**keftotifen** An antihistamine that may also have some of the properties of sodium cromoglycate. It is used in the prophylactic treatment of asthma.
**Dose:** 4 mg daily with food, continued for some weeks. Other anti-asthmatic therapy should be continued for at least 2 weeks to ensure maintenance of control. Side-effects include sedation and dryness of the mouth. (Zaditen). See page 110 and Table 2.

**Kogenate** A recombinant form of the human blood Factor VIII, given i.v. as replacement therapy in the treatment of haemophilia A.

60

K

**L** ·

**labetalol** A beta-adrenoceptor blocking agent with some alpha-blocking activity. Like related drugs, labetalol is indicated in all types of hypertension, including that following myocardial infarction.
**Dose:** 200 mg daily initially, with food, slowly increased up to a maximum of 2.4 g daily; by i.v. injection 50 mg repeated as required; for the rapid control of the hypertension of pregnancy 20–160 mg by i.v. infusion hourly. It should be used with care in asthma and heart block. Side-effects include weakness, nausea, brady-cardia and postural hypotension. Liver damage has been reported. (Trandate). See page 148 and Table 21.

**lacidipine** A calcium channel blocking agent with the actions and uses of nife-dipine. In hypertension it is given as a single morning dose of 2 mg with food, increased up to 6 mg as the response develops over 3–4 weeks. Half doses in hepatic impairment and the elderly. Early chest pain is an indication that the drug should be withdrawn. (Motens). See page 148 and Table 21.

**lactilol** A semi-synthetic sugar that is not absorbed orally, and acts as an osmotic laxative by retaining water in the intestinal tract. Also inhibits ammonia-producing organisms, and is of value in hepatic encephalopathy.
**Dose:** as laxative 20 mg daily mixed with food, together with 2 glasses of water. Dose in hepatic encephalopathy, 500–700 mg/kg daily.

**lactulose** An osmotic laxative. See lactilol.

**laevulose** Fructose. A sugar sometimes given i.v. as an alternative to glucose.

**lamivudine** An antiviral agent that acts like zidovudine by inhibiting reverse transcrip-tase, an enzyme essential for DNA formation and viral replication. It is used in HIV infections.
**Dose:** 300 mg daily, preferably with food, and combined with a protease inhibitor. (Epivir). See page 144 and Table 19.

**lamotrigine**∇ An anti-epileptic that allevi-ates the imbalance of neurotransmitters in the brain by inhibiting the influx of sodium ions. It is used both as primary treatment and as additional therapy (often with sodium valproate) for seizures not fully controlled by other drugs.
**Dose:** 25 mg daily initially for 14 days, slowly rising to 100–200 mg daily. See data sheet for details of combined therapy. (Lamictal). See page 136 and Table 15.

**lanolin** See wool fat.

**lansoprazole** An inhibitor of the enzyme $H^+K^+$–ATPase (the proton pump) used in the treatment of peptic ulcer.
**Dose:** 30 mg daily for 4–8 weeks. (Zoton). See omeprazole, page 162 and Table 27.

**Lassar's paste** A stiff ointment containing zinc oxide, starch and white soft paraffin with 2% salicylic acid. Used as protective in eczema.

**latanoprost** A prostaglandin alpha-analogue used once daily as eye drops (0.005%) in glaucoma. It increases the outflow of the aqueous humour, whereas other agents reduce its secretion. Continued use may cause changes in eye colour. (Xalantan). See page 138.

**lenograstim**∇ A recombinant form of the granulocyte colony stimulating factor (G–GSF) that governs the production of neutrophils. It is used as supplementary treatment in cancer chemotherapy to stimulate neutrophil production in drug-induced neutropenia.
**Dose:** under expert supervision by s.c. injection, in daily doses of 150 µg/m$^2$ until neutrophil count is satisfactory. Also used i.v. after bone marrow trans-plantation. (Granocyte). See filgrastim and molgramostim. See page 122 and Table 8.

**letrozole**∇ A non-steroid inhibitor of aromatase, the enzyme that controls the conversion of testosterone to oestrogen. It acts as an anti-oestrogen and is used in advanced breast cancer that has not responded to tamoxifen or similar therapy.
**Dose:** 2.5 mg once daily. Side-effects include musculoskeletal pain, arthralgia and hot flushes. (Femara). See page 122 and Table 8.

**leucovorin** See folinic acid.

61

**L** ·

**leuprorelin** A synthetic hormone that indirectly suppresses androgen and oestrogen production by inhibiting gonadotrophin activity. It is used in endometriosis and advanced prostatic cancer.
**Dose:** 3.75 mg by s.c. or i.m. injection every 4 weeks. Side-effects are impotence, flushing and local irritation. There may be an initial and temporary increase in pain. The injection site should be varied. (Prostap SR). See buserelin, goserelin, page 122 and Table 8.

**levamisole** A single-dose (150 mg) anthelmintic of value in round worm (*Ascaris*). It is also effective against hookworm (*Ancylostoma* and *Necator*).
**Dose:** 2.5–5 mg/kg daily for 2–5 days.

**levobunolol** A beta-blocker used as eye drops 0.5% in glaucoma. (Betagan). See carteolol.

**levocabastine** An antihistamine used as drops (0.05% twice a day in the symptomatic treatment of seasonal allergic conjunctivitis and rhinitis. (Livostin).

**levodopa** An amino acid that is converted to dopamine in the body. It is used in the treatment of Parkinson's disease, which is associated with a reduction in brain dopamine levels due to degeneration in the substantia nigra, thus causing an imbalance in the neurohormonal system of the brain. Levodopa is essentially replacement therapy, but as an oral dose is metabolized to some extent in the peripheral circulation It is often given with an enzyme inhibitor such as benserazide or carbidopa. Combined therapy permits a larger dose of active drug to reach the cerebral tissues, and at the same time reduces some of the general side-effects of levodopa.
**Dose:** 125–500 mg initially, increased according to need and response. Side-effects include nausea and cardiovascular disturbances, but psychiatric side-effects may be dose limiting. Close angle glaucoma is a contraindication. See page 160 and Table 26.

**lignocaine (lidocaine)** A local anaesthetic widely used for infiltration anaesthesia as a 0.25–0.5% solution, usually with adrenaline, as well as for epidural, caudal and nerve block anaesthesia. It is the local anaesthetic present in many dental cartridges. A 2–4% solution is used for surface anaesthesia, and a 2% gel is used to relieve the pain and discomfort of catheterization, but rapid absorption may cause side-effects. Lignocaine is also the drug of choice in the control of ventricular tachycardia following myocardial infarction.
**Dose:** 100 mg as an i.v. bolus, followed by a dose of 4 mg/min by i.v. infusion for 30 minutes, with subsequent doses of 2 mg/min. Side-effects include confusion, convulsions, bradycardia and hypotension. (Xylocard). Emla cream contains lignocaine and prilocaine. It is used for local anaesthesia and to relieve the pain associated with injections, especially in children. It is applied under an occlusive dressing 1–2 hours before the injection.

**lindane** A pesticide used as a 1% solution for the treatment of scabies.

**liothyronine (tri-iodothyronine)** A thyroid hormone with a rapid action, and probably a precursor of thyroxine. It is given orally in severe hypothyroid conditions when a rapid action is necessary, and by injection in hypothyroid coma.
**Dose:** 20–60 μg daily; 5–20 μg i.v. (Tertroxin).

**liquid paraffin** A lubricant laxative and faecal softener.
**Dose:** 10–30 ml. Its extensive use is now discouraged, as it may cause granulomatous reactions and reduce the absorption of fat-soluble vitamins.

**lisinopril** An ACE inhibitor similar to enalapril, but with a longer action that permits the use of a single daily dose.
**Dose:** in the treatment of hypertension, doses of 2.5 mg daily initially, slowly increased according to response up to 10–20 mg daily, occasionally up to 40 mg. In patients receiving diuretics, such therapy should be withdrawn for 2–3 days before lisinopril therapy and resumed later if necessary. (Carace; Zestril). See page 148 and Table 21.

**lithium carbonate** Lithium carbonate and citrate are used for their mood-regulating action in the prophylaxis and treatment of mania and depressive illness, but the mode of action is not known. The therapeutic/toxic range of lithium is very narrow, and continuous control of the plasma/lithium level is essential to avoid the many side-effects and hazards of therapy.

62

L

**Dose:** 0.25–2 g daily initially, then adjusted to maintain a lithium/plasma level of 0.4–1.0 mmol/l. Prolonged treatment may be required with an adequate fluid intake. Thiazide diuretics should be avoided. Some slow-release tablets are available, but different products *must not* be regarded as interchangeable. Lithium treatment cards giving advice can be obtained from a pharmacy. (Camcolit; Liskonum; Priadel).

**lithium succinate** Lithium succinate appears to have some antifungal and anti-inflammatory properties, and is used as an 8% ointment for seborrhoeic dermatitis. (Efalith).

**lodoxamide** A mast cell stabilizer similar to sodium cromoglycate. Used as eye drops (0.1%) in allergic conjunctivitis. (Alomide).

**lofepramine** An antidepressant of the imipramine group, with similar actions and uses, but reduced sedative and anticholinergic side-effects.
**Dose:** 140–210 mg daily. (Gamanil). See page 128 and Table 11.

**lofexidine** A narcotic antagonist. It has a selective blocking action on brain noradrenaline, and is used for the rapid relief of opioid withdrawal symptoms associated with central sympathetic activity.
**Dose:** 200 µg twice a day, slowly increased as required over 7–10 days, before withdrawal over 2–4 days. Care is necessary in cardiac insufficiency and bradycardia. (BritLofex).

**lomotil** A preparation of diphenoxylate with atropine, for the rapid control of diarrhoea.
**Dose:** 2 tablets 6-hourly.

**lomustine** A slow-acting cytotoxic agent used in Hodgkin's disease and solid tumours.
**Dose:** 130 mg/m² body surface at intervals of 6–8 weeks. Side-effects include anorexia, nausea, liver damage and myelodepression. Dosage should not be repeated until white cell and platelet counts have returned to an acceptable level. Reduced doses are given when lomustine forms part of a multi-drug dosage scheme. (CCNU). See page 122 and Table 8.

**loperamide** A synthetic inhibitor of peristalsis.

**Dose:** in acute diarrhoea, 4 mg initially, followed by 2 mg as required, up to a maximum of 16 mg daily. In chronic diarrhoea, 4–8 mg daily, but care is necessary in the elderly to avoid faecal impaction. Loperamide is not suitable for children under 4 years of age, nor in patients with liver disease, as it may cause undesirable sedation. (Imodium).

**loprazolam** A benzodiazepine hypnotic used mainly in the short-term treatment of insomnia and nocturnal arousal.
**Dose:** 1–2 mg at bedtime. Side-effects include drowsiness, dizziness, dry mouth and headache. See page 152 and Table 22.

**loratadine** An antihistamine with the general action of that group of drugs, but with reduced sedative side-effects.
**Dose:** 10 mg daily. (Clarityn). See page 110 and Table 2.

**lorazepam** A short-acting anxiolytic/hypnotic similar to diazepam, but less likely to cause next-day drowsiness.
**Dose:** 1–4 mg daily. It is also given in similar oral doses or by slow i.v. injection in doses of 50 µg/kg for preoperative sedation and amnesia. Occasionally used i.v. in status epilepticus in doses of 4 mg, but apnoea and hypotension are side-effects that may require resuscitation. (Ativan). See page 152 and Table 22.

**lormetazepam** A short-acting benzodiazepine hypnotic. It is useful in the treatment of insomnia in the elderly, but is less suitable for insomnia associated with early awakening.
**Dose:** 500 µg–1 mg at night. See page 152 and Table 22.

**losartan**∇ An angiotensin II receptor antagonist used in the treatment of hypertension.
**Dose:** 50 mg daily The use of potassium-sparing diuretics should be avoided with losartan. It has the advantage of not causing the persistent dry cough associated with ACE inhibitors. (Cozaar). See page 148 and Table 21.

**low molecular weight heparins** See heparin.

**loxapine** Antipsychotic agent with the actions and uses of chlorpromazine.
**Dose:** in acute and chronic psychoses,

63

L

25–50 mg daily, slowly increased as required. Maintenance doses range from 20–100 mg daily. Side-effects are those of other antipsychotic agents, but loxapine may cause nausea, vomiting and weight changes. (Loxapac). See page 168 and Table 30.

**Lugol's solution** An aqueous solution of iodine 5% and potassium iodide 10%. Used in the preoperative treatment of thyrotoxicosis.
**Dose:** 0.3–1 ml.

**lymecycline** A soluble complex of tetracycline and lysine. It has the action and uses and side-effects of tetracycline, but is absorbed more readily.
**Dose:** 800 mg daily. (Tetralysal).

**lypressin** An analogue of vasopressin used to control the polyuria of pituitary diabetes insipidus.
**Dose:** 2.5–10 units several times a day by nasal spray. Side-effects include nausea and abdominal pain. Lypressin has some vasoconstrictor properties, and desmopressin is sometimes preferred. (Syntopressin).

**lysuride (lisuride)** A bromocriptine-like drug for the treatment of parkinsonism. It acts by stimulating any surviving dopamine receptors in the brain.
**Dose:** 200 µg at night with food, increased at weekly intervals according to response up to a maximum of 5 mg daily. Side-effects include nausea, dizziness and initial hypotensive reactions which may affect driving ability. (Revanil). See page 160 and Table 26.

# M

**macrolides** A group of antibiotics that differ chemically from the penicillins, yet have a similar pattern of activity. They are active orally and are useful in the treatment of penicillin-sensitive patients. Erythromycin is the most widely used member of the group, with clarithromycin and azithromycin as more recent introductions.

**magnesium carbonate** A white, insoluble powder with antacid and laxative properties.
**Dose:** 0.6–4 g daily.

**magnesium hydroxide** A mild antacid laxative, usually given in aqueous suspension as Cream of Magnesia, although tablet forms are also available. Cream of Magnesia is a useful antidote in mineral acid poisoning.

**magnesium sulphate** Epsom salts. A powerful saline aperient, producing loose stools by preventing the reabsorption of water.
**Dose:** 5–15 g before breakfast. Used externally for the treatment of boils and carbuncles as a paste with glycerin. A marked loss of plasma magnesium may occur after severe diarrhoea or drug-induced diuresis, and may require the i.v. injection of magnesium sulphate in doses based on the degree of hypomagnesaemia. It has also been given i.v. in a dose of 8 mmol in the emergency treatment of severe arrhythmias associated with hypokalaemia.

**magnesium trisilicate** A white insoluble powder, with mild but prolonged antacid effects. It was formerly used widely in the symptomatic treatment of peptic ulcer; now used chiefly for dyspepsia.
**Dose:** 0.3–2 g.

**malathion** An organophosphorus insecticide. Used as a lotion 0.5% for lice and scabies as alternative to lindane or carbaryl.

**mannitol** A sugar that is not metabolized, and is used mainly as an osmotic diuretic.
**Dose:** (after a test dose of 200 mg/kg) 50–200 g by slow i.v. infusion over 24 hours. Mannitol has also been used by i.v. infusion as a short-term ocular hypotensive agent in the treatment of glaucoma. It is also useful in cerebral oedema, given by rapid i.v. injection in a dose of 1 g/kg as a 20% solution.

**maprotiline** A sedative antidepressant with a general action similar to that of the tricyclic drugs represented by amitriptyline.
**Dose:** 25–150 mg daily. If given at night as a single dose, the sedative action may reduce the need for other drugs. It has milder anticholinergic side-effects than some related compounds, although skin rash is more common. (Ludiomil). See page 128 and Table 11.

**mebendazole** An anthelmintic effective against most intestinal worms.

64

L

**Dose:** 100 mg once for threadworm, and 100 mg twice daily for 2 days against other infestations. Generally well tolerated, but it should not be given to children under 2 years of age. (Vermox).

**mebeverine** An antispasmodic agent which, unlike the anticholinergic drugs, appears to have a direct action on the intestinal smooth muscle. It is useful in the treatment of gastrointestinal spasm and in the irritable bowel syndrome.
**Dose:** 400 mg daily, before food. As with other antispasmodics, mebeverine should not be used in paralytic ileus. (Colofac).

**medroxyprogesterone** A synthetic progestogen.
**Dose:** in endometriosis 30 mg daily for 90 days; in dysfunctional uterine bleeding and secondary amenorrhoea: 2.5–10 mg daily for 5–10 days, starting on 16th–21st day of cycle and repeated for 2–3 cycles. Large doses of 400 mg–1.5 g daily are given in breast, endometrial, prostate and other hormone-dependent cancers, or 250 mg–1 g weekly by deep i.m. injection. (Farlutal; Provera). Depot-Provera is a long-acting product used by i.m. injection as a contraceptive, but only after full counselling.

**mefenamic acid** A non-steroidal anti-inflammatory analgesic agent used to relieve moderate pain in arthritic and rheumatoid conditions, and other states requiring mild analgesic therapy such as dysmenorrhoea.
**Dose:** 1.5 g daily after food. Side-effects are drowsiness and haemolytic anaemia. Diarrhoea is an indication that the drug should be withdrawn. (Ponstan). See page 165 and Table 29.

**mefloquine** A drug for the prophylaxis and treatment of chloroquine-resistant malaria.
**Dose:** for short-term prophylaxis 250 mg weekly, starting 1 week before exposure and for 4 weeks after return. Doses for treatment require specialist advice. Side-effects include gastrointestinal disturbances, dizziness and weakness. It is contraindicated in patients with a history of neuro-psychiatric disturbance, and is not suitable for use in severe renal or hepatic impairment. (Larium). See halofantrine.

**mefruside** A diuretic useful in the treatment of hypertension and oedema.
**Dose:** 25–50 mg daily in the morning, according to need and response; 25–100 mg

in oedematous states. A potassium supplement may be required. Care is necessary in renal and hepatic deficiency. (Baycaron). See page 148 and Table 21.

**megestrol** An orally active progestogen. It is used in oestrogen-dependent breast cancer, and acts by suppressing the uptake of oestrogens by the cancer cells.
**Dose:** 160 mg daily. Nausea and fluid retention with weight gain are occasional side-effects. (Megace). See page 122.

**meloxicam** A recently introduced non-steroidal anti-inflammatory drug (NSAID) indicated in the short-term treatment of acute osteo-arthritis and the longer-term treatment of rheumatoid conditions.
**Dose:** 7.5–15 mg once daily with food; half doses for the elderly. Suppositories of 15 mg are also available. The side-effects are basically those of the NSAIDs in general. Meloxicam has a more selective action on cyclo-oxygenase, the enzyme involved in the biosynthesis of prostaglandins, and is less likely to cause gastrointestinal disturbance, but it has no cytoprotective action, and is **not** suitable for patients with peptic ulcer. (Mobic). See page 165 and Table 29.

**melphalan** An alkylating agent of the mustine type. Used mainly in myelomas, lymphomas and some solid tumours.
**Dose:** 150–300 µg/kg daily for 4–6 days, repeated after 1–2 months. In myeloma it is also given by regional perfusion. The injection solution is highly irritant and contact should be avoided. Side-effects include myelo-depression, nausea, rash and pruritus. (Alkeran). See page 122 and Table 8.

**menadiol** A water-soluble form of vitamin K.
**Dose:** 10 mg daily. (Synkavit) Phytomenadione is now preferred.

**menotrophin** Human menopausal gonadotrophin containing follicle-stimulating hormone and luteinizing hormone. It is used in the treatment of anovulatory sterility. The dose depends on individual hormone assays and response. The use of the drug has resulted in multiple births. It is also given to males to stimulate spermatogenesis. (Humegon; Normegon).

**menthol** Colourless crystals obtained from oil of peppermint. Used as spray or drops for nasopharyngeal inflammation, and as

65

**M**

an inhalation, often with friar's balsam, for the relief of coryza and catarrh.

**mepacrine** A synthetic antimalarial. Now replaced by chloroquine and other powerful drugs. It is used occasionally in the treatment for *Giardia lamblia* infections.
**Dose:** 300 mg daily for 5–8 days.

**†meprobamate** A mild tranquilliser used in anxiety and tension states, but its extended use may lead to dependence.
**Dose:** 1.2–2.4 g daily. Side-effects are drowsiness, headache, gastrointestinal and visual disturbances. It has been largely replaced by benzodiazepine anxiolytics. (Equanil).

**meptazinol** An analgesic for the relief of moderate to severe pain. It has a more rapid and extended action than morphine, and is less likely to cause respiratory depression or induce dependence.
**Dose:** 800–1600 mg orally daily. In severe pain, 50–100 mg by injection, repeated as required; in obstetric analgesia, 2 mg/kg. The action can be partly antagonized by naloxone. Side-effects include dizziness and nausea. (Meptid).

**mequitazine** An antihistamine used for the symptomatic relief of allergic states such as hayfever and urticaria. It is less likely to cause sedation than some other antihistamines.
**Dose:** 10 mg daily. Side-effects may include dry mouth and blurred vision. (Primalan). See page 110 and Table 2.

**mercaptopurine** A cytotoxic agent used in the treatment of acute leukaemia.
**Dose:** 2.5 mg/kg daily. Close haematological control is essential, as the drug has a marked myelosuppressive action. Mercaptopurine is also hepatotoxic, and should be withdrawn if jaundice occurs. (Puri-Nethol). See page 122 and Table 8.

**meropenem** An antibiotic similar to imipenem, but more resistant to breakdown by renal enzymes, so combined use with an enzyme inhibitor is unnecessary.
**Dose:** given by i.v. infusion in doses of 500 mg–2 g 8-hourly according to the severity of the infection. Care is necessary in hepatic disease. (Meronem).

**mesalazine** The active metabolite of sulphasalazine. It is not suitable for oral use as such, but can be given as a resin-drug complex, so that the drug reaches and is released in the colon unchanged. It is used both for the acute attack and for the maintenance of remission of ulcerative colitis, particularly in patients unable to tolerate sulphasalazine.
**Dose:** 1.2–2.4 g daily. Side-effects include gastrointestinal disturbances, and care is necessary in patients hypersensitive to salicylates. Patients should be advised to report any bruising, bleeding or malaise. If a blood dyscrasia is suspected, a blood count should be done and the drug withdrawn. Lactulose should not be used as a laxative, as it may hinder the release of the active drug. Also used as enema and suppositories. (Asacol; Pentasa; Salofalk). See page 172 and Table 32.

**mesna** A compound used to prevent the haemorrhagic cystitis caused by the cytotoxic drugs cyclophosphamide and ifosfamide. The reaction is caused by the metabolite acrolein, and mesna reduces the toxicity by combining with acrolein in the urinary tract.
**Dose:** 20% of that of the cytotoxic drug, and should be given at the same time by i.v. injection. Subsequent supportive doses may be given orally or by injection 4–8 hours after therapy. (Uromitexan).

**mesterolone** An orally active androgen with the actions and uses of testosterone. It is used in androgen deficiency and male infertility but, unlike other androgens, it does not inhibit endogenous androgen production, and is less hepatotoxic.
**Dose:** 75–100 mg daily for some months. (Pro-Viron).

**mestranol** An orally active oestrogen present in some oral contraceptive products. See page 264.

**metaraminol** A sympathomimetic agent that increases the blood pressure by a general constriction of the peripheral blood vessels. It is used mainly in the acute hypotension that may occur with spinal anaesthesia. It has also been used in shock, but the use of vasoconstrictors has declined, as in shock the peripheral resistance may be already high, and the use of blood volume expanders and dopamine and dubotamine is now preferred.
**Dose:** 15–100 mg by i.v. infusion. Side-effects are tachycardia and reduced renal

blood flow. It is contraindicated in myocardial infarction. (Aramine).

**metformin** An orally active biguanide hypoglycaemic agent. Its action differs from that of the sulphonylureas, as it acts by increasing the peripheral uptake of glucose. It is used mainly in non-insulin-dependent diabetes not controlled by diet and sulphonylurea therapy.
**Dose:** 1.5–3 g daily according to need and response. Side-effects include nausea and transient diarrhoea. It may cause lactic acidosis and it should not be used in patients with renal impairment. (Glucophage). See page 131 and Table 13.

**†methadone** A morphine-like analgesic with reduced sedative effects. Of value in severe pain, and in the relief of useless cough in terminal disease.
**Dose:** 5–10 mg orally or by i.m. or s.c. injection, at intervals according to need. Prolonged treatment carries the risk of cumulative effects and overdose. (Physeptone).

**methenamine** See hexamine.

**methionine** A sulphur-containing amino acid essential for nutrition. It is used mainly in paracetamol poisoning, often with acetyl cysteine, and given within 10–12 hours.
**Dose:** 2.5 g 4-hourly up to a total of 10 g.

**methocarbamol** A skeletal muscle relaxant used in muscle injury and spasm.
**Dose:** 6 g daily orally; 1–3 g daily by slow i.v. injection. It may cause drowsiness, dizziness and allergic rash. Contra-indicated in epilepsy and myasthenia gravis. (Robaxin).

**methohexitone** A short-acting i.v. anaes-thetic similar to thiopentone. It is used mainly for the induction and maintenance of anaesthesia for short operative procedures, when the quick recovery may be an advantage. (Brietal).

**methotrexate** A cytotoxic agent that acts by inhibiting the synthesis of purines, and so indirectly interferes with cell proliferation. It is used chiefly for maintenance therapy in the remission of acute lymphoblastic leukaemia in children, but it has been used in choriocarcinoma as well as some lymphomas and solid tumours.

**Dose:** in children, 15 mg/m$^2$ weekly. It is sometimes effective in resistant psoriasis, and is given in oral doses of 10–25 mg weekly under specialist supervision. It is occasionally used in severe rheumatoid arthritis not responding to other treat-ment in doses of 7.5 mg once weekly. Side-effects are those of gastrointestinal toxicity, myelodepression, rash and cirrhosis. Blood counts and liver function tests during treatment are essential. Cough and dyspnea may indicate pulmonary toxicity. Aspirin and non-steroidal anti-inflammatory drugs (NSAIDs) should be avoided, as they delay the excretion of methotrexate and increase its toxicity. See page 122 and Table 8.

**methotrimeprazine** An antipsychotic agent of the chlorpromazine type, with similar actions, uses and side-effects. It is used in schizophrenia when a sedative effect is also required.
**Dose:** 25–50 mg daily, but much larger doses, up to 1 g daily, may be required, particularly for bedfast patients. It is of value as an adjunct to other therapy in terminal illness and is sometimes given by continuous s.c. infusion in doses of 25–200 mg over 24 hours. Postural hypotension may occur in elderly ambulant patients. (Nozinan). See page 168 and Table 30.

**methoxamine** A sympathomimetic agent that increases the blood pressure by con-striction of the peripheral vessels. It is used in the hypotension following spinal anaesthesia; to correct an excessive response to antihypertensive drugs; and to arrest supraventricular tachycardia.
**Dose:** 5–20 mg by i.m. injection; 5–10 mg by slow i.v. injection. Care is necessary in preexisting hypertension and cardio-vascular disease. (Vasoxine).

**methyl cellulose** A derivative of cellulose that is used as an emulsifying agent and bulk laxative.
**Dose:** 1.5–6 g with water, but not at night. It is sometimes given in diarrhoea, with a minimum amount of water.

**methyl salicylate** A pale yellow liquid with a characteristic odour. It has long been used as wintergreen liniment and oint-ment for the local relief of muscle pain and rheumatic conditions, but is now less popular.

**68**

**M**

**methylated spirit** Alcohol containing 5% of wood naphtha. Used for skin preparation and alcoholic applications. The methylated spirit used domestically differs, and is coloured violet to indicate its unsuitability for medicinal use.

**methylcysteine** A sputum-liquefier claimed to be of value in respiratory conditions where the sputum is viscid.
**Dose:** 600 mg daily. (Visclair).

**methyldopa** A centrally acting antihypertensive drug, usually given together with a diuretic. It has the advantage of being relatively safe in asthma, heart failure and pregnancy.
**Dose:** 750 mg–3 g daily; 250–500 mg by i.v. infusion. Side-effects are drowsiness, depression and diarrhoea. A systemic lupus erythematosus-like syndrome may also occur, and active liver disease is a contraindication. (Aldomet). See page 148 and Table 21.

**†methylphenidate** A central stimulant used occasionally under strict supervision for the treatment of hyperactive children.
**Dose:** 5–10 mg daily. (Ritalin).

**†methylphenobarbitone** An anticonvulsant with the actions, uses and side-effects of phenobarbitone.
**Dose:** in epilepsy, 100–600 mg daily. (Prominal). See page 136 and Table 15.

**methylprednisolone** A corticosteroid with the actions, uses and side-effects of prednisolone, and given in similar doses. (Medrone).

**methysergide** A synthetic drug related to ergometrine and used in the prevention of severe and recurrent migraine not responding to other drugs.
**Dose:** 2–6 mg daily. It is also given for the symptomatic treatment of the carcinoid syndrome in doses of 12–20 mg daily. Methysergide has many side-effects, including retroperitoneal and cardiac fibrosis, and its use requires expert supervision. (Deseril). See page 154 and Table 23.

**metipranolol** A beta-adrenoceptor blocking agent used as eye drops 0.1–0.6% for the treatment of chronic glaucoma.

**metirosine** An enzyme inhibitor that interferes with the synthesis of adrenaline and other pressor amines. It is used mainly in the preoperative control of adrenaline-producing tumours (phaeochromocytoma), and in the long-term treatment of patients unsuitable for surgery.
**Dose:** 1 g daily initially, increased if necessary up to 4 g daily. An adequate fluid intake is essential. Side-effects include sedation, which may be marked initially, diarrhoea, which may be severe, depression and confusion. (Demser).

**metoclopramide** A stimulant of gastric and small intestine transport. It is used in the treatment of nausea and vomiting generally, including that induced by drugs or migraine, in non-ulcer dyspepsia, and in accelerating the passage of a barium meal.
**Dose:** 15–30 mg daily orally or by i.m. or i.v. injection. A single dose of 10–20 mg is given by injection 10 minutes before radiological examination. Side-effects include extra-pyramidal reactions, facial spasms and oculogyric crises, mainly in young persons, and it is best avoided in patients under 20 years of age. (Maxolon). Some long-acting products are also available. See page 158 and Table 25.

**metolazone** A diuretic with the actions, uses and side-effects of bendrofluazide.
**Dose:** in hypertension, 5 mg daily initially; in oedematous states 5–20 mg or more daily may be given. The diuresis is increased by combined treatment with a loop diuretic such as frusemide, but monitoring of the response is necessary. (Metinex). See page 148 and Table 21.

**metoprolol** A beta-blocking agent used in the control of angina, but also of value in hypertension and the prophylaxis of migraine.
**Dose:** in angina, 100–300 mg daily; in hypertension, 100–400 mg daily; in migraine prophylaxis and thyrotoxicosis 200 mg daily. It is occasionally given by slow i.v. injection in acute cardiac arrhythmias; dose 1–2 mg/min up to a total of 10–15 mg. Care is necessary in heart block, bradycardia and pulmonary disease. (Betaloc; Lopresor). See page 114 and Table 4.

**metriphonate** An organophosphorus schistosomicide, but used only in infections of the hookworm *Schistosoma haemobium*, which is found in the genitourinary veins.

**Dose:** orally, in 3 doses of 7.5 mg/kg at intervals of 2–4 weeks. (Bilarcil).

**metronidazole** An orally effective drug used in trichomoniasis, amoebiasis and in infections due to anaerobic bacteria.
**Dose:** in bacterial and trichomonal vaginitis, 600 mg daily for 7 days, or as a single dose of 2 g. In acute intestinal amoebiasis, 2.4 g daily for 5 days. In surgical prophylaxis, and in the prophylaxis and treatment of infections caused by colonic anaerobic pathogens such as *Bacteriodes fragilis*, as well as infections by some Gram-negative organisms, metronidazole is given in doses of 1.2 g daily orally, or as 1 g suppositories. In severe infections, doses of 1.5 g are given daily by i.v. infusion, replaced by oral therapy as soon as possible. In *Giardia lamblia* infections, 2 g daily for 3 days; 600 mg daily for 3 days in ulcerative gingivitis. Metronidazole is also valuable in pseudomembranous colitis (see clindamycin). Side-effects are mainly gastrointestinal disturbances and can be reduced by giving the dose with food, but epileptiform seizures may occur with high doses, and the drug may cause a disulfiram-type reaction if alcohol is taken. (Flagyl). Metronidazole is also used as a 0.75% gel (Metrogel; Rosex) in rosacea and as Anabact and Metrotop to deodorize malodorous tumours.

**metyrapone** An inhibitor of glucocorticoid synthesis.
**Dose:** 750 mg 4-hourly for 6 doses as a test of anterior pituitary function, as following such doses the plasma concentration of corticosteroids falls. The fall stimulates the production of steroid precursors by the adrenal glands, and a rise in the urinary excretion of such precursors is indicative of an active anterior pituitary gland. Metyrapone is also used in resistant oedema due to an increased production of aldosterone, and in the symptomatic control of Cushing's syndrome. Nausea and vomiting are side-effects. (Metopirone).

**mexiletine** An anti-arrhythmic drug that is useful in the control of ventricular arrhythmias, particularly those following myocardial infarction, or when lignocaine is ineffective.
**Dose:** as a loading dose, 100–250 mg i.v. under ECG control, followed by i.v. infusion of a 0.1% solution until a further 250 mg have been given. Oral therapy: a

loading dose of 400 mg, followed by 600 mg–1 g daily. Side-effects are nausea, drowsiness, confusion and blurred vision. Contraindicated in bradycardia, hypotension, and hepatic or renal failure. (Mexitil).

**mianserin** An antidepressant of the amitriptyline type, with reduced anticholinergic and cardiovascular side-effects, and well tolerated by the elderly. It is of value in all types of depression, including those associated with anxiety.
**Dose:** 30–90 mg daily, which may be taken as a single dose at night, although higher doses have been given. Care is necessary in recent myocardial infarction and heart block. Severe hepatic disease is a contraindication. Side-effects include aplastic anaemia, and blood counts during treatment are essential. The drug should be withdrawn if any signs of infection occur. See page 128 and Table 11.

**miconazole** An antifungal agent of value in systemic and alimentary fungal infections.
**Dose:** 1 g daily orally, or up to 1.8 g daily by i.v. infusion, and the duration of treatment largely depends on the response. Pessaries of 100 mg and a cream (2%) are used for vaginal candidiasis. A gel is available for oral fungal infections. Side-effects after systemic use include nausea, pruritus and rash. Miconazole may potentiate the action of anticoagulant, anticonvulsant and hypoglycaemic drugs, requiring an adjustment of dose. Combined use with astemizole, terfenadine and cisapride should be avoided. (Daktarin).

**midazolam** A sedative of the benzodiazepine group, used mainly for sedation before and during gastroscopy, endoscopy and other investigations. The action is rapid, and an anterograde amnesia often follows.
**Dose:** by slow i.v. injection 70 μg/kg up to a total of 2.5–7 mg. Premedication, 2.5–5 mg i.m. For the induction of anaesthesia in poor-risk patients, 100–300 μg/kg by slow i.v. injection. Side-effects after i.v. injection include respiratory depression and, occasionally, severe hypotension. (Hypnovel).

**mifepristone** An antiprogestational agent used as an alternative to surgery for the termination of pregnancy, up to 63 days' gestation.
**Dose:** a single oral dose of 600 mg. For hospital use only. (Mifegyne).

69

**M**

**milrinone** An inhibitor of phosphodi-esterase, an enzyme concerned in cardiac function. It has a digoxin-like effect on the myocardium, and may be effective in congestive heart failure not responding to other drugs.
**Dose:** by i.v. infusion as an initial dose of 50 µg/kg, with maintenance doses of 0.5 µg/min up to a total of 1.13 mg/kg over 24 hours. Side-effects are anginal pain, hypotension and headache. (Primacor). See enoximone, page 141 and Table 18.

**minocycline** A tetracycline with the general properties of that group of antibiotics, with the advantage of being useful in meningococcal prophylaxis. The absorp-tion of minocycline is little influenced by food. It is also suitable for use when the renal function is impaired, as accumula-tion of the drug is unlikely.
**Dose:** 200 mg daily. In acne treatment half-dose should be given for 6 weeks. The side-effects are those of the tetracyclines generally, although monocycline may also cause dizziness, vertigo and rash. (Minocin).

**minoxidil** A vasodilator used in severe hypotension resistant to other drugs.
**Dose:** 5–50 mg daily. Side-effects are weight gain, breast tenderness and tachy-cardia. Almost all patients experience hypertrichosis, and should be warned accordingly. (Loniten). A 2% solution is used as a lotion in the local treatment of male-pattern baldness. (Regaine).

**mirtazapine** An alpha$_2$-receptor antagonist. It is used in depression as it increases central noradrenergic and serotenergic neurotransmission.
**Dose:** 15–45 mg at night for 4–6 months. Side-effects are weight gain and drowsi-ness. (Zispin).

**misoprostol** A synthetic prostaglandin with an inhibitory action on gastric secretion. It is used in the control of peptic ulcer, and in the prophylaxis of ulcers induced by non-steroidal anti-inflammatory drugs (NSAIDs).
**Dose:** 800 µg daily with food, with a last dose at night, and continued for some weeks. Dose in prophylaxis, 400–800 µg daily. Side-effects are usually transient, and include diarrhoea, nausea and abdominal pain. (Cytotec). See page 162. Contraindicated in pregnancy.

**mitobronitol** A cytotoxic agent used mainly in chronic myeloid leukaemia.
**Dose:** 250 mg daily until the white cell count falls, then 125 mg daily according to need. May cause gastrointestinal disturbance, alopecia and bone marrow depression. Haematological control is necessary. (Myelobromal). See page 122 and Table 8.

**mitomycin** A cytotoxic antibiotic used in breast, gastrointestinal and other cancers.
**Dose:** 4–10 mg by i.v. infusion at intervals of 1–6 weeks. Great care must be taken to avoid extravasation. Also used in bladder cancer by the weekly instillation of a solution of 10–40 mg in 20–40 ml of water. Side-effects include bone marrow and renal damage, and lung fibrosis.

**mitozantrone** A cytotoxic drug related to doxorubicin, and indicated in advanced breast cancer.
**Dose:** 14 mg/m$^2$ once i.v., repeated after 21 days, provided the white cell and platelets counts have returned to normal. It is highly irritant, and contact of the drug with the skin must be avoided. Side-effects are nausea, vomiting, alopecia, myelosuppression and cardiac weakness. (Novantrone). See page 122 and Table 8.

**mivacurium** A non-depolarizing muscle relaxant with the short action and uses of atracurium.
**Dose:** initial dose 70–250 µg/kg i.v., followed by doses of 100 µg/kg/min at intervals of 15 minutes as required. Smaller doses are given by i.v. infusion. (Mivacron).

**moclobemide**∇A short-acting, reversible inhibitor of monoamine oxidase (MAO) for the treatment of **severe** depression. The older MAO-inhibitors act on both the A- and B-forms of the enzyme, and have a long and irreversible action. Moclobemide has a rapid and selective action on MAO-B, but the duration is short and fades after about 24 hours, as the drug is soon metabolized. The risks of reactions with other drugs (common with old MAO-inhibitors) are correspondingly reduced.
**Dose:** 300 mg daily initially (after with-drawal of other therapy), slowly increased up to 600 mg daily. Side-effects are dizziness and sleep disturbances. (Manerix). See page 128 and Table 11.

**moexepril** An ACE-inhibitor.

**Dose:** (when given alone) 7.5 mg daily initially, increasing if required up to 30 mg daily. When given as a second-line therapy with a diuretic (which should be avoided), initial dose is 3.75 mg under supervision until the blood pressure has stabilized. Side-effects are hypotension and cough. Hyperkalaemia may occur if potassium supplements or potassium-sparing diuretics are also given. (Perdix). See page 148 and Table 21.

**molgramostim**∇A recombinant form of human granulocyte macrophage colony stimulating factor (GM–CSF). It is used in the neutropenia following cytotoxic and bone marrow transplant therapy.

**Dose:** 60 000–100 000 units by s.c. injection or i.v. infusion, under haematological control. (Leucomax). See filgrastim and lenograstim.

**mometasone**∇A potent corticosteroid used as 0.1% cream/lotion once a day in severe eczema, psoriasis and other skin conditions not responding to other therapy. (Elocon). Also used as a nasal spray in allergic rhinitis. (Nasonex).

**monoamine oxidase inhibitors**

Monoamine oxidase is an enzyme concerned with the breakdown of dopamine, serotonin, noradrenaline and adrenaline. Those substances are stored in many organs of the body, including the brain, where they function as transmitters of nerve impulses. The period for which they act is very short, as they are rapidly metabolized by monoamine oxidase. An inhibition of the enzyme could permit an increase in the brain levels of such amines, and on that basis some monoamine oxidase inhibitors (MAOIs) have been used in the treatment of depression. Therapy is complicated by the fact that these drugs can increase the response to pressor drugs, anaesthetics and many other agents, including the mild sympathomimetics present in some cough mixtures and decongestive nasal sprays. Even certain foods, particularly cheese, may cause a dangerous rise in blood pressure during MAOI therapy and patients should always carry the MAOI warning card. Great care is necessary during combined therapy, and ideally 10–14 days should elapse after ceasing

MAOI treatment before using other potent drugs. Examples of MAOIs are isocarboxazid, phenelzine and tranylcypromine. Their use has declined as more effective antidepressants of the amitriptyline type, with fewer side-effects, have become available. See moclobemide, page 128 and Table 11.

**moracizine** A potent cardiac membrane-stabilizing agent used like lignocaine to control ventricular arrhythmias.

**Dose:** 600–900 mg daily initially, adjusted later according to need and response. Side-effects include dizziness, palpitations and chest pain. (Ethmozine).

†**morphine** The principal alkaloid of opium. It is widely used as a narcotic analgesic for the relief of severe pain and the associated anxiety and stress, and in shock.

**Dose:** in acute pain, 10 mg by injection as required; in chronic pain it may be given orally or by injection according to need in doses varying from 5–10 mg. Some long-acting oral forms of morphine are available (MST Continus; Oramorph SR) designed to reduce the frequency of dosing in conditions of severe pain. Side-effects include nausea and vomiting, which can often be controlled by small doses of chlorpromazine, or a similar antiemetic. Morphine may cause respiratory depression, and severe respiratory depression is a contraindication. The possibility of tolerance to and dependence on morphine should be kept in mind if treatment is prolonged, but in terminal conditions is of little importance.

**moxisylyte (thymoxamine)** An alpha$_2$-adrenergic blocking agent, given by intracavernous injection for the induction of erection.

**Dose:** 10 mg not more than 3 times a week. Side-effects are drowsiness, dizziness and flushing. (Erecnos).

**moxonidine** A centrally acting antihypertensive agent of the clonidine type. It has a greater affinity for certain receptors in the brain stem that reduce the peripheral resistance and so indirectly lowers the blood pressure.

**Dose:** in mild to moderate hypertension, 200 µg daily in the morning, rising after 3 weeks to 400 µg daily, and rarely up to

71

**M**

600 µg daily. Side-effects are dry mouth, dizziness and sleep disturbances. Contra-indicated in cardiac disorders and renal/hepatic dysfunction. (Physiotens). See page 148 and Table 21.

**mupirocin** An antibacterial agent that is effective against most of the pathogens responsible for skin infections. It is used as a 2% ointment in impetigo, folli-culitis and similar conditions. It should not be used for longer than 10 days to avoid the development of resistance. (Bactroban).

**mustine** A cytotoxic drug used mainly in the treatment of Hodgkin's disease and related conditions.
**Dose:** 0.1 mg/kg daily for 3 days as a fast-running i.v. infusion, or as a single dose of 0.4 mg/kg. The solution is highly irritant, and extra venous injection causes very severe local necrosis. Side-effects include severe vomiting, bone marrow depression and alopecia. Close haematological control during treatment is essential. Now in less frequent use. See page 122 and Table 8.

**mycophenolate mofetil** An immuno-suppressant used together with cyclosporin and corticosteroids to prevent acute renal transplant rejection. It acts on a specific enzyme concerned with T- and B-lymphocyte proliferation, as well as inhibiting antibody formation.
**Dose:** 2 g daily, starting within 24 hours of transplantation. Blood counts are necessary during treatment, and, as with other immunosuppressants, there is an increased risk of opportunistic infection. (CellCept).

# N

**nabilone** A cannabinoid antiemetic used in the treatment of nausea and vomiting associated with cancer chemotherapy.
**Dose:** 2–4 mg daily, beginning the day before cytotoxic treatment is commenced, and continued for a day after the end of the course. Side-effects are drowsiness, confusion and tremor. Care is necessary in liver dysfunction or any history of psy-chotic illness. See page 158.

**nabumetone** A non-acidic anti-inflamma-tory agent of the naproxen type. It is effective in rheumatoid and osteoarthritis and has reduced gastric irritant properties.
**Dose:** 1 g at night. Reduced doses are necessary in renal impairment, and the dose of any oral anticoagulant or hypogly-caemic agent may require adjustment. (Relifex). See page 165 and Table 29.

**nadolol** A beta-blocking agent with the actions and uses of propranolol.
**Dose:** in angina, 40 mg daily, or more; in hypertension, 80 mg daily, increased slowly as required; in the prophylaxis and treatment of migraine, 80–160 mg daily. Maximum daily dose 240 mg. (Corgard). See pages 114 & 148, and Tables 4 & 21.

**nafarelin** A synthetic suppressant of steroid production by the gonads, and used in the treatment of endometriosis.
**Dose:** given as a once-only course of treatment by nasal spray in doses of 200 µg twice a day, starting between 2 and 4 days of the menstrual cycle, and continued for up to 6 months. Side-effects are numerous and of the menopausal type. (Synarel). See buserelin, goserelin and leuprorelin.

**naftidrofuryl** A peripheral and cerebral vasodilator. Claimed to be of value in cerebrovascular disorders.
**Dose:** 300–600 mg daily. (Praxilene).

**nalbuphine** An opioid analgesic, compara-ble with morphine in potency, but with reduced side-effects and a reduced dependence potential.
**Dose:** by injection, 10–20 mg as required. It may cause nausea and dizziness, and care is necessary in respiratory, renal or hepatic dysfunction. (Nubain).

**nalidixic acid** A quinolone antibacterial agent used in cystitis and infections of the lower urinary tract, especially those due to Gram-negative bacteria (except *Pseudomonas*). It is not suitable for systemic infections as the blood levels reached with nalidixic acid are too low to be effective.
**Dose:** 4 g daily for 7 days, with subse-quent doses of 2 g daily. Side-effects are nausea, visual disturbance, rash, jaundice and phototoxicity. Exposure to sunlight should be avoided; epilepsy is a contra-indication. (Mictral; Negram). See ciprofloxacin and norfloxacin.

72

M

**naloxone** A powerful and rapidly acting opioid narcotics antagonist. It is used immediately after operation to reduce any narcotic-induced respiratory depression.
**Dose:** 100–200 μg i.v. initially, followed by 100 μg at 2-minute intervals, as required. For neonates, 10 μg/kg by injection are given. In narcotic analgesic overdose, 800 μg–2 mg may be given, up to a total dose of 10 mg. (Narcan).

**naltrexone** A long-acting narcotic antagonist used only to prevent relapse and maintain recovery after treatment for opioid addiction. It prevents re-addiction only whilst the drug is being taken.
**Dose:** 25 mg initially, later up to 50 mg daily. It must not be given to patients who are still opioid-dependent as an acute withdrawal syndrome may be precipitated. (Nalorex).

**nandrolone** An anabolic steroid related to testosterone, with markedly reduced virilizing properties. It has anabolic or tissue-building properties and has been used in postoperative convalescence, osteoporosis and wasting diseases but the response is poor. It is sometimes effective in aplastic anaemia.
**Dose:** 50 mg by deep i.m. injection every 3 weeks. (Deca-Durabolin).

**naproxen** A widely used non-steroidal anti-inflammatory agent (NSAID) for the relief of rheumatic and musculoskeletal disorders and acute gout.
**Dose:** 0.5–1 g daily, increased up to 2 g daily in severe conditions. Suppositories of 500 mg are useful at night to reduce morning stiffness. Side-effects include headache, dizziness, and dyspepsia with occasional bleeding. Blurred vision may also occur, as well as hypersensitivity reactions such as rash and bronchospasm. Care is necessary in renal and hepatic impairment; peptic ulcer is a contraindication. (Naprosyn; Synflex). See page 165 and Table 29.

**naratriptan**∇A serotonin (5–HT$_1$) receptor agonist for the treatment of acute migraine.
**Dose:** 2.5 mg. A second dose may be given after at least 4 hours if the symptoms recur. (Naramig). See page 154 and Table 23.

**nedocromil** An inhibitor of the release of inflammatory mediators in the respiratory tract. It is used like sodium cromoglycate in the prophylactic treatment of asthma, but it is not effective in an established attack.
**Dose:** by aerosol inhalation, 8 mg (4 puffs) daily. Side-effects are transient nausea and headache. (Tilade). See page 118. It is also used as eye drops in allergic conjunctivitis. (Rapitil). See page 118 and Table 2.

**nefazodone**∇ A new antidepressant of the selective serotonin-re-uptake inhibitor (SSRI) type.
**Dose:** 200–600 mg daily. (Dutonin).

**nefopam** An analgesic for moderate, acute and chronic pain before using more potent drugs.
**Dose:** 90–270 mg daily; 20 mg by i.m. injection. Side-effects include drowsiness, headache and tachycardia. Care is necessary in hepatic or renal disease. (Acupan).

**neomycin** An antibiotic with a wide range of activity against Gram-positive and Gram-negative bacteria, but it is too toxic for systemic use. It is used mainly as an ointment or cream (0.5%), often with an anti-inflammatory steroid, in infected skin conditions. It is also used locally for ear and eye infections as drops (0.5%), and it is occasionally given orally in doses of 6 g daily before bowel surgery. Extended local use may cause allergic reactions, and occasionally ototoxicity. (Mycifradin; Nivemycin).

**neostigmine** An inhibitor of cholinesterase which thus indirectly prolongs the action of acetylcholine released at nerve endings. It is used mainly in the treatment of myasthenia gravis.
**Dose:** 75–300 mg daily; 1–2.5 mg by injection. Side-effects are nausea, salivation, diarrhoea and abdominal cramp, and supplementary treatment with an anticholinergic drug may be required. It is also used postoperatively to antagonize the residual effects of muscle relaxants. Dose: 1–5 mg i.v., after a preliminary injection of 0.5–1 mg of atropine. It is contraindicated in urinary or intestinal obstruction. (Prostigmin).

**netilmicin** An aminoglycoside antibiotic, less toxic than related drugs. Used mainly in severe infections of the urinary and respiratory tracts that are resistant to gentamicin.
**Dose:** 4–6 mg/kg daily by i.v. injection; in urinary tract infections a single oral daily dose of 150 mg is given for 5 days. Side-effects are dizziness, vertigo, malaise and rash; ototoxicity may also occur. (Netillin).

73

N

**neuromuscular blocking agents** Drugs used to induce adequate muscle relaxation under a light plane of anaesthesia to facilitate surgery. The non-depolarizing agents such as vercuronium compete with acetylcholine at the neuromuscular receptor site, and have a relatively long action that can be reversed by neostigmine. The depolarizing relaxants, such as suxamethonium, have an acetylcholine-like action on the receptor site, but as they are broken down less rapidly than acetylcholine, they delay the return of the ability of the muscle to contract again. The action of suxamethonium cannot be reversed by neostigmine.

**niacin** See nicotinic acid.

**nicardipine** A calcium channel blocking agent with a coronary vasodilator action similar to that of verapamil, but with reduced anti-arrhythmic activity. It is used mainly in angina and hypertension, and unlike verapamil it may be given to patients already receiving beta-blockers.
**Dose:** 60–120 mg daily. Side-effects are dizziness, flushing, nausea and palpitations. If chest pain occurs early, the drug should be withdrawn. Marked aortic stenosis is a contraindication. (Cardene). See page 114 and Table 4.

**niclosamide** A synthetic anthelmintic of value in the elimination of tapeworm.
**Dose:** after fasting 2 g followed 2 hours later by a purge. The tablets should be chewed or crushed, and taken with a glass of water. Side-effects are nausea and abdominal pain, and occasionally pruritus. (Yomesan).

**nicorandil** A cardiac drug that has an action mediated by the activation of potassium channels. It reduces the excitability of cardiac muscle and promotes coronary circulation, and is used in the prophylaxis and treatment of angina.
**Dose:** 5–10 mg twice daily initially, rising to a maximum of 60 mg daily. Side-effects are initial headache, palpitations, dizziness. (Ikorel). See page 114 and Table 4.

**nicotinamide** A compound derived from nicotinic acid, possessing similar properties, but differing in that it has little vasodilator action. It is useful in deficiency states as well as in pellagra when the vasodilator action of nicotinic

acid limits the dose. It is also used locally as a 4% gel (Papulex) for the treatment of inflammatory acne vulgaris.

**nicotinic acid** An essential food factor, occurring in yeast, liver, etc., but now prepared synthetically. It is a specific in the treatment of pellagra. It causes vasodilation, and has been used in Ménière's disease and chilblains, but with variable results. In large doses it reduces the plasma levels of some lipoproteins.
**Dose:** 10–30 mg daily for prophylaxis; therapeutic dose in pellagra, 250–500 mg daily. In hyperlipidaemia up to 6 g daily have been given. Side-effects include flushing, dizziness and pruritus, which may sometimes be reduced by taking aspirin 75 mg half an hour before a dose. See page 146.

**nicotinyl alcohol** A derivative with the vasodilator properties of nicotinic acid, but they are less intense. Useful in peripheral circulatory disturbances such as Raynaud's disease and acrocyanosis.
**Dose:** 100–200 mg daily. (Ronicol).

**nicoumalone** A synthetic anti-coagulant similar to warfarin, and used mainly in the treatment of deep-vein thrombosis.
**Dose:** 8–12 mg initially; subsequent doses are based on the response, as shown by determination of the blood prothrombin time, expressed as the International Normalized Ratio (INR). Haemorrhage is a potential side-effect. (Sinthrome).

**nifedipine** A calcium channel blocking agent similar to verapamil, but with a more powerful peripheral and coronary vasodilator action. It is used in the treatment of angina, hypertension and Raynaud's disease, and may be given if required in association with a beta-blocking agent.
**Dose:** in angina, 15–60 mg daily; in hypertension 40–80 mg daily. Side-effects are flushing and headache, which are usually transient, and some ankle oedema may occur. It should be withdrawn if anginal pain develops. Severe aortic stenosis is a contraindication. (Adalat; Coracten; Nifensar). See pages 114 & 148, and Tables 4 & 21.

**nimodipine** A calcium channel blocking agent that acts preferentially on the cerebral vessels. It is used in subarachnoid haemorrhage to prevent ischaemic sequelae.

**Dose:** within 4 days of onset: 60 mg 4-hourly, continued for 21 days. Dose for treatment: 1 mg/hrly initially by i.v. infusion, increased later to 2 mg/hr for 5 days. Side-effects are flushing, hypotension and gastrointestinal disturbances. (Nimotop).

**nisoldipine** A calcium channel blocking agent of the nifedipine type. Used in mild to moderate hypertension and in the prophylaxis of chronic angina.
**Dose:** 10 mg once daily before breakfast with adequate fluid, slowly increased as required up to 40 mg daily. Tablets to be swallowed whole, not chewed or crushed. It may react with some other drugs in common use, and grapefruit juice should be avoided. (Syscor). See pages 114 & 148, and Tables 4 & 21.

**nitrazepam** A benzodiazepine used as a mild hypnotic when some degree of daytime sedation is acceptable.
**Dose:** 5–10 mg at night, with reduced doses for elderly patients, and in renal and hepatic dysfunction. Care is necessary in respiratory depression. Some dependence on nitrazepam may occur, so extended treatment should be avoided. The combined use of alcohol increases the hypnotic action. (Mogadon; Remnos). See page 152 and Table 22.

**Nitrocine** A solution of glyceryl trinitrate, for i.v. infusion in myocardial ischaemia and refractory angina.

**nitrofurantoin** An antibacterial agent with a wide range of activity against the majority of urinary pathogens. It is of value in cystitis and pyelitis, and in renal infections that have become resistant to other drugs. It is also used prophylactically but extended use requires care.
**Dose:** 400 mg daily; 50–100 mg at night for prophylaxis. It is ineffective in an alkaline urine. Nausea, rash and peripheral neuropathy are side-effects, and acute and chronic pulmonary reactions have been reported. (Furadantin; Macrobid).

**nitroglycerine** See glyceryl trinitrate.

**nitroprusside** See sodium nitroprusside.

**nitrous oxide** The oldest inhalation anaesthetic. Supplied in blue cylinders, it is widely used for induction and as part of a mixed anaesthetic system. It is also used as a 50% oxygen mixture as an inhalation analgesic in obstetrics.

**nizatidine** A potent and selective $H_2$-receptor antagonist chemically distinct from cimetidine or ranitidine.
**Dose:** in the treatment of benign duodenal and gastric ulcer, single doses of 300 mg daily, taken in the evening, or 150 mg twice a day, and continued for 4 weeks, or for 8 weeks in gastric ulcer including non-steroidal anti-inflammatory agent (NSAID)-induced ulceration. Occasionally given by i.v. infusion in doses of 300 mg daily. For prophylactic maintenance, doses of 150 mg daily may be given for up to a year. Reduced doses should be given in renal impairment. Side-effects include headache, myalgia, cough, pruritus and abnormal dreams. (Axid; Zinga). See page 162 and Table 27.

**non-steroidal anti-inflammatory drugs (NSAIDs)** A group of drugs with analgesic anti-inflammatory properties widely used in arthritic, rheumatoid and related conditions. The response to a NSAID and the incidence and severity of side-effects such as gastric irritation and renal toxicity vary considerably, and the best NSAID for an individual patient is the one that gives optimum relief with minimal side-effects. The NSAIDs, of which aspirin is the oldest example, act by interrupting the biosynthesis of prostaglandins from arachidonic acid, in which process the enzyme cyclooxygenase (COX) plays a key role. It is now known that COX exists in two forms identified as COX-1 and COX-2. The anti-inflammatory action of the NSAIDs appears to be linked with the inhibition of COX-2, whereas the unwanted side-effects are associated with COX-1 inhibition. Different NSAIDs have varying degrees of activity against the different forms of COX, which may explain the differences in the therapeutic response and the incidence of side-effects. Recently, a NSAID (meloxicam) has been introduced that has a more selective inhibitory action on COX-2, with which the incidence of side-effects appears to be lower than with the older drugs, and so may have therapeutic advantages. In general, the response to a NSAID may take 1–3 weeks to develop fully, but monitoring for gastrointestinal bleeding may be advisable if treatment is extended. A NSAID should not be given to a patient with a history of asthma or hypersensitivity, nor when peptic ulcer is

75

**N**

suspected or present. In all cases, treatment should be commenced with the lowest recommended dose, and caution is necessary in the elderly, and when renal or hepatic function is impaired. See page 165 and Table 29.

**noradrenaline (norepinephrine)** The pressor hormone released at sympathetic nerve endings when such nerves are stimulated. It is also present with adrenaline in the medulla of the adrenal gland. It raises blood pressure mainly by a general vasoconstriction, whereas adrenaline acts by constricting the peripheral vessels and increasing the cardiac output. Noradrenaline is given by slow i.v. infusion in the treatment of shock, peripheral failure, and low blood pressure states, but the response may fluctuate with small variations in dose. The value of vasoconstrictors in shock is now questioned, as in shock the peripheral resistance may well be high, and the blood supply to essential organs such as the kidneys may be reduced.
**Dose:** 2–20 µg/min, based on need and response. Great care must be taken to avoid extra-venous injection. (Levophed).

**norethisterone** An orally active progestogen. Used in amenorrhoea, functional uterine bleeding and dysmenorrhoea.
**Dose:** 5–20 mg daily. In breast cancer, large doses up to 60 mg daily have been used. To postpone menstruation, 15 mg daily for 3 days have been used. In small doses, and in association with an oestrogen, norethisterone and related drugs are widely used as oral contraceptives. See page 264.

**norfloxacin** A quinolone antibacterial with the actions, uses and side-effects of cinoxacin and other quinolones.
**Dose:** in acute urinary tract infections, 800 mg daily for 3–10 days: in chronic infections continued for up to 12 weeks. (Utinor).

**norgestrel (levonorgestrel)** An orally active progesterone-like drug and inhibitor of ovulation. Used as a constituent of mixed oral contraceptive products, and as a 'progestogen-only' oral contraceptive. See page 264.

**nortriptyline** A tricyclic antidepressant with actions, uses and side-effects similar to those of amitriptyline, but with a reduced sedative activity.

**Dose:** 20–100 mg daily. It is given in nocturnal enuresis in doses of 10–20 mg nightly, but the duration of treatment should not exceed 3 months. (Allegron). See page 128 and Table 11.

**NSAIDs** See non-steroidal anti-inflammatory drugs, page 168 and Table 29.

**nystatin** A fungicidal antibiotic, used in the treatment of intestinal, vaginal and superficial candidiasis. Oral tablets contain 500 000 units, pessaries contain 100 000 units; cream and ointment 1%.
**Dose:** (oral) 2 million units daily. It is also used as pastilles of 100 000 units for mouth infections.

# O

**octreotide** A synthetic compound that inhibits the release of the growth hormone. It is used in acromegaly, which is caused by an overproduction of the growth hormone by a pituitary tumour and it is given in doses of 100–200 µg 8-hourly by s.c. injection. It is also used in the symptomatic treatment of the carcinoid syndrome, in which the release of vasoactive substances by a gastro-pancreatic tumour causes flushing and severe diarrhoea.
**Dose:** 50 µg by s.c. injection, increased as needed up to 600 µg daily. It has no action on the cause of the syndrome. It is used occasionally in terminal care to reduce intestinal secretions and vomiting. Dose: 300–600 µg by s.c. infusion. (Sandostatin).

**oestradiol** The oestrogenic hormone controlling ovulation and menstruation. It has been used to control menopausal symptoms in doses of 10–20 µg daily, but skin patches are now preferred for hormone replacement therapy (HRT). It is used occasionally as s.c. implants for long-term treatment. Oestradiol is also present in some cream preparations for menopausal atrophic vaginitis.

**oestriol** A natural oestrogen used in intravaginal cream to relieve the atrophic vaginitis and kraurosis vulvae associated with the menopause. Also given in doses of 1–32 mg daily for the genito-urinary symptoms linked with infections in oestrogen deficiency states. (Ovestin).

**ofloxacin** A fluorinated quinolone with the actions, uses and side-effects of other quinolones such as ciprofloxacin and norfloxacin. It is used mainly in urinary and lower respiratory tract infections.
**Dose:** 400 mg daily as a single morning dose. Dose in severe infections 200–400 mg daily by i.v. injection. An occasional side-effect is tendon damage with pain and inflammation, which requires immediate withdrawal of the drug. Exposure to strong sunlight should be avoided. (Tarivid). Also used as eye drops (0.3%) for superficial eye infections. (Exocin).

**olanzapine**∇ An antipsychotic agent for the treatment of schizophrenia. It has a more selective action on certain 5–HT-receptors, and is less likely to cause extra-pyramidal side-effects.
**Dose:** 10 mg as a single daily dose, slowly increased as required. Maintenance dose 5–20 mg daily. Side-effects include sedation and weight gain. (Zyprexa). See page 168 and Table 30.

**olsalazine** A compound formed from mesalazine, and used in the treatment of ulcerative colitis. It is more slowly absorbed, and reaches the colon largely unchanged, where it is broken down by intestinal bacteria to release the active metabolite mesalazine.
**Dose:** 1–3 g daily in acute mild ulcerative colitis; 1 g daily for maintenance, often for long periods. The common side-effect is a watery diarrhoea. Salicylate sensitivity is a contraindication. Patients are now advised to report any bruising, bleeding or malaise. If a blood dyscrasia is suspected, a blood count should be made and the drug withdrawn. (Dipentum). See page 172 and Table 32.

**omeprazole** An inhibitor of the enzyme $H^+K^+ATPase$. That enzyme controls the final stage of gastric acid production, and its inhibition by omeprazole is of value in peptic ulcer resistant to $H_2$ receptor antagonists, and in reflux oesophagitis, where such agents are not always effective.
**Dose:** in benign gastric and duodenal ulcer, 20–40 mg as a single daily dose for 4–8 weeks. Larger doses may be required in the Zollinger–Ellison syndrome. Side-effects such as nausea, gastro-intestinal disturbances and headaches are usually mild. (Losec). See page 162 and Table 27.

**ondansetron** A potent antiemetic, of value in the nausea and vomiting associated with cancer chemotherapy. Such vomiting appears to be induced by the release of serotonin, which acts on receptors in the gut as well as stimulating the chemoreceptor trigger zone in the brain. Ondansetron is a specific $(5–HT_3)$ serotonin blocking agent, and is given before the commencement of cytotoxic treatment or radiotherapy.
**Dose:** 24 mg daily; in severe vomiting an initial dose of 8 mg is given by slow i.v. injection, followed by 1 mg/hrly for 24 hours by continuous i.v. infusion, followed by oral therapy. Side-effects are an initial sense of warmth, headache and constipation. (Zofran). See page 158.

**†opium** The dried juice from the capsules of the opium poppy. See morphine.

**orciprenaline** A sympathomimetic agent with the bronchodilator properties of isoprenaline. It is used for the relief of obstructive airway conditions, although more selective drugs of the salbutamol type are often preferred.
**Dose:** up to 80 mg daily; by aerosol inhalation up to 12 puffs (9 mg) daily. Side-effects include tremor and tachycardia. (Alupent). See page 118 and Table 6.

**orphenadrine** A spasmolytic drug, used in the treatment of parkinsonism, and for the relief of voluntary muscle spasm.
**Dose:** 150–400 mg daily. It may also be given by i.m. injection in doses of 60 mg. In parkinsonism it tends to control the rigidity more than the tremor. Side-effects are anticholinergic and include dryness of the mouth, dizziness and visual disturbances. Weight gain has occurred with high doses. (Disipal; Norflex). See page 160 and Table 26.

**oxazepam** A benzodiazepine with the actions, uses and side-effects of diazepam. It is useful in acute anxiety and panic states.
**Dose:** 45–120 mg daily. See page 117 and Table 5.

**oxerutins** A mixture of rutosides (flavonoid derivatives) which is claimed to reduce capillary fragility and permeability. It has been used in venous disorders of the lower limbs.
**Dose:** 750–1000 mg daily. (Paroven).

**oxitropium** An anticholinergic broncho-dilator similar to ipratropium, and used by aerosol inhalation in stable chronic asthma and related conditions.
**Dose:** 200–300 µg (4–6 puffs) daily. (Oxivent). See page 118 and Table 6.

**oxpentifylline** An aminophyline-like drug used mainly as a vasodilator in peripheral vascular disorders.
**Dose:** 800–1200 mg. It may cause nausea, flushing and dizziness. Care is necessary in hypotensive states. (Trental).

**oxprenolol** A beta-adrenoceptor blocking agent with the actions, uses and side-effects of propranolol. It also has anxiolytic properties, and may reduce the symptoms of transient stress such as tremor and palpitations.
**Dose:** 60–480 mg daily. (Slow-Trasicor). See page 148 and Table 21.

**oxybuprocaine** A local anaesthetic for ophthalmic use, including tonometry, as a 0.4% solution.

**oxybutynin** An anticholinergic anti-spasmodic that promotes relaxation of the detrusor muscle of the bladder.
**Dose:** in urinary incontinence, 10–20 mg daily; 10 mg daily for children with neuro-genic bladder instability. Side-effects are those of anticholinergic drugs generally. (Cystrin; Ditropan). See page 174.

**†oxycodone** A powerful narcotic analgesic with a prolonged action. Used as supposi-tories of 30 mg in terminal care.

**oxypertine** A tranquillizer with a chlorpro-mazine-like action, and used in anxiety neuroses, psychoses and schizophrenic states.
**Dose:** 30–60 mg daily in anxiety states; up to 300 mg daily in schizophrenia. In higher doses it may cause nausea, dizzi-ness and drowsiness. See page 168 and Table 30.

**oxytetracycline** (Terramycin). See tetracy-cline.

**oxytocin** The oxytocic fraction of pituitary extract, but now made synthetically. Used for the induction and maintenance of labour, and to control post-partum haemorrhage, either alone or in associa-tion with ergometrine.

**Dose:** 1–3 mega-units/min by i.v. infu-sion only, with monitoring. Excessive doses may cause severe uterine contrac-tions with the risk of fetal asphyxiation. (Syntocinon).

# P

**paclitaxel**∇ A new cytotoxic agent origi-nally obtained from the bark of the Pacific Yew. It prevents mitosis and inhibits cell growth by stabilizing microtubule produc-tion. It is used by specialists for metastatic ovarian cancer not responding to platinum therapy. Premedication is necessary to prevent severe hypersensitivity reactions. (Taxol). See page 122 and Table 8.

**pamidronate disodium** A bisphosphonate with the actions and uses of etidronate. It is used mainly in the hypercalcaemia of malignancy, as it inhibits the development of active osteoclasts.
**Dose:** by i.v. infusion 10–90 mg or more according to the degree of hypercalcaemia. The initial response may occur within 24–48 hours. Dose in Paget's disease of bone, 30 mg weekly. Care is necessary in marked renal impairment. (Aredia).

**pancreatin** A preparation containing the pancreatic enzymes, trypsin, lipase and amylase. It is used to aid the digestion of fats, proteins and carbohydrates in cystic fibrosis and pancreatitis. Some high-strength products have caused fibrotic strictures of the large bowel.

**pancuronium** A non-depolarizing or competitive muscle relaxant that has little histamine-releasing or cardiovascular action.
**Dose:** 50–100 µg/kg i.v. initially with supplementary doses of 10–20 µg/kg as required. (Pavulon).

**pantoprazole**∇ A proton pump inhibitor similar to omeprazole, used in peptic ulcer and reflux oesophagitis.
**Dose:** 40 mg daily with breakfast. The tablets must be swallowed whole with water, and not chewed or crushed. (Proteum). See page 162 and Table 27.

**papaveretum** A preparation of the alka-loids of opium, containing approximately

50% of morphine together with papaverine and codeine. Used mainly by injection, often in association with hyoscine (scopolamine) for premedication.
**Dose:** 7.7–15.4 mg repeated as required.

**papaverine** One of the alkaloids of opium. It has little analgesic action, and has been used mainly as a smooth muscle relaxant in peripheral vascular diseases. More recently it has been used by intracavernosal injection in the treatment of impotence.

**paracetamol** A widely used mild analgesic with few side-effects except in large doses. It differs from aspirin in the absence of any anti-inflammatory action.
**Dose:** 2–4 g daily. Paediatric suppositories of 125 mg are available. Overdose may cause severe liver damage (see acetylcysteine).

**paraffin** A generic name for hydrocarbon mixtures. Soft paraffin is the common ointment base; liquid paraffin is a lubricant laxative. Hard paraffin was used in the wax bath treatment of rheumatic conditions.

**paraldehyde** A colourless liquid with a strong characteristic odour. It was once used as a chloral-like sedative causing little respiratory depression; now given by deep i.m. injection in status asthmaticus.
**Dose:** 5–10 ml. Occasionally given in similar doses by rectum, diluted with saline or arachis oil. Discoloured paraldehyde must **not** be used.

**paroxetine** A selective inhibitor of serotonin uptake in the central nervous system, and indicated in the treatment of depression.
**Dose:** 20 mg daily, initially in the morning, with food, slowly increased as required to 50 mg daily. It should not be given with any other drug likely to increase serotonin uptake. Side-effects are nausea, drowsiness and insomnia. Extrapyramidal reactions may occur more often with paroxetine. (Seroxat). See page 128 and Table 11.

**penciclovir** An antiviral agent used as a 1% cream for cold sores (*Herpes labialis*). Treatment should be started as soon as possible by applying the cream every 2 hours for 4 days. (Vectavir). See page 144 and Table 19.

**penicillamine** A breakdown product of penicillin which has the power of combining with certain metals to form a water-soluble, non-toxic complex that is excreted in the urine. It is used in Wilson's disease, which is due to the retention of copper in the body, in poisoning by lead and mercury, in chronic active hepatitis (after the condition has been controlled), in cystinuria, and in severe rheumatoid arthritis in which it has an action similar to that of gold.
**Dose:** in Wilson's disease, 1.5–2 g daily before food for some months. In chronic hepatitis, 500 mg daily initially, slowly increased over some weeks to 1.25 g daily. In rheumatoid arthritis, 125–250 mg daily initially before food, slowly increased at monthly intervals with maintenance doses of 500–750 mg daily. Patients should be warned that the response in rheumatoid arthritis is slow. In cystinuria, 1–3 g daily with adequate fluids, adjusted later to maintain the urinary cysteine level below 200 mg/l. Dose in heavy metal poisoning, 2 g daily. Side-effects include nausea, loss of taste, rash and thrombocytopenia. Blood counts during treatment are essential and patients should be advised to report most side-effects. A late onset rash may require cessation of treatment. (Distamine; Pendramine). See page 165 and Table 29.

**penicillin, benzyl penicillin, penicillin G** The first of the antibiotics. It acts by preventing the development of the bacterial cell wall, but some groups of organisms vary widely in the degree of sensitivity to penicillin, and it is inactivated by penicillinase-producing organisms. Penicillin is inactive orally, and so is given by i.m. injection, but as it is rapidly excreted the action is relatively brief. Derivatives such as procaine-penicillin have a longer action (penicillin V is an orally active derivative). The main side-effect is hypersensitivity, and sensitivity to one penicillin extends to any other penicillin, and may also include sensitivity to the related cephalosporins. High doses of penicillin, especially in patients with renal insufficiency, may occasionally cause cerebral irritation and encephalopathy. Cloxacillin and amoxycillin are derivatives of penicillin active against resistant staphylococci; ampicillin has a wide range of activity against Gram-positive and Gram-negative organisms; piperacillin and ticarcillin are active against *Pseudomonas aeruginosa*.

79

P

**pentaerythitol tetranitrate** A vasodilator with properties resembling those of glyceryl trinitrate, but with a more prolonged action. Used mainly in the prophylaxis of angina as side-effects are relatively infrequent.
**Dose:** 60–240 mg daily. (Mycardol). See page 114 and Table 4.

**pentamidine** A synthetic drug used in the treatment of *Pneumocystis carinii* pneumonia in AIDS and other immuno-compromised patients, as an alternative to co-trimoxazole.
**Dose:** 4 mg/kg daily by i.v. infusion for 14 days or more, or by inhalation of a nebulized solution. Other dosage schemes are used in the treatment of trypano-somiasis and leishmaniasis. Severe reactions, particularly hypotension, may occur, and pentamidine should be used only under expert supervision. (Pentacarinat).

**pentastarch** A starch-derived plasma substitute used as a 10% solution in burns and septicaemia.
**Dose:** by i.v. infusion 500 ml–2 L. (Haes, Pentaspan). See hetastarch.

**†pentazocine** A powerful analgesic of the morphine type, but less likely to cause addiction, although dependence may occur with long treatment.
**Dose:** 100–400 mg daily after food, up to 360 mg daily by injection. Suppositories of 50 mg are available. Hallucinations are an occasional side-effect. It should be avoided after myocardial infarction as it may increase the cardiac load. Other side-effects include dizziness, nausea, tachycardia and rash. It should be avoided in opioid-dependent patients. (Fortral).

**pentostatin** A potent cytotoxic agent used in hairy cell leukaemia. It is an inhibitor of adenosine deaminase, and may affect RNA synthesis and cause DNA breakdown.
**Dose:** i.v. under specialist supervision, 4 mg/m$^2$ every other week, continued up to 6 months unless a remission has been achieved. Side-effects include myelo-suppression, leukopenia, renal and liver toxicity and rash. Blood counts are necessary during treatment. (Nipent). See page 122.

**peppermint oil** Aromatic carminative.
**Dose:** 0.2–0.4 ml. (Colpermin; Mintec).

**pergolide** A dopamine agonist with a stimulating action on both $D_1$ and $D_2$ receptors. It is used in the auxillary treatment of parkinsonism, and combined treatment may permit a reduction in the dose of levodopa and its side-effects.
**Dose:** 100 µg daily initially, slowly increased at 3-day intervals according to response, with care taken to avoid initial hypotension. Other side-effects include nausea, diarrhoea, confusion and hallucinations. (Celance). See page 160 and Table 26.

**pericyazine** A tranquillizer of the chlorpromazine type with similar uses and side-effects. It is used mainly in schizophrenia and severe anxiety states.
**Dose:** 15–75 mg daily, slowly increased according to need up to 300 mg. (Neulactil). See page 168 and Table 30.

**perindopril** A long-acting ACE inhibitor used in the control of essential hypertension not responding to other drugs.
**Dose:** initially, a single daily dose of 2 mg (before food), subsequently adjusted up to a maximum of 8 mg daily. Diuretic therapy should first be withdrawn for 2–3 days, and renal function should be assessed before and during treatment. It is also used as supplementary therapy in heart failure in doses of 2–4 mg. (Coversyl). See page 148 and Table 21.

**permethrin** An insecticide used as 1% cream for head lice, and 5% cream for scabies. (Lyclear).

**perphenazine** A tranquillizer with the actions, uses and side-effects of chlorpromazine, but it is less sedating, and effective in lower doses.
**Dose:** psychiatric and antiemetic, 12–24 mg daily. It is sometimes useful in the control of intractable hiccup. (Fentazin). See page 168 and Table 30.

**†pethidine** A synthetic analgesic with spasmolytic properties. Widely employed as an alternative to morphine for pre- and post-operative use. Of value in obstetrics as it has a less depressant action than morphine on the respiration.
**Dose:** 300–600 mg daily; by s.c. or i.m. injection doses of 25–100 mg at intervals according to need. Occasionally pethidine is given by slow i.v. injection in doses of 25–50 mg. As a supplementary analgesic in

general anaesthesia, 10–25 mg i.v. Side-effects include dizziness, nausea and palpitations.

**†phenazocine** A synthetic morphine-like analgesic, with similar properties and uses, but with a more rapid and prolonged action. It is of value in biliary colic, as it is less likely to cause a rise in biliary pressure.
**Dose:** 20–30 mg daily, orally or sublingually, although single doses as high as 20 mg are sometimes given. The side-effects are similar to those of morphine and related drugs, but sedation and the risk of dependence is less. (Narphen).

**phenelzine** A monoamine oxidase inhibitor, used in the treatment of depression.
**Dose:** 45–60 mg daily, according to need and response. It has many side-effects, including dizziness, dry mouth and blurred vision. Very severe hypertension has been precipitated by some foods, notably cheese. Care is necessary in cardiovascular disease and epilepsy. It may also potentiate the action of other drugs on the central nervous system. (Nardil). See monoamine oxidase inhibitors, page 128 and Table 11.

**phenindamine** An antihistamine of medium potency. It differs from most antihistamines in having a mild central stimulant action, and so rarely causes drowsiness.
**Dose:** 75–200 mg daily. (Thephorin). See page 110 and Table 2.

**phenindione** An orally active anticoagulant used in the control of deep-vein thrombosis.
**Dose:** 200 mg initially; maintenance, 25–100 mg daily, depending on laboratory reports of the prothrombin time. Side-effects include hypersensitivity reactions and haemorrhage. Patients should be warned that the drug may colour the urine. Phenindione has now been largely replaced by warfarin. (Dindevan).

**pheniramine** An antihistamine similar to but less potent than chlorpheniramine.
**Dose:** 150 mg daily. (Daneral SA). See page 110 and Table 2.

**†phenobarbitone** A powerful sedative, hypnotic and anticonvulsant drug. It is mainly of value in epilepsy, as it is effective in most types of seizure except petit mal (absence seizures).

**Dose:** 60–180 mg daily, at night, adjusted to need and response. In severe conditions, doses of 50–200 mg may be given by i.m. or i.v. injection. Side-effects include drowsiness and skin reactions. In the elderly it may cause confusion, and paradoxically it may give rise to hyperkinesia in some children. See page 136 and Table 15.

**phenol** Once widely used as a general antiseptic. Weak solutions relieve itching, and phenol is present in Calamine Lotion. A 5% solution in almond oil is used for the injection treatment of haemorrhoids.

**phenolphthalein** A synthetic laxative. It is sometimes given with emulsion of liquid paraffin.
**Dose:** 50–100 mg daily. It may occasionally cause a rash, and its use has declined.

**†phenoperidine** A narcotic analgesic, often used in association with droperidol in neuroleptanalgesia. It is also used as a supplementary analgesic in general anaesthesia.
**Dose:** 0.5–1 mg i.v. with subsequent doses as required. It may cause respiratory depression, which can be controlled by doxapram or naloxone. (Operidine).

**phenothrin** An insecticide used as 0.2% lotion for head and crab lice. (Full Marks).

**phenoxybenzamine** An alpha-adrenoceptor blocking agent used in the severe, episodic hypertension associated with phaeochromocytoma.
**Dose:** orally and by injection, 10–20 mg according to need and response. Side-effects include dizziness and tachycardia; rapid and marked hypotension after injection. (Dibenyline).

**phenoxymethylpenicillin** An orally active, acid-stable penicillin, also known as penicillin V. It is used mainly in respiratory infections in children, in tonsillitis, and to supplement injection treatment. It is not suitable for use in severe infections.
**Dose:** 1–2 g daily, before food. Doses of 500 mg daily are given in rheumatic fever and pneumococcal prophylaxis.

**†phentermine** An appetite depressant given in the short-term treatment of obesity.
**Dose:** 15–30 mg before breakfast. (Duramine; Ionamin).

81

P

**phentolamine** An alpha-adrenoceptor blocking agent that can temporarily reverse the vasoconstrictive action of adrenaline and noradrenaline. It is used mainly in the diagnosis and control of the episodic hypertension of phaeochromocytoma, and during surgical removal of the tumour.
**Dose:** 2–5 mg i.v. repeated as required. Side-effects are tachycardia, hypotension, dizziness, nausea and diarrhoea. (Rogitine).

**phenylbutazone** A powerful, non-steroidal anti-inflammatory agent, formerly used in the treatment of rheumatic and arthritic conditions. Because of blood dyscrasias, which may occur suddenly, the drug is now used only for the treatment of ankylosing spondylitis under hospital supervision.
**Dose:** 400–600 mg daily. (Butacote). See page 165 and Table 29.

**phenylephrine** A vasoconstrictor similar to adrenaline, but less toxic. Given in acute hypotensive states.
**Dose:** 5 mg by i.m. injection, or 100–500 µg by slow i.v. injection. Sometimes valuable in paroxysmal atrial tachycardia. It is also used locally as 1:400 solution as nasal decongestive, and as eye drops, 2.5–10%.

**phenylpropanolamine** A sympatho-mimetic agent used with other drugs in preparations for the symptomatic relief of nasal congestion.

**phenytoin** An anticonvulsant used in all forms of epilepsy with the exception of petit mal (absence seizures). It has little hypnotic effect and combined treatment with phenobarbitone may evoke the best response.
**Dose:** 150–600 mg daily with or after food. In status epilepticus it is given under ECG control in doses of 10–15 mg/kg by slow i.v. injection. It is also given to control ventricular tachycardias in doses of 3.5–5 mg/kg by slow i.v. injection via a caval catheter. The side-effects of extended treatment are numerous, and include rash, dizziness, blood dyscrasias, hirsutism and gingival hypertrophy. (Epanutin). See page 136 and Table 15.

**pholcodine** A cough centre depressant resembling codeine, but it lacks any anal-gesic properties. It is present in a range of

products used for the relief of useless cough, and has the advantage over codeine of not causing constipation.
**Dose:** 10–60 mg daily.

**physostigmine** A plant alkaloid, also known as eserine, once used as a miotic (0.25–1%) to counteract the effects of atropine.

**phytomenadione** Vitamin $K_1$. The form of vitamin K used in the prophylaxis and treatment of neonatal haemorrhage due to vitamin K deficiency.
**Dose:** 1 mg by i.m. injection. It is also of value in the haemorrhage due to overdose of oral anticoagulants. Dose: 10–40 mg by slow i.v. injection. In less severe condi-tions, 10–20 mg orally, according to the base-line prothrombin time. (Konakion).

**pilocarpine** A plant alkaloid with a miotic action similar to, but less intense than that of physostigmine.
**Dose:** in glaucoma as eye drops of 0.5–4%, 3–6 times a day. Occasionally given in doses of 15–30 mg daily with food to reduce the dry mouth associated with irradiation of the head and neck. (Salagen). See page 138 and Table 16.

**pimozide** A tranquillizer with the actions and uses of chlorpromazine. It is used mainly in the treatment of schizophrenia, as it reduces the delusions without causing drowsiness.
**Dose:** 10 mg daily initially, adjusted up to a maximum of 20 mg daily, with mainte-nance doses according to response. Similar doses are given in mania and psycho-motor agitation. The side-effects are similar to those of chlorpromazine. (Orap). See page 168 and Table 30.

**pindolol** A beta-receptor blocking agent, with actions and uses similar to those of propranolol. Less likely to cause bronchospasm.
**Dose:** 7.5–45 mg daily. (Visken). See page 148 and Table 21.

**piperacillin** A semi-synthetic penicillin with a wide range of activity that extends to *Pseudomonas* and anaerobes. It can be used in association with other antibiotics in life-threatening and multiple infections.
**Dose:** in severe infections, 200–300 mg/kg daily by i.m. or slow i.v. injection or infu-sion, increased in life-threatening infections

to 16 g daily. In less severe infections, 100–150 mg/kg i.m. daily, with a maximum single dose of 2 g. (Pipril). Sometimes given with the beta-lactamase inhibitor tazobactam as the mixed product Tazocin.

**piperazine** An effective anthelmintic against threadworms and roundworms.
**Dose:** 2–4 years, 750 mg; 5–12 years, 1.5 g; in children over 12 years and in adults, 2 g; as a single daily dose for 7 days, repeated if necessary after 1 week. For roundworm, a single dose of 4 g is given, but as the worms are narcotized, and not killed, a purgative is necessary to ensure expulsion. Side-effects are nausea, diarrhoea and occasional dizziness. Care is necessary in renal impairment, epilepsy and psychiatric conditions.

**pipothiazine** A chlorpromazine-like drug, with similar uses and side-effects, but given mainly as a depot preparation for the maintenance treatment of schizophrenia.
**Dose:** (after a test dose of 25 mg) 50–100 mg by deep i.m. injection every 4 weeks, increased if necessary up to a maximum of 200 mg per dose. (Piportil Depot). See page 168 and Table 30.

**piracetam**∇ A new drug used for the treatment of the spasmodic condition cortical myoclonus.
**Dose:** 7–20 g daily. Side-effects include diarrhoea, nervousness and rash. (Nootropil).

**piroxicam** A non-steroidal anti-inflammatory agent (NSAID) with an extended action, and used in arthritis, spondylitis, gout and musculoskeletal disorders.
**Dose:** 20–30 mg daily; up to 40 mg daily in gout and other acute conditions. It is also used for local application as a 3% gel. As with related drugs, side-effects include gastrointestinal disturbances of varying severity, especially with higher doses. (Feldene). See page 165 and Table 29.

**pivampicillin** A derivative of ampicillin, with similar actions and uses. Is hydrolyzed to ampicillin after absorption, but gives higher blood levels. Much is excreted in the urine, so it is of value in urinary infections.
**Dose:** 1–2 g daily. (Pondocillin).

**pizotifen** A serotonin antagonist used in the prophylaxis of migraine, and vascular headache.

**Dose:** 1.5–3 mg daily. Side-effects include drowsiness, nausea, dizziness and weight gain. (Sanomigran). See page 154 and Table 23.

**podophyllum resin** A plant extract used topically as a paint (0.5–25% in alcohol) for anogenital and plantar warts. It is very irritant to normal tissues, and its use requires care. (Condyline; Warticon).

**polygeline** A modified gelatin, used with sodium chloride and other electrolytes as a blood volume expander.
**Dose:** 500–1000 ml by i.v. infusion. (Haemaccel).

**polymyxin B** An antibiotic used by local application for infections of the ear, eye and skin. It is too toxic for systemic use.

**polymyxin E** See colistin.

**polystyrene resin** An ion-exchange resin for the removal of potassium in conditions associated with hyperkalaemia, as in oliguria and anuria.
**Dose:** 15 g 3–4 times a day according to the plasma level of potassium. When the drug is not tolerated orally, 30 g daily as a suspension may be given per rectum. Care is required in renal or hepatic impairment. (Resonium).

**polythiazide** A potent diuretic with the actions, uses and side-effects of the thiazide diuretics but effective in the low dose of 1–4 mg daily. (Nephril).

**poractant** A lung surfactant used in the respiratory distress syndrome of premature infants. It is given by endotracheal tubing with mechanical ventilation. (Curosurf).

**potassium** One of the most important ions of the body, mainly present in intracellular fluid. Many diuretics increase loss of potassium as well as sodium; with extended treatment the potassium balance may be disturbed, with acute muscle weakness, cardiac arrhythmias, and an increased sensitivity to digitalis. Potassium loss can be treated with potassium chloride orally (often as Slow-K, but may cause peptic ulceration), or by effervescent potassium tablets. Mixed diuretic and potassium products are also available. In acute potassium deficiency, various potassium-containing i.v. solutions are available, but dose and rate of administration require care, as in excess potassium can cause cardiac arrest. Intravenous solutions should not contain more than 3.2 g/l of potassium chloride.

**potassium citrate** A diuretic useful in cystitis and other inflammatory conditions of the urinary tract. It relieves discomfort by making the urine alkaline. It is also given in gout to increase the excretion of uric acid.
**Dose:** 9–24 g daily.

**potassium permanganate** Purple crystals, soluble in water. A powerful oxidizing and deodorizing agent used 1:1000 as lotion, 1:10 000 to 1:5000 as mouthwash, douche, bladder washout and bath.

**povidone-iodine** A complex of iodine with an organic carrier. When applied to the skin it slowly releases iodine, and has an extended antiseptic action. Used for local application to the skin and mucous membranes as solution containing the equivalent of 0.75–1% of iodine.

**pralidoxime** A reactivator of cholinesterase. Organophosphorus insecticides inhibit that enzyme, and poisoning by such insecticides is an occupational hazard. Their toxicity can be reversed in part by the injection of 2 mg atropine, but the enzyme can be reactivated and muscle power restored by pralidoxime (30 mg/kg) given by slow i.v. injection, repeated as required. It is effective only if given within 24 hours of exposure to the insecticide.

**pravastatin** A blood lipid-lowering agent with the specific enzyme-inhibiting properties of simvastatin, and used in primary hypercholesterolaemia not responding to the other drugs.
**Dose:** 10–40 mg daily as a single dose. Side-effects include myalgia, rash and gastrointestinal disturbances. (Lipostat). See page 146 and Table 20.

**prazinquantel** A schistosomicide of low toxicity, effective against *Schistosoma haematobium*, *S, mansoni* and *S. japonicum*. It is also active against tapeworm.
**Dose:** 10–20 mg/kg as a single oral dose. (Biltricide).

**prazosin** An alpha-adrenoceptor blocking agent and vasodilator used in the treatment of hypertension and congestive heart failure.

**Dose:** 1 mg daily initially, increased as required up to a maximum of 20 mg daily. The initial dose may cause marked hypotension, and it should be taken at night, in bed. Prazosin is also given in benign prostatic hypertrophy in maintenance doses of 4 mg daily. Side-effects are drowsiness, nausea and postural hypotension. (Hypovase). See page 148 and Table 21.

**prednisolone** A glucocorticosteroid with the actions and uses of hydrocortisone, but effective in much lower doses. It is often the preferred drug for oral use, and is given in a wide range of conditions including asthma, severe allergic reactions, rheumatoid arthritis, collagen disorders and inflammatory skin conditions. Prednisolone is also of value in leukaemia, ulcerative colitis, the nephrotic syndrome, pemphigus, sarcoidosis, myasthenia gravis, haemolytic anaemia, agranulocytosis and other blood dyscrasias. Large doses are given in the immunosuppressive control of transplant surgery. The dose varies with the nature and severity of the condition being treated, and in every case the lowest dose required to evoke an adequate response should be used, after which the dose should be reduced in stages.
**Dose:** in rheumatoid arthritis, 7.5–10 mg daily initially; other conditions may require doses up to 100 mg daily. Dose by i.m. injection 25–100 mg once or twice a week. As a retention enema, 20 mg to relieve the inflammation of colitis and Crohn's disease; as eye drops and ear drops, 0.5% solution. The side-effects are those of the corticosteroids generally, and include salt and water retention, hypertension, muscle weakness and peptic ulcer.

**prednisone** A glucocorticosteroid that is converted to prednisolone in the body, and so has the actions and uses of that drug.

**prilocaine** A local anaesthetic with the actions, uses and side-effects of lignocaine. (Citanest).

**primaquine** An antimalarial drug used mainly to prevent a relapse of benign tertian malaria after treatment with chloroquine, as it kills the malarial parasites that may still be present in the liver.
**Dose:** 15 mg daily, for 2–3 weeks after chloroquine treatment. Side-effects are nausea and abdominal pain.

**primidone** An anticonvulsant used in the treatment of grand mal and psychomotor epilepsy.
**Dose:** 125 mg daily initially, slowly increased as required up to a maximum of 1.5 g daily. Side-effects include drowsiness, nausea, blurred vision and rash. (Mysoline). See page 136 and Table 15.

**probenecid** A uricosuric agent that increases the excretion of uric acid, and so is useful in the treatment of gout and hyperuricaemia.
**Dose:** 0.5–2 g daily. An adequate fluid intake and an alkaline urine are necessary for the best response. Probenecid also delays the excretion of penicillin and some cephalosporins, and is given in doses of 2 g daily to raise the plasma level of those antibiotics. Side-effects include occasional nausea, flushing and dizziness. (Benemid). See page 140 and Table 17.

**procainamide** A procaine derivative occasionally of value in the treatment of ventricular arrhythmias.
**Dose:** up to 50 mg/kg daily. It is also given by slow i.v. injection under ECG control in doses of 25–50 mg/minute up to a maximum of 1 g. Side-effects are gastrointestinal disturbances, fever and rash. (Pronestyl).

**procaine** A local anaesthetic now largely replaced by lignocaine.

**procaine penicillin** An old long-acting form of penicillin, given together with penicillin G to obtain a high initial blood level. It is now used mainly in early syphilis.
**Dose:** 900 mg daily by i.m. injection for 10 days. (Bicillin).

**procarbazine** A cytotoxic drug used mainly as part of a multi-drug treatment of Hodgkin's disease. It is also used to treat other lymphomas no longer responding to other therapy.
**Dose:** 50 mg initially, increasing to a maximum of 300 mg daily. Side-effects include nausea, anorexia and bone marrow depression. Alcohol may cause a disulfiram reaction. (Natulan). See page 122 and Table 8.

**prochlorperazine** A tranquillizer with the actions, uses and side-effects of chlorpromazine.
**Dose:** in schizophrenia, 25–100 mg daily; in severe anxiety, 15–20 mg daily. In

severe nausea and vomiting, 20 mg orally, or 12.5 mg by deep i.m. injection. It is also used as suppositories of 25 mg. (Stemetil). See page 168 and Table 30.

**procyclidine** An anticholinergic drug similar to benzhexol, used mainly in the treatment of parkinsonism. Reduces rigidity more than tremor.
**Dose:** 7.5–30 mg daily. In acute states it is given by i.m. injection in doses of 5–10 mg, or 5 mg doses i.v. (Arpicolin; Kemadrin). See page 160 and Table 26.

**progesterone** The hormone of the corpus luteum, responsible for the preparation of the uterus to receive a fertilized ovum. It is used in dysfunctional uterine bleeding and in the premenstrual syndrome.
**Dose:** 200–400 mg daily *per vagina* on a cyclic basis. (Cyclogest). Also a constituent of some oral contraceptives. See dydrogesterone and norethisterone.

**proguanil hydrochloride** A synthetic antimalarial of high potency and low toxicity, used in the prophylaxis and suppressive treatment of malaria, often in association with chloroquine.
**Dose:** 100–200 mg daily, and continued for 6 weeks after leaving the infected area. (Paludrine).

**promazine** A tranquillizer with the actions, uses and side-effects of chlorpromazine, but less potent. It is used mainly to control agitation in the elderly, and in other minor conditions of psychiatric disturbance.
**Dose:** 50–800 mg daily, adjusted to need and response; by injection 25–50 mg. (Sparine).

**promethazine** A long-acting antihistamine with sedative properties. It is used for the relief of a wide range of allergic conditions, in mild insomnia and for pre-operative sedation. It is also of value as an antiemetic in the prophylaxis and treatment of travel sickness, vertigo and drug-induced nausea.
**Dose:** 25–50 mg daily; 25–100 mg by deep i.m. injection. In anaphylaxis, sometimes given by slow i.v. injection in doses up to 100 mg to supplement previously injected adrenaline. The side-effects are those of the antihistamines generally. (Phenergan). See page 110 and Table 2.

**85**

**P**

**propafenone** An anti-arrhythmic agent of the lignocaine type, used in the prophylaxis and treatment of ventricular arrhythmias.
**Dose:** under ECG control 450 mg daily initially, after food, increased at 3-day intervals up to a maximum of 900 mg daily. Side-effects are dizziness, gastrointestinal disturbances and postural hypotension. (Arythmol).

**propantheline** An anticholinergic agent used as a spasmolytic in gastrointestinal disorders, in urinary frequency associated with bladder neck weakness, and in nocturnal enuresis.
**Dose:** 45–120 mg daily at least 1 hour before food. Side-effects include dryness of the mouth and blurred vision. (Pro-Banthine). See page 174 and Table 33.

**propofol** A non-irritant short-acting i.v. anaesthetic for smooth induction and maintenance of general anaesthesia for up to 1 hour.
**Dose:** 2–2.5 mg/kg initially, followed by supplementary doses of 0.1–0.2 mg/kg/min as required but some local pain may occur. Side-effects include mild hypotension, transient apnoea and bradycardia. Recovery is normally rapid and uneventful but delayed recovery, convulsions and anaphylaxis have been reported. Care is necessary in cardiovascular, respiratory or renal impairment. (Diprivan).

**propranolol** A beta-adrenoceptor blocking agent that reduces the cardiac response to circulating adrenaline and noradrenaline. It reduces the load on the heart during exercise and stress, and is used in the treatment of angina, coronary insufficiency, cardiac arrhythmias, hypertension, and after myocardial infarction. It also ameliorates the tremor and palpitation of transient anxiety and stress, and is useful in the prophylactic treatment of migraine.
**Dose:** 160–320 mg daily according to need. In arrhythmias and thyrotoxic crisis, propranolol is given by slow i.v. injection in doses of 1 mg, repeated up to a maximum of 10 mg. Side-effects are bradycardia, bronchospasm and gastrointestinal disturbances. Care is necessary in renal and hepatic deficiency; asthma is a contraindication. (Inderal). See page 146 and Table 21.

**propylthiouracil** A thyroid inhibitor occasionally used as an alternative to carbimazole in hyperthyroidism.
**Dose:** 300–450 mg daily.

**prostacyclin** See epoprostenol.

**prostaglandin** A generic term applied to a series of closely related hormone-like fatty acid derivatives, originally extracted from the prostate gland, but now prepared synthetically. Prostaglandins are widely distributed in animal tissues, and have a complex and varying range of biological activity. Thus they may have a smooth muscle stimulating or relaxant action, pressor, vasodilator, inflammatory or other properties. The anti-inflammatory action of aspirin and related drugs is due to an inhibition of prostaglandin synthesis. See alprostadil, carboprost, dinoprostone and gemeprost.

**protamine sulphate** A simple protein obtained from fish sperm. It neutralizes the anticoagulant effect of heparin, and it is used in controlling the haemorrhage that may occur during heparin therapy.
**Dose:** 1% solution i.v. according to need; 1 mg will neutralize 80–100 units of heparin.

**prothionamide** A second-line antitubercular drug that has been used in resistant tuberculosis. See page 170 and Table 31. It has also been used in the treatment of leprosy.

**protirelin** The thyrotrophin-releasing hormone (TRH) of the hypothalamus.
**Dose:** in the diagnosis of hyperthyroidism, as a single i.v. dose of 200 µg. It normally induces a rapid rise in the plasma levels of thyrotrophin, but in thyrotoxicosis that rise does not occur. Side-effects include nausea, flushing, a strange taste and urinary urgency.

**protriptyline** A tricyclic antidepressant with actions and uses similar to amitriptyline. It is used in depression associated with apathy, as it has some stimulant action.
**Dose:** 15–40 mg daily. Side-effects are cardiovascular disturbance, rash and photosensitivity. (Concordin). See page 128 and Table 11.

**proxymetacaine** A local anaesthetic used as 0.5% drops in ophthalmology. (Ophthaine).

**pseudoephedrine** A drug very closely related to ephedrine, but now used mainly as a respiratory decongestant. It has been used in nocturnal enuresis, but may cause hallucinations in some children.

**pumactant** A lung surfactant with the actions and uses of poractant. (Alec).

**pyrazinamide** An antituberculous drug that is active against the intracellular and dividing forms of *M. tuberculosis*, and is most effective in the early stages of the disease. It penetrates the meninges, and is of value in tuberculous meningitis.
**Dose:** in combination with other drugs, 2 g 3 times a week. Side-effects include fever, jaundice and hepatotoxicity. Liver function tests should be carried out before and during treatment. (Zinamide). See page 170 and Table 31.

**pyridostigmine** An anticholinesterase similar to neostigmine. It has a slower and more prolonged action that is useful in some cases of myasthenia gravis.
**Dose:** 300–720 mg daily. The side-effects are similar to those of neostigmine, but may be less severe. (Mestinon).

**pyridoxine** (vitamin $B_6$) This vitamin plays an essential part in protein metabolism. Apart from its use in deficiency states, which are uncommon, pyridoxine has been used in isoniazid-induced neuropathy.
**Dose:** 25–150 mg daily; in some sideroblastic anaemias, up to 400 mg daily.

**pyrimethamine** An antimalarial drug used with dapsone as Maloprim or with sulphadoxine as Fansidar in the prophylaxis of malaria. The use of these mixed products is not without risk, as they may have severe and sometimes fatal side-effects.

**Q**

**quetiapine** A new 'atypical' antischizophrenic drug of the clozapine type with a high affinity for serotonin (5–$HT_2$) and dopamine D1 and D2 receptors.
**Dose:** in schizophrenia, initital doses of 25 mg twice a day, slowly increased up to 150–750 mg daily. Initial doses may cause hypotension. Care is necessary in cardiovascular disease. Side-effects include drowsiness and dizziness. The routine blood monitoring necessary with clozapine is not required. (Seroquel). See page 168 and Table 30.

**quinagolide** A dopamine agonist used in the treatment of hyperprolactinaemia.

**Dose:** 25 µg at bedtime initially, increased at 3-day intervals to 75–100 µg daily. Side-effects include hypotension, and the blood pressure should be monitored after a change of dose. (Norprolac). See bromocriptine and cabergoline.

**†quinalbarbitone sodium** A short-acting barbiturate. Used in mild insomnia and anxiety states.
**Dose:** 50–100 mg. (Seconal).

**quinapril** An ACE inhibitor with the actions, use and side-effects of that group of drugs.
**Dose:** in hypertension, 5–10 mg daily initially, slowly increased to 20–40 mg as a single daily dose. (Accupro). See ACE inhibitors, page 148, and Table 21.

**quinidine** An alkaloid of cinchona, similar to quinine, that has been used in the preventive treatment of ventricular arrhythmias, but beta-blocking agents are now preferred.
**Dose:** (after a test dose of 200 mg) 200–400 mg 3–4 times a day. Side-effects are tinnitus, vertigo and confusion. Treatment should be stopped if response does not occur within 10 days.

**quinine** The principal alkaloid of cinchona bark. It was once used extensively in the treatment of malignant tertian malaria, and recently it has regained some of its value with the emergence of chloroquine-resistant malaria.
**Dose:** 1.8 g daily for 7 days; in serious infections it is given by i.v. infusion in doses of 10 mg/kg for up to 3 doses, followed by oral therapy. Side-effects include tinnitus, nausea, rash and visual disturbances. See specialist literature.

**R**

**raltitrexed**∇ A selective enzyme inhibitor used in the palliative treatment of advanced colorectal cancer. It has advantages over fluorouracil, as treatment is less complicated and the incidence of leucopenia, mucositosis and other side-effects is less severe.
**Dose:** 3 mg/m² by slow i.v. injection, repeated at intervals of 3 weeks if tolerated. Blood counts and liver function tests are necessary. (Tomudex). See page 122 and Table 8.

**ramipril** An ACE inhibitor with the general
properties of such drugs.
**Dose:** in mild hypertension, 1.25 mg daily,
increased at intervals of 1–2 weeks up to a
maximum of 10 mg, given with food and
adequate fluid. Prophylactic dose after
myocardial infarction 5–10 mg daily.
(Tritace). See page 148 and Table 21.

**ranitidine** A powerful and selective
histamine H₂ antagonist of the cimetidine
type, but with a longer action. It reduces
the volume, acidity and pepsin content of
gastric secretion, and is of value in peptic
ulcer, reflux oesophagitis and similar
conditions.
**Dose:** 300 mg daily for at least 4 weeks,
maintenance doses, 150 mg daily. In
severe conditions, 50 mg by i.m. or slow
i.v. injection repeated at intervals of
6–8 hours. In suspected gastric ulcer,
malignancy should be excluded before
treatment is commenced. (Zantac). See
cimetidine, page 162 and Table 27.

**ranitidine bismuth citrate**▽ It has the
general action of ranitidine, but it also has
a protective effect on the ulcerated area,
and inhibits digestive action of pepsin on
the gastric mucosa. It is given with
amoxycillin and clarithromycin to promote the elimination of *Helicobacter
pylori*.
**Dose:** 800 mg daily. (Pylorid). See
page 162.

**razoxane** A cytotoxic agent occasionally
used in the treatment of leukaemias.
**Dose:** 150–500 mg/m² daily for 3–5 days,
under laboratory control. Side-effects are
nausea and myleosuppression. (Razoxin).

**reboxetine**▽ An inhibitor of noradrenaline
reuptake used in depression.
**Dose:** 4 mg twice a day, half-doses for the
elderly. Side-effects are those of other
antidepressants. Care in renal/hepatic
impairment. (Edronax). See page 128 and
Table 11.

**remifentanil**▽ An analgesic of the fentanyl
type used as an adjunct in doses of
0.5–1 µg/kg/min for the induction of
anaesthesia. Its use reduces the amount of
general anaesthetic required. (Ultiva).

**reproterol** A bronchodilator with the
actions, uses and side-effects of
salbutamol.

**Dose:** by aerosol inhalation; 0.5–1 mg
(1–2 puffs), repeated up to 3 times a day.
Side-effects include tremor and mild
tachycardia. (Bronchodil). See page 118
and Table 6.

**resorcinol** A keratolytic agent used mainly
as an ointment in acne, and as a hair
lotion for removing dandruff. Myxoedema
has been reported following the prolonged
use of resorcin preparations.

**reteplase** A thrombolytic agent used in
acute myocardial infarction.
**Dose:** 10 units by slow i.v. injection
within 2 hours of the infarction. A second
dose may be given 36 hours later, together
with heparin, to reduce the risk of
rethrombosis. Side-effects are arrhythmias
and gastrointestinal bleeding. (Rapilysin).
See page 156 and Table 24.

**retinol** See vitamin A.

**riboflavine (vitamin B₂)** Part of the
vitamin B complex, it is concerned with
the oxidation of carbohydrates and amino
acids. A deficiency causes several characteristic effects, including angular stomatitis
and 'burning feet'.
**Dose:** 1–10 mg in deficiency states
associated with restricted diets or poor
absorption.

**rifabutin**▽ A derivative of rifampicin used
in the multi-drug treatment of pulmonary
tuberculosis.
**Dose:** 150–450 mg daily. It is also used
prophylactically against opportunistic
infection with *Mycobacterium avium*.
(Mycobutin). See page 170 and Table 31.

**rifampicin** An antibiotic now considered to
be the first-choice drug in the treatment of
tuberculosis, and given together with
isoniazid and pyrazinamide.
**Dose:** 600 mg before breakfast. It is also
used with dapsone and clofazimine in the
initial treatment of severe leprosy.
Combined therapy is also used in brucel-
losis, legionnaire's disease and severe
staphylococcal infections. Side-effects
include gastrointestinal disturbances, rash,
an influenza-like syndrome and hepatic
reactions. Jaundice is a contraindication.
Patients should be warned that rifampicin
gives a red colour to the urine, sputum
and tears, and to soft contact lenses.
It may decrease the response to oral

anticoagulants such as warfarin, and the failure of oral contraceptives has also been reported in patients receiving rifampicin. (Rifadin; Rimactane). See page 170 and Table 31.

**riluzole**▽ A new drug used only for motor neurone disease (a myotrophic lateral sclerosis–ALS). ALS is a degenerative disease and may be due to the local accumulation of the neurotransmitter glutamate, with consequent neurone damage. Riluzole slows down the progressive nature of the disease, and improves the response to mechanical ventilation.
**Dose:** 100 mg daily. See specialist literature. (Rilutek).

**rimiterol** A bronchodilator similar in actions and uses to salbutamol, but with a shorter duration of effect. It is largely free from any cardiac stimulant activity. Rimiterol is used mainly for the relief of bronchospasm in bronchitis, bronchial asthma and similar conditions.
**Dose:** by aerosol inhalation, 200–600 μg (1–3 puffs) up to a maximum of 8 puffs daily. (Pulmadil). See page 118 and Table 6.

**Ringer's solution** An electrolyte replacement solution containing sodium chloride, potassium chloride and calcium chloride.

**risperidone** An antischizophrenic agent of the clozapine type, with a selective affinity for serotonin and dopamine receptors. It may relieve the aggressive symptoms of schizophrenia as well as the negative aspects such as apathy.
**Dose:** 6–10 mg. daily. Side-effects are headache, dizziness and agitation. Agranulocytosis is uncommon, and the close blood monitoring required with clozapine is not necessary. (Risperdal). See page 168 and Table 30.

**ritonavir**▽ An HIV-protease inhibitor used in HIV infections in association with a nucleoside analogue.
**Dose:** 1.2 g daily with food. (Norvir). See page 144 and Table 19.

**ritodrine** A beta₂-adrenoceptor stimulant with a relaxant action on uterine muscle, used to inhibit premature labour.
**Dose:** 50 μg/min initially by i.v. infusion (avoiding fluid overload), slowly increased

up to 350 μg/min, or 10 mg by i.m. injection and continued until the contractions have ceased; then orally up to 120 mg daily to prevent relapse. Side-effects include tremor, nausea and hypotension. (Yutopar).

**rocuronium** A muscle relaxant similar in actions and uses to vercuronium.
**Dose:** 600 μg/kg initially, followed by 300–600 μg/kg/hrly as required. (Esmeron).

**ropinirole**▽ A potent and selective dopamine D₂-receptor agonist used in the treatment of Parkinson's disease, a condition basically due to a deficiency of dopamine in the brain. It is well absorbed orally, and reaches the central nervous system where it functions as dopamine replacement therapy.
**Dose:** first week 750 μg daily with food; second week 1.5 mg daily, third week 2.25 mg daily, then 3 mg daily. Ropinirole may be given as monotherapy or together with levodopa. Side-effects are somnolence, hypotension, leg oedema and gastrointestinal disturbances. Caution in severe cardiac, renal and hepatic conditions. (Requip). See page 160 and Table 26.

**ropivacaine** A local anaesthetic with the actions and uses of lignocaine. (Naropin).

**Rose bengal** A dye used as eye drops (1%) to stain and detect damaged conjunctival cells, and in the diagnosis of dry eye.

**rubella vaccine** A suspension of a live, attenuated strain of rubella virus. It is used for active immunization in girls of 10–14 years, and in seronegative women of childbearing age.
**Dose:** 0.5 ml by s.c. injection. It is contraindicated in pregnancy, and pregnancy within 3 months of vaccination should be avoided. A combined measles/mumps/rubella (MMR) vaccine is now recommended for all children.

**89**

**S**

# S

**saccharin** A synthetic sweetening agent widely used as a non-calorific substitute for sugar. Has been used by rapid i.v. injection (2.5 g in 4 ml) for arm-tongue circulation time.

**salbutamol** A selective beta$_2$-adrenoceptor stimulant. It is widely used to relieve bronchospasm in airway obstruction, including bronchial asthma and status asthmaticus, with the advantage of being largely free from cardiac side-effects.
**Dose:** up to 16 mg orally daily; by aerosol inhalation (in which patients should be carefully instructed) 100–200 µg (1–2 puffs) up to 4 times a day; by s.c. or i.m. injection 500 µg as required; 250 µg by i.v. injection. Salbutamol also relaxes uterine muscle, and is given in premature labour in doses of 10 µg/min initially by i.v. infusion, increased to 45 µg/min until contractions have ceased, when oral therapy may be given. Side-effects include tremor, headache, peripheral vasodilation and tachycardia. Care is necessary in ischaemic heart disease, hypertension and hyperthyroidism. (Ventolin). See page 118 and Table 6.

**salcatonin** A synthetic form of calcitonin, preferred for extended use, as it is less likely to provoke allergic reactions.
**Dose:** in hypercalcaemia, 5–10 units/kg daily by s.c. or i.m. injection according to need; in Paget's disease 60 units 3 times a week up to 100 units daily. It is also used in post-menopausal osteoporosis and for the bone pain of malignancy. (Calcynar; Miacalcic).

**salicylic acid** Has useful keratolytic and fungicidal properties. Used as ointment (2%) for skin conditions, and as ointments and plasters (up to 40%) for corns and warts.

**salmeterol** A beta$_2$-adrenoceptor stimulant of the salbutamol type, but with a longer action. It is used for the extended prophylaxis of asthma, bronchitis and other forms of obstructive airway disease, and together with corticosteroid therapy if required. It is not indicated in acute conditions.
**Dose:** 50 µg twice daily, either from a metered dose aerosol or by a 'Diskhaler'. Salmeterol is well tolerated, but headache, tremor and tachycardia may occur with doses above 200 µg daily. (Serevent). See page 118 and Table 6.

**saquinavir**∇ An antiviral agent that inhibits the enzyme HIV-protease, and prevents the development of immature virus particles into the infective virus. Used in HIV infection together with a nucleoside analogue that has a different action.
**Dose:** 1.8 g daily. (Invirase). See page 144 and Table 19.

**scopolamine** See hyoscine.

**selective serotonin re-uptake inhibitors (SSRIs)** A small group of drugs that inhibit the re-uptake of serotonin in the central nervous system, and are used in the treatment of depression. They differ from the tricyclic antidepressants in being less likely to cause sedation or cardiac disturbances, or have anticholinergic side-effects. Care remains necessary with machine-related activities, and before and after monoamine oxidase inhibitors (MAOI) therapy. See page 128 and Table 11.

**selegiline** A selective enzyme inhibitor that prevents the inactivation of dopamine in the brain. It is used to supplement the action of levodopa in the treatment of parkinsonism, and combined use may give a smoother response, and permit a reduction in the dose of levodopa.
**Dose:** 5–10 mg daily. It may cause nausea and hypotension, and may possibly increase the side-effects of levodopa. (Eldepryl). See page 160 and Table 26.

**selenium sulphide** Used as a shampoo in the treatment of dandruff. Prolonged use may cause alopecia. (Selsun).

**senna** The leaves and pods of *Cassia* sp., used as a purgative. Standardized preparations such as Senokot are now preferred.

**sermorelin**∇ A synthetic analogue of somatorelin, the growth hormone releasing factor (GHRH). It is used in the diagnosis of growth hormone deficiency as a single i.v. dose of 1 µg/kg. (Geref 50).

**sertindole**∇ An antipsychotic agent with a selective action on the limbic system, and used in acute and chronic schizophrenia.
**Dose:** 4 mg once daily initially, increased after 2–4 days up to 20 mg daily according to need. Blood pressure should be monitored initially as hypotension may occur. Side-effects include extension of the QT interval. Contraindicated in patients receiving itraconazole, ketoconazole, quinidine, terfanidine, or any drug known to affect the QT interval. (Serdolect). See page 168 and Table 30.

**serotonin** A substance present in many body cells, which also acts as a neurotransmitter in the central nervous system. A reduction in the brain serotonin levels may be associated with depression and the cranial vasodilation associated with migraine. (See page 154). Some allergic reactions may also be linked with the action of serotonin on sensitized cells (see cyproheptadine).

**sertraline** A selective serotonin-re-uptake inhibitor (SSRI) antidepressant used both for the treatment of depression and the prevention of relapse.
**Dose:** 50 mg daily initially with food, increased at weekly intervals up to a maximum of 200 mg daily. Not to be given with monoamine oxidase inhibitors (MAOIs). Side-effects are tremor and a dry mouth. (Lustral). See page 128 and Table 11.

**silicones** Synthetic water-repellent substances present in barrier creams and other skin protective products. Dimethicone is a silicone used as an anti-foaming agent in some antacid preparations.

**silver nitrate** Used mainly as silver nitrate sticks (caustic points) for cauterizing warts. It has also been used as a 0.5% lotion for suppurating lesions. It was once used prophylactically as eye drops (0.1%) in the newborn, and is still used for that purpose in the USA.

**silver sulphadiazine** Sulphadiazine combined with silver. It is used topically as a 1% cream for its wide-range antibacterial properties in burns and infected skin conditions, especially when an extended action is required. It is active against *Pseudomonas aeruginosa* and other Gram-negative organisms. (Flamazine).

**simvastatin** A selective inhibitor of a specific enzyme (HMGC0A reductase) concerned with the synthesis of cholesterol in the liver. It is used in the treatment of primary hypercholesterolaemia in patients not responding to other drugs.
**Dose:** 10–40 mg at night. Liver function tests should be carried out regularly. Side-effects include gastrointestinal disturbances. (Zocor). See page 146 and Table 20.

**snake-bite antivenom** A bite from an adder, the only poisonous snake indigenous to the UK, can cause local pain and swelling as well as systemic effects such as colic and vomiting, but death from adder bite is very rare. If the reaction to an adder bite is severe, European viper anti-venom, if available, should be given by i.v. infusion within 4 hours of the bite.

**soda-lime** A mixture of calcium and sodium hydroxides, used in closed-circuit anaesthetic apparatus to remove carbon dioxide.

**sodium acetrizoate** An iodine compound used as a contrast agent in i.v. pyelography.

**sodium aurothiomalate** A gold compound used in the treatment of active rheumatoid arthritis. It is no value in other forms of the disease, or where bone change has already occurred.
**Dose:** 10 mg by deep i.m. injection weekly initially, slowly increased to 50 mg weekly, and continued until a remission occurs, or until a total dose of 1 g has been given. Blood and urine tests are essential after each injection. After remission, 20–50 mg may be given every 2–4 weeks for many months. Side-effects are common, and include blood disorders, skin reactions, mouth ulcers and oedema, and may require withdrawal of the drug. It is contraindicated in renal and hepatic disease, blood dyscrasias and hypertension. (Myocrisin). See auranofin, page 165 and Table 29.

**sodium bicarbonate** A soluble antacid, often used in association with less soluble antacids such as magnesium carbonate or trisilicate.
**Dose:** 1–4 g. In severe metabolic acidosis it is given by slow i.v. injection as an 8.4% solution. For alkalization of the urine, up to 3 g orally 2-hourly with further 10 g doses daily as required.

**sodium calcium edetate** A chelating or binding agent used in poisoning by lead and other heavy metals.
**Dose:** 80 mg/kg daily by i.v. infusion in glucose/saline solution. Nausea and cramp are side-effects, and care is necessary in renal impairment. (Ledclair).

**sodium cellulose phosphate** An ion-exchange compound that binds with calcium in the intestines, and so reduces calcium absorption. Used in the oral treatment of hypercalcaemia and renal stones, and as an adjunct to low-calcium diets.
**Dose:** 15 g daily. Diarrhoea is an occasional side-effect. (Calcisorb).

91

S

**sodium chloride** An important constituent of blood and tissues. It is widely used by i.v. infusion as normal saline solution (0.9%), or as glucose-saline in the treatment of dehydration, shock and other conditions of sodium depletion. It is also useful when given orally as Sodium Chloride with Glucose Oral Powder (BNF) (after solution in water), for children with diarrhoea to offset any loss of salt. Its use as an emetic in the treatment of poisoning is no longer recommended. It is used externally as saline solution when a simple cleansing lotion is required.

**sodium citrate** An alkaline diuretic similar to potassium citrate and given for similar purposes.
**Dose:** 1–4 g. For citrating milk, 100 mg to each feed may be used. A 3% solution is used by bladder irrigation for the dissolution of blood clots.

**sodium clodronate** See clodronate, editronate and pamidronate.

**sodium cromoglycate** An antiallergic agent with a specific action and used for the prophylactic treatment of asthma by inhalation. It stabilizes mast cells and inhibits the release of histamine and other spasmogens that cause bronchospasm.
**Dose:** by powder inhalation from a 'Spinhaler' 20 mg up to 8 times a day; by aerosol inhalation, 10 mg (2 puffs) up to 8 times a day. Dose in the treatment for food allergy associated with local inflammation, 800 mg daily orally. It is also of value as eye drops (2%) and eye ointment (4%) in allergic conjunctivitis, and as nasal drops or spray (2%) in the prophylaxis of allergic rhinitis. (Intal; Rynacrom). See page 110 and Table 2.

**sodium fluoride** The fluoride present in dentifrices used to reduce dental caries. It may also be given orally when more intensive treatment is required.
**Dose:** 250–500 μg daily.

**sodium fusidate** An antibiotic used mainly in penicillin-resistant staphylococcal infections, although a secondary anti-staphylococcal antibiotic is often given to increase the response and inhibit drug-resistance. It is useful in osteomyelitis and similar conditions as it penetrates into bone tissues.
**Dose:** 2 g daily. In severe infections, 1.5 g

daily by i.v. infusion. Side-effects include nausea, rash and jaundice. Liver function tests should be carried out during treatment. (Fucidin).

**sodium hypochlorite** A weak solution of sodium hypochlorite containing 0.25% of available chlorine is used as eusol, for the cleansing of wounds and ulcers. The solution is unstable and should be freshly prepared. Its value has recently been questioned. Stronger, stabilized solutions are used for the general disinfection of surfaces contaminated with blood and other body fluids. Their use reduces the risk of transmission of hepatitis and other viral infections.

**sodium ironedetate (sodium feredetate)** A soluble iron complex available as a solution containing 27.5 mg of iron per 5 ml. It is used in the oral treatment of iron-deficiency anaemias, and is of value when other iron preparations are not tolerated.
**Dose:** 15–30 ml daily. (Sytron). See page 112 and Table 3.

**sodium lactate** Has been used as M/6 solution, or as Hartmann's solution, by i.v. infusion for metabolic acidosis, but sodium bicarbonate is now preferred.

**sodium nitrite** A cyanide antidote.
**Dose:** as a 3% solution by i.v. injection of 10 ml, followed by the slow injection of 25 ml of sodium thiosulphate solution (50%). Early treatment is essential. See kelocyanor.

**sodium nitroprusside** A short-acting arteriovenous vasodilator used in hypertensive crisis and for controlled hypotension during anaesthesia.
**Dose:** by i.v. infusion, 0.3–1 μg/kg/min, the lower doses being used to obtain hypotension during surgery. It is also used in acute heart failure in doses of 10–15 μg/min, increased as required to 200 μg/min.

**sodium perborate** White powder soluble in water, with antiseptic and deodorant properties similar to hydrogen peroxide. A 2% solution is used as a mouthwash.

**sodium phosphate** A solution of sodium phosphate with sodium acid phosphate is sometimes used by enema as a laxative. These phosphates are also occasionally added to i.v. electrolyte solutions when a phosphate deficiency is present or suspected.

**sodium picosulphate** A synthetic laxative similar to bisacodyl, but with a slower action.
**Dose:** 5–15 mg at night.

**sodium stibogluconate** An organic antimony drug used in the treatment of visceral leishmaniasis or kala-azar.
**Dose:** 20 mg/kg daily by i.m. or i.v. injection for 30 days. Side-effects include anorexia, vomiting, cough and sub-sternal pain. (Pentostam).

**sodium tetradecyl sulphate** A venous-occluding agent used in the injection sclerotherapy of varicose veins.
**Dose:** 0.5–1 ml at any one site, followed by compression bandaging for some weeks. The local irritant action of the drug brings about an occlusive venous fibrosis at the injection site. Extra-vascular injection may cause necrosis. Care is necessary in allergic subjects.

**sodium thisulphate** A 50% solution is given by i.v. injection in cyanide poison-ing. See sodium nitrite and kelocyanor.

**sodium valproate** An anticonvulsant effective in most forms of epilepsy.
**Dose:** 600 mg daily in adults initially, increased if required up to a maximum of 2.5 g daily. It may also be given by slow i.v. injection in doses of 400–800 mg, followed by similar doses given by i.v. infusion. Liver function tests before and during treatment are essential. Severe side-effects such as vomiting, drowsiness or jaundice require withdrawal of the drug, as does spontaneous bleeding or bruising. (Epilim). See page 136 and Table 15.

**somatropin** A form of human growth hormone obtained by biosynthesis. It is used to stimulate growth in hormone-deficient young patients whilst the epiphyses are still open.
**Dose:** 0.07 units/kg daily by i.m. or s.c. injection. Subcutaneous injection sites should be varied. (Genotropin; Humat-rope; Norditropin; Salzen).

**sorbitol** A saccharide that after absorption is converted in the liver almost entirely to laevulose. It has been used as a sugar-substitute in diabetes, and it is sometimes

given by i.v. injection as a 50% solution to promote diuresis and to reduce cerebral oedema.

**sotalol** A beta-adrenergic blocking agent used in the treatment of hypertension, angina, cardiac arrhythmias and thyrotoxicosis.
**Dose:** 120 mg initially, increased as required; maintenance, 160–600 mg daily. For prophylaxis after infarction, 320 mg daily. In acute cardiac arrhythmias, 20–60 mg by slow i.v. injection under ECG control. Care is necessary in heart block, asthma, hepatic and renal impairment. (Beta-Cardone; Sotacor). See pages 114 & 148, and Tables 4 & 21.

**spectinomycin** An antibiotic used in the treatment of penicillin-resistant gonorrhoea.
**Dose:** 2–4 g by deep i.m. injection. Side-effects include nausea, dizziness and urticaria. (Trobicin).

**spironolactone** An aldosterone antagonist which potentiates the action of thiazide and loop diuretics in some resistant conditions. It is of value in the oedema of liver cirrhosis, as well as in the nephrotic syndrome and congestive heart failure.
**Dose:** 100 mg daily up to a maximum dose of 400 mg daily. Side-effects include drowsiness, gastrointestinal disturbances, gynaecomastia and an increased sensitivity to warfarin. The combined use of potas-sium-sparing diuretics or potassium supplements is contraindicated. (Aldactone; Spiroctan).

**SSRIs** See selective serotonin re-uptake inhibitors.

**stanozolol** An anabolic steroid with actions and uses similar to those of nandrolone.
**Dose:** 5 mg daily. It also has fibrinolytic properties, and is used in lipodermatoscle-rosis (a complication of deep-vein sclerosis), and in some forms of vasculitis. It may also be of some value in hereditary angioneurotic oedema and in the relief of itching due to biliary obstruction. Also used in some aplastic anaemias, 2.5–10 mg daily. Some androgenic side-effects may occur, but are usually mild and reversible on stopping treatment. (Stromba).

**starch** Carbohydrate granules obtained from maize, rice, wheat or potato. Widely used as absorbent dusting powder.

**stavudine**∇ An antiviral agent that inhibits the enzyme reverse transcriptase, and so indirectly blocks the synthesis of viral DNA. It is used in HIV infections resistant to or not responding to zidovudine.
**Dose:** 60 mg daily, 1 hour before food. Side-effects include malaise, peripheral neuropathy and pancreatitis. (Zerit). See page 144 and Table 19.

**sterculia** A natural gum that swells in water to a gelatinous mass. It is used as a bulk laxative as when taken with plenty of water it increases faecal volume and promotes peristalsis. It is also used in diverticulitis and irritable bowel syndrome, and as an appetite suppressant.
**Dose:** 5–10 g daily but not at night. (Normacol).

**stilboestrol** A synthetic oestrogen with the actions and uses of oestradiol.
**Dose:** 0.1–0.5 mg daily for menopausal symptoms, but it is now prescribed less frequently. Dose in breast cancer, 10–20 mg daily; in prostatic carcinoma, 3 mg daily or more, although fosfestrol is often preferred. Side-effects include nausea, fluid retention, thrombosis, impotence and gynaecomastia.

**streptokinase** An enzyme preparation obtained from cultures of haemolytic streptococci. It has fibrinolytic properties, and is of value in deep vein thrombosis, pulmonary embolism, myocardial infarction and other conditions requiring fibrinolytic therapy.
**Dose:** by i.v. infusion, 250 000 units or more initially, followed by maintenance doses of 100 000 units hourly for up to 72 hours. For myocardial infarction 1 500 000 units over 1 hour. Side-effects are fever, rash, haemorrhage and allergic reactions. (Kabikinase; Streptase).

**streptokinase-streptodornase** A mixture of enzymes obtained from cultures of haemolytic streptococci. It brings about the dissolution of blood clots and the liquefaction of purulent exudates, and it is used as a solution to clean foul wounds, pressure sores and ulcers. (Varidase).

**streptomycin** The first of the aminoglycoside antibiotics, but now used mainly as part of the multi-drug treatment of tuberculosis.

**Dose:** 1 g daily by deep i.m. injection. Its use requires care, as it is both ototoxic and nephrotoxic, especially in full doses and in renal impairment. Measurement of the plasma concentration of streptomycin is advisable during treatment. Cutaneous sensitization has followed contact of the drug with the skin.

**sucralfate** An aluminium sucrose sulphate used in the treatment of peptic ulcer. It is not an antacid, but forms a barrier over the ulcer that is resistant to peptic attack and so promotes healing.
**Dose:** 4 g daily for at least 4 weeks. Antacids should not be taken immediately before or after sucralfate. (Antepsin). See page 162.

**sulconazole** A synthetic antifungal agent similar in actions and uses to miconazole. Applied as a 1% cream twice daily. (Exelderm).

**sulfadoxine** A long-acting sulphonamide, with the general antibacterial action of the group. It has been used in the treatment of leprosy.
**Dose:** 1–1.5 g weekly. In association with pyrimethamine, it is used in the treatment of malaria, but the use of such mixed products requires great care, as severe, sometimes fatal side-effects have occurred. It is no longer used for malaria prophylaxis. (Fansidar).

**sulfametopyrazine** A very long-acting sulphonamide used mainly in chronic bronchitis and urinary tract infections.
**Dose:** 2 g once a week. Side-effects and toxic reactions, although mainly those of the sulphonamides generally, may be linked with the slow excretion of the drug. (Kelfizine).

**sulindac** A non-steroidal anti-inflammatory analgesic agent (NSAID) with actions, uses and side-effects similar to naproxen. It is of value in the pain and inflammation of rheumatoid disease and acute gout.
**Dose:** 200–400 mg daily with food. It may cause gastrointestinal disturbance and occasional bleeding. (Clinoril). See page 165 and Table 29.

**sulphadiazine** One of the more active and less toxic sulphonamides. It is used mainly in the treatment of severe conditions such as meningococcal meningitis.

94
S

**Dose:** 6–9 g daily by deep i.m. injection or i.v. infusion for 2 days, followed by 2 g or more orally daily. Dose in the prevention of rheumatic fever 1 g daily. Side-effects are nausea, rash and blood dyscrasias.

**sulphadimidine** One of the least toxic of the sulphonamides, now used mainly in urinary infections.
**Dose:** 2 g initially, with maintenance of 1.5–4 g daily orally. Side-effects include nausea, drug fever, rash and leucopenia.

**sulphamethoxazole** A sulphonamide present with trimethaprim in co-trimoxazole.

**sulphasalazine** A sulphonamide derivative that is taken up selectively by the connective tissues of the intestines. It is used in the treatment and maintenance of remission in ulcerative colitis and Crohn's disease.
**Dose:** 4–8 g daily initially; maintenance, 1.5–2 g daily. It is also given as a 3 g enema and as 500 mg suppositories. Occasionally given in rheumatoid arthritis in doses of 0.5–3 g daily. Side-effects include nausea, rash, drug fever and blood dyscrasia. If a blood dyscrasia is suspected, a blood count should be done and the drug withdrawn. (Salazopyrin). See mesalazine, olsalazine, page 172 and Table 32.

**sulphathiazole** One of the early sulphonamides, and survives in a few mixed products.

**sulphinpyrazone.** A uricosuric agent with the selective action of increasing the excretion of uric acid, hence used in the treatment of chronic gout and hyperuricaemia.
**Dose:** 100–200 mg initially with food, increased according to the plasma uric acid levels up to 600–800 mg daily, with lower maintenance doses according to need and response. Side-effects are nausea, abdominal pain and rash. Care is necessary in peptic ulcer and renal impairment, and blood counts are necessary during treatment. Salicylates antagonize the action of the drug. (Anturan). See page 140 and Table 17.

**sulphonamides** A group of drugs that have an antibacterial action by preventing the uptake and use of folic acid. They are thus bacteriostatic and not bactericidal in action. The use of the sulphonamides has

declined, and they are now used mainly in urinary tract infections due to sulphonamide-sensitive bacteria. The side-effects of the sulphonamides include nausea, dyspepsia, diarrhoea and allergic reactions. Bone marrow depression may occur if treatment is prolonged. The uncommon Stevens–Johnson syndrome is a very serious reaction. See sulphadiazine and co-trimoxazole.

**sulphonylureas** A group of orally active drugs represented by chlorpropamide that promote the release of insulin from the beta-cells of the pancreas. They are used in mild diabetes not controlled by diet, and in the late-onset diabetes of middle age, but they are not suitable for the treatment of juvenile diabetes. The presence of some still-functioning beta-cells is essential for sulphonylurea activity. Side-effects include weight gain, rash, fever and jaundice. During illness and pregnancy, insulin treatment should replace sulphonylurea therapy. See page 131 and Table 13.

**sulpiride** An antipsychotic drug with a central action on dopamine receptors. It is used in the treatment of acute and chronic schizophrenia, as in low doses it increases awareness in apathetic and withdrawn patients, and in larger doses controls the active forms of the illness.
**Dose:** 400–800 mg daily: in severe conditions up to 2.4 g daily. The side-effects are similar to those of chlorpromazine. (Dolmatil; Sulparex; Sulpitil). See page 168 and Table 30.

**sumatriptan** A serotonin agonist used in the treatment of acute migraine. (It is not suitable for prophylaxis.)
**Dose:** 50–100 mg orally as soon as possible after onset of an attack, but a second dose should not be given for the same attack, but may be repeated once if migraine symptoms recur. In severe migraine and cluster headache 6 mg by **s.c.** injection, but not more than 12 mg in 24 hours. (Pre-filled syringes and an auto-injector are available.) It should not be given until 24 hours after other antimigraine treatment, or any other drug that influences the re-uptake of serotonin. Side-effects include tingling and tightness in any part of the body, and an angina-like chest pain that may be severe. (Imigran). See page 154 and Table 23.

**95**

**S**

**suramin** A drug used in the early treatment of trypanosomiasis, but it is of no value in the later stages of the disease as it does not enter the cerebrospinal fluid.
**Dose:** 1 g i.v. weekly for 5 weeks, after a tolerance test dose of 200 mg. Side-effects are gastrointestinal disturbances, dermatitis, hyperaesthesia and kidney damage.

**suxamethonium** A short-acting, depolarizing muscle relaxant, with an action lasting 3–5 minutes. A preliminary injection of thiopentone should first be given, as the initial effect of suxamethonium is a painful muscle contraction before the relaxant action supervenes.
**Dose:** 20–100 mg i.v. during surgery, with further doses according to need. Suxamethonium may also be given as a 0.1% solution by i.v. infusion. Exceptionally, the muscle relaxant action of the drug may be prolonged with marked apnoea. Unlike non-depolarizing muscle relaxants, the action of suxamethonium cannot be reversed. Severe hepatic disease is a contraindication. (Anectine; Scoline).

**sympathomimetics** Drugs that have an action similar to adrenaline, and act on both alpha- and beta-adrenoceptors. More selective compounds, such as salbutamol, act on the beta$_2$-adrenoceptors in the lungs and have an increased bronchodilator action. They also relax uterine muscle, and are used to prevent premature labour. Others such as dobutamine and dopamine have a more selective action on the beta$_1$-receptors in the heart, and are referred to as inotropic sympathomimetics.

# T

**tacalcitol** A vitamin D$_3$ derivative used in the treatment of psoriasis as an ointment containing 4 µg/g of the drug. It is applied sparingly once daily at night, and continued as required. Not more than 2 treatments over 8 weeks per year. (Curatoderm).

**tacrolimus**∇ A macrolide derivative with marked immunosuppressant properties. It is used in liver and kidney transplantation, and appears to act by suppressing T-cell activation. It may also inhibit the formation of cytotoxic lymphocytes that are concerned

with graft rejection. See Drug Data Sheet for details of dose and extensive side-effects including neurotoxicity and hypertrophic cardiomyopathy. (Prograf).

**talc** A form of magnesium silicate, widely used as a skin dusting powder. It has also been used as a lubricant for surgeons' gloves, but it may cause a talc granuloma if any reaches the tissues during operation, and glove powders prepared from starch are preferred.

**tamoxifen** An oestrogen-receptor antagonist used mainly in breast cancer, particularly when metastases are present.
**Dose:** 20 mg daily. It is usually well tolerated, but side-effects include hot flushes, dizziness, rash, hypercalcaemia and an increase in tumour pain. Unlike other oestrogen-antagonists, tamoxifen has no androgenic properties. It has also been used in some forms of anovulatory sterility. (Nolvadex). See page 122 and Table 8.

**tamsulosin**∇ A relatively selective alpha adrenoceptor antagonist. It lowers the tone of bladder and prostatic smooth muscle, and is used in benign prostatic hyperplasia.
**Dose:** 400 mg daily after breakfast with a glass of water. The first dose should be taken in bed to avoid postural hypotension. Other side-effects include palpitations and dizziness and hypotension. (Flomax). See page 164 and Table 28.

**tazabactam** An inhibitor of beta-lactamases. It is used in association with some antibiotics to extend the activity against resistant beta-lactamase-producing bacteria. Tazacin is a mixed product containing piperacillin and tazabactam.

**tazarotene** A retinoid used as an aqueous gel (0.05–0.1%) in psoriasis. Applied once daily to the affected skin area only. (Zorac).

**teicoplanin** An antibiotic that acts by interfering with bacterial cell wall development. It has a wide range of activity, but is used mainly in the treatment of severe staphylococcal infections that fail to respond to other antibiotics.
**Dose:** 400 mg initially by i.v. injection, followed by 200 mg as a single daily dose, which may be given by i.m. injection. Double doses in severe infections. Side-effects include gastrointestinal disturbances, dizziness, fever and rash (Targocid).

**†temazepam** A mild hypnotic of the nitrazepam type, but with a shorter duration of action. It is useful in the insomnia of the elderly, and is also of value as a preoperative anxiolytic agent.
**Dose:** 10–20 mg. Daytime drowsiness is less common than with related drugs. See page 152 and Table 22.

**temocillin** A penicillin-type of antibiotic active chiefly against infections due to penicillinase-producing Gram-negative bacteria, with the notable exception of pseudomonas. It is used in respiratory and urinary tract infections due to susceptible organisms.
**Dose:** 2–4 g daily by injection, but in simple urinary tract infections a single daily dose of 1 g may be effective. (Temopen).

**tenoxicam** A non-steroidal anti-inflammatory drug (NSAID) with the actions, uses and side-effects of that group.
**Dose:** 20 mg as a single daily dose. (Mobiflex). See page 165 and Table 29.

**terazocin** An alpha-receptor antagonist used in hypertension. It produces a peripheral vasodilation by a blockade of post-synaptic alpha-receptors.
**Dose:** 1 mg *at night* initially, slowly increased up to 10 mg as a single daily dose. Small initial doses are necessary to avoid episodes of syncope during early treatment. Reduced doses are indicated when terazocin is given with thiazide diuretics or other anti-hypertensive agents. Side-effects are dizziness, drowsiness and peripheral oedema. It is also used in benign prostatic hypertrophy. (Hypovase). See page 148 and Table 21.

**terbinafine** An antifungal agent that acts by interfering with the synthesis of ergosterol, an essential constituent of fungal cell membranes. It is used in fungal infections of the skin and nails, but it is not effective in pityriasis (*Tinea versicolor*).
**Dose:** 250 mg daily for 2–6 weeks; half-doses in severe liver or renal impairment. Side-effects are rash, loss of appetite and gastrointestinal disturbances. (Lamisil).

**terbutaline** A selective beta-adrenoceptor stimulant and bronchodilator, with the actions, uses and side-effects of salbutamol.
**Dose:** 7.5–15 mg orally daily, by aerosol inhalation; 250–500 µg by s.c., i.m. or i.v.

injection. (Bricanyl). See page 118 and Table 6.

**terfenadine** An antihistamine with reduced sedative and other side-effects on the central nervous system. It is effective in hay fever, allergic skin conditions and other allergic states.
**Dose:** 120 mg daily. Best given alone, as combined use with imidazole antifungal agents or with many other drugs may cause severe reactions. See Drug Data Sheet for details. (Triludan). See page 110 and Table 2.

**terlipressin** A synthetic form of vasopressin, used to control bleeding from oesophageal varices.
**Dose:** 1–2 mg i.v., repeated if required 4–6-hourly. (Glypressin).

**testosterone** The androgenic hormone of the testes, which controls the development of the male sex characteristics. It is used mainly in the treatment of hypogonadism by the i.m. injection of depot preparations of long-acting testosterone derivatives. Subcutaneous implantation of testosterone pellets (200–600 mg) has been used in the treatment of metastatic breast cancer. Side-effects are weight gain, virilism and hypercalcaemia.

**tetanus vaccines** Preparations of tetanus toxin that has been modified by treatment with formaldehyde. They stimulate the formation of protective antitoxin. They are used for active immunization against tetanus, but for young children a combined diphtheria, pertussis and tetanus vaccine is usually preferred.

**tetrabenazine** A drug of the haloperidal type, but used mainly in the treatment of Huntington's chorea and similar disorders of movement.
**Dose:** 75–200 mg daily. It may cause drowsiness and extra-pyramidal side-effects.

**tetracosactrin** A synthetic form of corticotrophin.
**Dose:** a single injection of 250 µg as a test of adrenal cortex function, as after such an injection the level of cortisol in the plasma should rise within an hour. It is also given as single 1 mg i.m. depot preparation in the 5-hour diagnostic test. (Synacthen; Synacthen Depot).

97

T

**tetracycline** A wide-range antibiotic very similar both chemically and pharmacologically to chlortetracycline, oxytetracycline, clomocycline, and related compounds referred to generically as the tetracyclines. They all have the same type of action against both Gram-positive and Gram-negative organisms, but exhibit certain differences in solubility, absorption and excretion. These differences are reflected in the different doses, as tetracycline is given in doses of 250 mg 4 times a day, whereas with doxycycline a single daily dose of 100 mg may be adequate. Long treatment with a tetracycline may lead to gastrointestinal disturbance owing to changes in the normal bacterial population of the intestinal tract. The use of the tetracyclines has declined with the emergence of bacterial resistance. They also have the disadvantage of being taken up and staining growing teeth and bone, and so should not be given to children or used during pregnancy. The absorption of the tetracyclines is reduced by antacids, calcium, iron and milk. See page 249 and Table 35.

**theophylline** A bronchodilator used in the less severe forms of asthma and respiratory disease. (In severe and acute asthma aminophylline is usually preferred.)
**Dose:** 180 mg–1 g daily. Side-effects include gastrointestinal disturbances and tachycardia, but are less frequent when long-acting preparations of theophylline are used. Such preparations are also useful in the control of nocturnal asthma. These long-acting forms differ, and a patient stabilized on one preparation should not be transferred to another without good cause. See page 118 and Table 6.

**thiabendazole** An anthelmintic effective against a wide range of intestinal parasites. Also useful in creeping eruption.
**Dose:** 2.5 mg/kg daily, up to a maximum of 3 g daily for 2–3 days. Side-effects (more marked in the elderly) are nausea, diarrhoea, rash, yellow vision and jaundice. (Mintezol).

**thiamine (vitamin B₁)** Essential for carbohydrate metabolism, but is used clinically in cases of deficiency, as in beri-beri, or when the diet is restricted. Also of value in the neuritis of pregnancy and alcoholism.
**Dose:** 2–5 mg daily; therapeutic 25–100 mg daily, in severe deficiency 200–300 mg daily. Severe allergic reactions have followed the i.v. injection of thiamine in high-dose mixed vitamin products such as Pabrinex. Anaphylactic treatment must be immediately available. (Benerva).

**thiazides** See diuretics and page 150.

**thioguanine** A cytotoxic agent similar in action and uses to mercaptopurine, and used to induce and maintain remission in acute myeloblastic and other leukaemias.
**Dose:** 2 mg/kg daily. Side-effects are bone marrow depression, nausea and jaundice. (Lanvis). See page 122 and Table 8.

**thiopentone** A widely used, short-acting i.v. anaesthetic.
**Dose:** 100–150 mg initially, repeated at intervals of 10–15 seconds as required. Solutions should be freshly prepared, and great care must be taken to avoid extravasation, as the solution is very alkaline and may cause tissue necrosis. Intra-arterial injection is even more dangerous. (Intraval Sodium).

**thioridazine** A tranquillizing drug related to chlorpromazine, and used in similar doses for the treatment of schizophrenia and other psychiatric conditions. Unlike most related drugs, it has no antiemetic properties.
**Dose:** 30–600 mg daily. (Melleril). See page 168 and Table 30.

**thiotepa** A cytotoxic agent used mainly by intra-cavity instillation, particularly for recurrent superficial tumours of the bladder.
**Dose:** 15–60 mg dissolved in 60 ml of water, instilled weekly for 4 weeks, followed by a rest period of 2 weeks before further doses are given.

**thymoxamine** A peripheral vasodilator that is useful in vasospasm and other peripheral ischaemic conditions.
**Dose:** 160–240 mg daily. Side-effects such as headache and facial flushing are usually mild and transient. Treatment should be discontinued after 2 weeks if there is no response. (Opilon). See moxisylyte.

**thyroxine** The active constituent of thyroid, but now prepared synthetically. Thyroxine is a powerful metabolic stimulant, specific in neonatal hypothyroidism (cretinism) and myxoedema. In the former, early diagnosis

and treatment are essential to ensure normal development, and therapy can be commenced with an initial dose of 10 µg/kg.
**Dose:** in thyroid deficiency states generally, 100 µg daily may be given initially, with subsequent maintenance doses of up to 200 µg daily. Overdose or too-rapid treatment may cause palpitations, flushing and diarrhoea.

**tiaprofenic acid** A non-steroidal analgesic and anti-inflammatory agent with the actions, uses and side-effects of related NSAIDs such as naproxen.
**Dose:** 600–800 mg daily. Mild oedema may occur with extended treatment. Peptic ulcer and asthma are contra-indications. Severe cystitis is an occasional side-effect. It should not be given to patients with urinary tract disorders, and should be withdrawn at once if any urinary symptoms develop. (Surgam). See page 165 and Table 29.

**tibolone** A compound described as an gonadomimetic steroid as it has oestrogenic and progestogenic properties. It is used to control the vasomotor symptoms of the menopause, including those surgically induced as well as those occurring naturally.
**Dose:** 2.5 mg daily for some months. Similar doses in the prophylaxis of osteoporosis. Side-effects are headache, dizziness and vaginal bleeding. Treatment should be withdrawn if any thrombo-embolic symptoms or jaundice appear. (Livial).

**ticarcillin** An antibiotic with an increased activity against *Pseudomonas aeruginosa*. In pseudomonal septicaemia, combined treatment with an aminoglycoside antibiotic such as gentamicin may evoke an increased response.
**Dose:** 15–20 g daily by slow i.v. injection or infusion in systemic infections; 3–4 g daily by i.m. injection in urinary infections. (Ticar). It is sometimes given together with clavulanic acid as Timentin, but a delayed post-treatment reaction with Timentin is cholestatic jaundice, thought to be due to clavulanic acid.

**tiludronic acid** A bisphosphonate that inhibits the bone resorbing activity of osteoclasts, and so reduces the excessive demineralization of bone that occurs in Paget's disease.

**Dose:** 400 mg as a single daily dose for 12 weeks, to be taken with water at least 2 hours before or 2 hours after meals. Antacids and milk should be avoided. The improvement in serum alkaline phosphatase activity may persist, and a second course needed only after an interval of at least 6 months. Gastrointestinal side-effects are common, but renal function should be monitored regularly. (Skelid).

**timolol** A beta-andrenergic blocking agent of the propranolol type, used in the control of angina and hypertension.
**Dose:** 10–60 mg daily. In the prophylactic treatment of migraine, 10–20 mg daily. Care is necessary in bradycardia, cardiac insufficiency and bronchial disease. It is also of value as eye drops (0.25%–0.5%) in simple chronic glaucoma, as it reduces intra-ocular pressure by reducing the formation of the aqueous humour. (Betim; Blocadren; Timoptol). See pages 148 & 154, and Table 21.

**tinidazole** A drug similar to metronidazole, and used mainly in the prophylaxis and treatment of anaerobic infections and amoebiasis.
**Dose:** 2 g initially, followed by 1 g daily for 5 days. A single oral dose of 2 g is given 12 hours before abdominal surgery, and a similar single dose is given in amoebiasis and giardiasis. Side-effects are nausea, vomiting and diarrhoea. A disulfiram-like reaction may occur if alcohol is taken. (Fasigyn).

**tinzaparin** A low-molecular weight heparin used in the prevention of thrombo-embolism.
**Dose:** by s.c. injection 2500–3000 units daily for 7–10 days. It is also used to prevent clotting in haemodialysis apparatus. (Innohep; Logiparin). See dalteparin and enoxaparin. With these products laboratory control is not necessary.

**tioconazole** An antifungal agent used in tinea infections of the nails by the extended application of a 28% solution. Treatment for 6 months or more may be necessary. (Trosyl).

**titanium dioxide** A metallic oxide, similar to zinc oxide, with mild astringent properties. It is present in some sunburn protection preparations.

**tizanidine** A central alpha$_2$ receptor agonist used in the spasticity associated with multiple sclerosis and spinal injury.
**Dose:** 2 mg weekly, increased according to response up to 24 mg daily. Monitor liver function monthly for 4 months. (Zanaflex).

**tobramycin** An aminoglycoside antibiotic with the actions, uses and side-effects of gentamicin, but considered to be more active against *Pseudomonas aeruginosa.*
**Dose:** 3–5 mg/kg daily by i.m. injection or i.v. infusion. It may be given together with a penicillin or metronidazole in serious mixed infections. Care is necessary to avoid the ototoxic and nephrotoxic effects of aminoglycosides. (Nebcin).

**tocainide** An anti-arrhythmic agent similar in action to lignocaine. It is a powerful drug, and may cause severe blood disturbances, and its use is largely restricted to the control of life-threatening arrhythmias not responding to other drugs.
**Dose:** 1.2–2.4 g daily. Blood counts during treatment are essential. Side-effects include bradycardia, hypotension, rash, tremor and aplastic anaemia. (Tonocard).

**tocopherol** A synthetic form of vitamin E.

**tolazamide** An oral hypoglycaemic agent related to tolbutamide, with similar actions, uses and side-effects.
**Dose:** 100–250 mg daily, increased if necessary up to a maximum dose of 1 g daily. (Tolanase). See page 131 and Table 13.

**tolbutamide** A sulphonylurea used like chlorpropamide in the treatment of maturity-onset diabetes, but it has a shorter action, and twice-daily doses are usually necessary. It is effective only when some insulin-secreting cells of the pancreas are still functioning, and a return to insulin therapy may be necessary during illness and infection. Tolbutamide is not suitable for the treatment of juvenile or severe diabetes.
**Dose:** 0.5–2 g daily. Side-effects include hypoglycaemia, rash, jaundice and blood dyscrasias, but are uncommon with low doses. (Rastinon). See page 131 and Table 13.

**tolcapone** An inhibitor of the enzyme concerned with the biosynthesis of dopamine. It is used with other drugs in the treatment of parkinsonism in initial doses of 100 mg 3 times a day. Side-effects are dyskinesia, nausea and sleep disturbances. (Tasmar). See page 160 and Table 26.

**tolfenamic acid** A non-steroidal anti-inflammatory drug (NSAID) but exceptional in being used in the treatment of migraine, on the basis that prostaglandins are involved in the pathology of migraine.
**Dose:** 200 mg at the onset of an attack, repeated once after 2–3 hours if necessary. Close monitoring is required if anticoagulants also given; caution in peptic ulcer. (Clotam). See page 154 and Table 23.

**tolmetin** An anti-inflammatory analgesic agent used in rheumatoid and musculoskeletal conditions. As with related non-steroidal anti-inflammatory drugs (NSAIDs) it may cause gastrointestinal disturbances in some patients, and should be taken after food. Hypersensitivity reactions may occur occasionally.
**Dose:** 0.6–1.8 g daily. (Tolectin). See page 165 and Table 29.

**topiramate**▽ A new anti-epileptic that differs chemically from related drugs. It is used as adjunctive therapy in partial seizure patients not adequately controlled by standard treatment.
**Dose:** initial dose 100 mg daily, slowly increased at weekly intervals as required up to 800 mg daily. Patients receiving digoxin should be monitored. Not recommended for children. (Topamax). See page 136 and Table 15.

**topotecan**▽ A new advance in cancer chemotherapy is the use of topoisomerase inhibitors. Topoisomerase I is necessary for DNA replication, and topotican acts by binding with super-coiled DNA and so preventing further DNA development.
**Dose:** 1.5 mg/m$^2$ by i.v. infusion daily for 5 days under expert supervision. Side-effects are myelosuppression and severe neutropenia. (Hycamptin). See page 122 and Table 8.

**torasemide** A loop diuretic of the frusemide type.
**Dose:** in oedema, 5–20 mg once daily; in pulmonary oedema 10–20 mg daily by slow i.v. injection but much larger doses are sometimes necessary. In hypertension, 5–20 mg daily. (Torem). See page 148 and Table 21.

**toremifene**∇ An anti-oestrogen used in hormone-dependent metastatic breast cancer.
**Dose:** 60 mg as a single daily dose. Side-effects are linked with the mode of action and include hot flushes, dizziness and sweating. Care is necessary in severe hepatic deficiency, angina and cardiac weakness. (Fareston). See page 122 and Table 8.

**tramadol**∇ An analgesic used in the short-term treatment of moderate to severe pain. It has reduced affinity for opioid receptors, and the action may be mediated by inhibiting the neuronal re-uptake of noradrenaline and related amines.
**Dose:** 300–400 mg; in severe pain it may be given by i.m. injection or i.v. injection/infusion in doses of 50–100 mg 4–6-hourly. (Tramake; Zamadol; Zydol).

**trandolapril** An ACE inhibitor used in mild to moderate hypertension.
**Dose:** 500 µg daily initially, increased at intervals of 2–3 weeks up to 1–2mg once daily. If hypotension occurs, reduce supportive therapy before lowering the trandolopril dose. Prophylactic dose after myocardial infarction 500 µg–4 mg daily. Diuretic therapy should be stopped before starting with trandolapril, to reduce the risks of initial hypotensive side-effects. Care with monitoring in patients with renal and hepatic impairment. (Gopten; Odrik). See page 148 and Table 21.

**tranexamic acid** An antifibrinolytic agent used to check haemorrhage after prostactectomy, in surgery generally and in the control of menorrhagia.
**Dose:** 2–8 g daily; 3 g daily by slow i.v. injection. Side-effects are nausea, diarrhoea and dizziness. (Cyklokapron).

**tranquillizers** These drugs were once separated into the major tranquillizers, represented by chlorpromazine, and the minor tranquillizers exemplified by diazepam, but are now often referred to as antipsychotic drugs and anxiolytics respectively. The antipsychotics are used mainly in the control of disturbed patients, and in schizophrenia, although they have some anti-anxiety properties, and long-term treatment is often necessary. The anxiolytic drugs are intended mainly for the short-term treatment of acute anxiety states, as extended use may cause dependence. See pages 117 & 168, and Tables 5 & 30.

**Transiderm-Nitro** A medicated patch containing glyceryl trinitrate designed to have an action over 24 hours in the prophylaxis of angina.

**tranylcypromine** A monoamine oxidase inhibitor (MAOI), of use in severe depression not responding to other drugs.
**Dose:** 20 mg daily initially, increased to 30 mg daily or more according to need. The use of tranylcypromine requires care, as the drug has a stimulant action that may complicate therapy, and phenelzine may be preferred. Side-effects are dizziness, dry mouth and insomnia. Liver damage may also occur, and a hypertensive crisis with throbbing headache requires withdrawal of the drug. Hyperthyroidism is a contra-indication. (Parnate). See page 128 and Table 11.

**trazodone** An antidepressant chemically distinct from other drugs with a similar action, and with reduced anticholinergic and cardiovascular side-effects. It is indicated mainly in depression associated with anxiety when a sedative action is also required.
**Dose:** 150–300 mg daily. The side-effects are those of the tricyclic antidepressants such as amitriptyline. (Molipaxin). See page 128 and Table 11.

**treosulfan** A cytotoxic agent related to busulphan, but used mainly in ovarian cancer.
**Dose:** 1 g daily for 28 days, repeated after a 4-week rest period; 5–15 g by i.v. injection at intervals of 1–3 weeks. In all cases the dose is adjusted according to the degree of bone marrow depression that occurs. Other side-effects are those of cytotoxic drugs generally. Extravasation causes pain and local tissue damage. See page 122 and Table 8.

**tretinoin** A derivative of vitamin A. It is used locally for acne (Retin-A) and also for the treatment of photodamage to the skin (Retinova). A new use is the induction of remission in acute promyelocytic leukaemia.
**Dose:** 22.5 mg/m$^2$ twice daily with food. Combined therapy may reduce the risk of relapse (Vesanoid).

**triamcinolone** A glucocorticosteroid with the actions, uses and side-effects of hydrocortisone, but differing by promoting sodium excretion, and so is of no value in adrenal cortex deficiency states. It is used in a wide range of inflammatory, allergic and respiratory states, and in inflammatory skin conditions.
**Dose:** 8–24 mg daily. It is also given as triamcinolone acetonide in doses of 40 mg by deep i.m. injection for a depot action. The acetonide is also given by intra-articular injection in doses of 2.5–40 mg in local inflammation of the joints, and by intra-lesional injection in doses of 2–3 mg at any one site for the treatment of skin lesions. Triamcinolone actonide is also used as a 1% cream or ointment in severe inflammatory skin conditions. The side-effects are those of the corticosteroids (see hydrocortisone), but triamcinolone may also cause myopathy with high dose treatment. (Kenalog; Ledercort).

**triamterene** A potassium sparing diuretic, used mainly in association with more powerful drugs. It is indicated in oedematous conditions generally, and, as it causes some retention of potassium, its use avoids the need for supplementary potassium therapy.
**Dose:** 150–250 mg daily, with lower doses for the elderly and when given in association with other diuretics. Rash and gastrointestinal disturbances are side-effects. (Dytac). See page 148 and Table 21.

**tribavarin** An inhibitor of viral replication used in severe viral bronchiolitis in infants.
**Dose:** by aerosol inhalation of a solution (20 mg/ml) for 12–18 hours daily for 3–7 days, together with supportive therapy. (Virazid).

**triclofos** A derivative of chloral, with the sedative properties of the parent drug, but less irritant to the gastric mucosa.
**Dose:** 1–2 g daily.

**triclosan** A chlorinated phenolic antiseptic, used mainly in surgical scrubs and similar preparations. (Manusept; Ster-Zac).

**trientine** A copper-chelating agent used in Wilson's disease, but only for patients unable to tolerate penicillamine.
**Dose:** 1.2–2.4 g daily. It is not an alternative to penicillamine in other conditions. The main side-effect is nausea.

**trifluoperazine** A powerful tranquillizing drug of the chlorpromazine type. It is used mainly in schizophrenia and similar psychoses, and in severe anxiety.
**Dose:** 10–20 mg or more daily according to need. In severe anxiety, 2–6 mg daily. In acute conditions, 1–3 mg daily by deep i.m. injection. As an antiemetic, it is given in doses of 2–4 mg or 1–3 mg by injection. The side-effects are similar to those of chlorpromazine, including extra-pyramidal symptoms, but the anticholinergic and sedative side-effects are less severe. (Stelazine). See page 168 and Table 30.

**tri-iodothyronine** See liothyronine.

**trilostane** An inhibitor of enzyme systems concerned with production of mineralo- and glucocorticosteroids by the adrenal cortex, and so resembles metyrapone to some extent. It is used to control adrenal cortex hyperfunction and the excessive production of aldosterone.
**Dose:** 240 mg initially, adjusted up to a maximum of 480 mg daily, according to the plasma corticosteroid levels. Care is necessary in liver and kidney dysfunction. (Modrenal).

**trimeprazine** A sedative antihistamine used in the treatment of pruritus and allergic itching conditions, and for pre-medication.
**Dose:** 30–100 mg daily; pre-medication dose: 3 mg/kg. (Vallergan).

**trimetaphan** A short-acting ganglionic-blocking agent. It is used to produce a controllable reduction in blood pressure during neuro- and vascular surgery when a relatively bloodless field is necessary.
**Dose:** by i.v. infusion, 3–4 mg/min initially, with subsequent doses carefully adjusted to the response. Side-effects are tachycardia and respiratory depression. Frequent determination of blood pressure during use is essential.

**trimethoprim** An antibacterial agent similar in action to the sulphonamides. It is used in the prophylaxis and treatment of urinary tract and respiratory infections due to sensitive bacteria.
**Dose:** in chronic infections, 200–400 mg daily; prophylactic dose, 100 mg daily. In

severe infections, 150–250 mg twice daily by slow i.v. injection. Side-effects are nausea, vomiting, rash and pruritus, and possible bone marrow depression. (Ipral; Monotrim). See co-trimoxaole.

**trimetrexate**∇ An antibacterial agent used like atovaquone in AIDS patients with *Pneumocystis carinii* pneumonia.
**Dose:** 45 mg/m$^2$ daily by i.v. infusion for 21 days, followed by calcium folinate 80 mg/m$^2$ daily for 28 days, orally or i.v. (Neutrexin).

**trimipramine** A sedative anti-depressant with the action and side-effects of amitriptyline. It is valuable in depression complicated by anxiety.
**Dose:** 75–300 mg daily. (Surmontil).

**triple vaccine** Diphtheria, tetanus and pertussis vaccine for the primary immun-ization of children.
**Dose:** 0.5 ml by i.m. or deep s.c. injection.

**triptorelin** A synthetic form of gonadorelin, used in the treatment of advanced prostatic cancer. Such cancers are testosterone-dependent, and triptorelin acts by depressing pituitary function, and so indirectly reduces the plasma level of testosterone.
**Dose:** It has been formulated so that a single i.m. injection of 4.2 mg depresses testosterone production for 28 days. Initially there may be a temporary flare-up of symptoms, which can be prevented by giving an anti-androgen for 3 days before treatment, and continued for 2–3 weeks. Patients should be monitored for uteric obstruction and spinal cord compression during the first months of treatment. (Decapeptyl Sr). See page 122.

**trisodium edetate** A chelating or binding agent that is sometimes used in hypercal-caemia. The calcium complex so formed is excreted in the urine.
**Dose:** slow i.v. infusion up to 70 mg/kg daily according to need and response, as shown by plasma calcium measurement. It is also used as a 0.4% solution for ophthalmic use in lime burns of the eyes. Side-effects after injection are nausea, diarrhoea and cramp. Contraindicated in renal impairment. (Limclair).

**troglitazone** A new drug for non-insulin dependent diabetes. It differs from other oral antidiabetic drugs by increasing the sensitivity to endogenous insulin, and so acts as an insulin enhancer.
**Dose:** 200 mg daily with breakfast, increased if required by 200 mg at intervals of 2–4 weeks up to 600 mg daily. Side-effects are diarrhoea, fatigue and malaise. (Romozin). See page 131 and Table 13.

**tropicamide** A short-acting mydriatic agent similar to homatropine. Used as 0.5% and 1% solution.

**tropisetron** A 5–HT$_3$-receptor antagonist, similar to ondansetron but with a longer action. It is used to control the nausea and vomiting induced by cancer chemotherapy.
**Dose:** initially as a 5 mg dose i.v. shortly before such therapy, and followed by oral doses of 5 mg daily, 1 hour before food, for 5 days. Side-effects are dizziness, headache and gastrointestinal disturbance. (Navoban). See page 122.

**tryparsamide** Used in late trypansomiasis when the CNS is involved.
**Dose:** 1–3 g by injection weekly, up to a maximum of 24 g. May damage optic nerves.

**tryptophan**∇ An amino acid involved in the biosynthesis of serotonin. It is used in specialist centres for the treatment of severe and prolonged depression resistant to other drugs, and where a deficiency of serotonin may be a factor. (Optimax). See page 128 and Table 11.

**tuberculin** A product obtained from cultures of *Mycobacterium tuberculosis*. It is used in the diagnosis of tuberculosis. See BGC vaccine.

**tulobuterol** A selective beta$_2$-adrenergic agonist of the salbutamol type, used in the prophylaxis and treatment of broncho-spasm in asthma and related conditions.
**Dose:** 4–6 mg daily. (Respacal). See page 118 and Table 6.

**tyrothricin** A minor antibiotic used as lozenges for mouth infections.

**103**

**T**

# U

**undecenoic acid** An organic acid with useful antimycotic properties. It is used mainly as powder or ointment (5%), often with zinc undecenoate in the treatment of athlete's foot and associated conditions.

**urea** An osmotic diuretic. It has been used orally in doses of 5–15 g. Applied locally as a 10% solution, it promotes granulation and reduces odour from foul ulcers.

**urofollitrophin** A preparation of human follicle-stimulating hormone (FSH) used with menotrophin for the induction of ovulation. Dose and duration of treatment require careful control to avoid over-stimulation. (Metrodin; Orgafol).

**urokinase** A plasmin activator obtained from human urine. It is used mainly in the thrombolysis of blocked i.v. shunts, and in the lysis of blood clots in the eye.
**Dose:** 5000–37 500 units, instilled into the shunt; similar doses are injected into the anterior chamber of the eye for the resolution of blood clots. (Ukidan).

**104**

**U**

**ursodeoxycholic acid** The acid appears to be a solvent of cholesterol, and is given orally to promote the dissolution of cholesterol-containing gall stones.
**Dose:** 8–12 mg/kg as a single daily dose, but prolonged treatment is required, which should be continued after the disso-lution of the stones to inhibit recurrence. The dissolution of calcium-containing or radio-opaque stones is unlikely to occur. (Destolit; Ursofalk).

# V

**vaccines** Bacterial vaccines are suspensions or extracts of dead bacteria, but some anti-viral vaccines are also available. They may be given by s.c. or i.m. injection, and are used mainly for prophylaxis against a particular infection. The most commonly used vaccines include those for typhoid, cholera, diphtheria, influenza, tetanus and polio. Protection against mumps, measles, pertussis, rubella, yellow fever and hepati-tis can also be obtained. The so-called

allergen vaccines, used for desensitization to various allergens such as grass pollens, are not true vaccines, but weak solutions of allergen extracts. They may precipitate allergic reactions in susceptible patients, and should be used only when emergency resuscitation measures are immediately available.

**valaciclovir**∇ A pro-drug of acyclovir used in herpes zoster. It is well absorbed orally, and quickly converted to the parent drug and promotes an improved response.
**Dose:** 3 g daily for 7 days, reduced in severe renal impairment. Dose in herpes simplex 1 g daily. Side-effects are headache and nausea. (Valtrex). See page 144 and Table 19.

**valproic acid** (Convulex). See sodium valproate.

**valsartan** An angiotensin II receptor antag-onist used in hypertension. It has a more selective action than the ACE-inhibitors.
**Dose:** 80 mg daily. Combined treatment with a potassium-sparing diuretic is not advisable. (Diovan). See page 148 and Table 21.

**vancomycin** An antibiotic used in severe antibiotic-associated staphylococcal colitis (pseudomembranous colitis).
**Dose:** 0.5 g daily for 7–10 days. It is also given by injection in resistant bacterial endocarditis; 1 g twice a day by slow i.v. infusion over 1–2 hours, as rapid injection may cause anaphylactic shock. Blood concentrations of the antibiotic should be monitored, as the many side-effects include renal damage, ototoxicity and neutropenia. Pruritus and upper body flushing may occur, and tinnitus is an indication that the drug should be with-drawn. (Vancocin).

**vasoconstrictors** Drugs such as noradren-aline that constrict the peripheral vessels, and so cause a temporary rise in blood pressure. They are useful in hypotensive conditions when the blood volume is still adequate, and in controlling the fall in blood pressure that occurs in spinal and general anaesthesia. They were widely used in the treatment of cardiogenic shock, but the rise in blood pressure that they produce is linked with a fall in pres-sure in vital organs such as the kidneys, and in shock reliance is now largely based on drugs such as dobutamine and dopamine, together with plasma expanders such as dextran.

**vasodilators** Traditional vasodilators used in the prophylaxis and treatment of angina include glyceryl trinitrate and other nitrates. They have a general effect on the venous system but newer and more selectively acting antihypertensive drugs are the beta-adrenoceptor blocking agents represented by propranolol, and the calcium channel blocking agents such as nifedipine. Other vasodilator drugs are the alpha-adrenoceptor blocking agents (indoramin, prazosin) and the ACE inhibitors (captopril). Cerebral vasodilators are represented by isoxsuprine. Peripheral vasodilators include cinnarizine and thymoxamine. See pages 114 & 148.

**vasopressin** A preparation of the blood pressure-raising and antidiuretic factors of the pituitary gland. It has been used in doses of 5–20 units twice daily by s.c. or i.m. injection in diabetes insipidus, but has been largely superseded by demopressin. (Pitressin).

**vecuronium** A non-depolarizing muscle relaxant of the rocuronium type. It has a medium duration of action, with the advantage of not causing histamine release.
**Dose:** 80–100 µg/kg/min initially, with supplementary doses as required. (Norcuron).

**venlafaxine** An antidepressant that inhibits the re-uptake of both serotonin and noradrenaline.
**Dose:** in depressive illness, 75 mg daily, rising if necessary after some weeks to 150 mg daily, or exceptionally to 375 mg daily. Prolonged treatment is necessary for an adequate response and reduce potential relapse. Reduced doses are given in hepatic disease and the elderly. Care is necessary in epilepsy, and before and after monoamine oxidase inhibator (MAOI) therapy. Many side-effects have been noted, but any skin reaction should be reported to the prescriber. (Efexor). See page 128 and Table 11.

**verapamil** A calcium channel blocking agent that reduces the movement of calcium ions in cardiac tissues. It reduces the oxygen demand as well as the contractility of the myocardium, and it is used in angina, arrhythmias and hypertension.

**Dose:** 120–480 mg daily according to the condition and degree of response. In severe arrhythmias, 5–10 mg i.v. under ECG control. Contraindicated in bradycardia, heart failure and heart block. Side-effects include nausea, hypotension and heart block. It should be used with caution in a patient already receiving a beta-adrenoceptor blocking agent. (Cordilox; Securon). See page 148 and Table 21.

**vigabatrin** A new anti-epileptic drug. GABA (a gamma aminobutyric acid) is an inhibitor of neurotransmission, and epileptic seizures may be linked with a GABA deficiency. Vigabatrin has an inhibitory action on the GABA-metabolizing enzyme, and so indirectly permits a rise in the brain level of GABA. It is used in the treatment of epilepsy not responding to other anticonvulsants.
**Dose:** 2 g daily initially, with adjustments up to 4 g daily together with current antiepileptic therapy. Side-effects are numerous, and include drowsiness, fatigue, dizziness and weight gain. Sudden withdrawal is inadvisable. (Sabril). See page 136 and Table 15.

**viloxazine** An antidepressant with the general action, uses and side-effects of amitriptyline, but with a reduced sedative activity. It is given in depression associated with apathy, and in the depression of epilepsy.
**Dose:** 150–400 mg daily. It may increase the action of phenytoin and antihypertensive agents. (Vivalan). See page 128 and Table 11.

**vinblastine** An alkaloid of periwinkle that has cytotoxic properties. It is used in the control of acute leukaemias, lymphomas and other malignant conditions, and in mycosis fungoides.
**Dose:** 100 µg/kg weekly i.v., increased by 50 µg/kg weekly, up to 500 µg/kg weekly according to response. Side-effects include myelosuppression, neurotoxicity and abdominal disturbances. The drug should be handled with care as it is a tissue irritant. (Velbe). See page 122 and Table 8.

**vincristine** A vinca alkaloid with the action and uses of vinblastine, but much less likely to cause myelodepression. It is used mainly in the treatment of acute leukaemias in children, Hodgkin's disease and other malignant lymphomas.

**Dose:** 50 µg/kg by i.v. injection weekly initially, adjusted according to need up to a maximum of 150 µg/kg weekly. Neuromuscular side-effects may limit the dose. Other side-effects are abdominal disturbance and alopecia. The injection of the drug requires care as it is a tissue irritant. (Oncovin). See page 122 and Table 8.

**vindesine** A vinca alkaloid with an action similar to that of vincristine. It is used mainly in acute lymphoblastic leukaemia in children, and in other malignant conditions not responding to treatment.
**Dose:** 3 mg/m$^2$ weekly by i.m. injection, subsequently increased up to 5 mg/m$^2$ according to response. The side-effects are similar to those of other vinca alkaloids, but granulocytopenia may be a dose-limiting factor. Extravasation should be avoided, as it may cause considerable local irritation. (Eldesine). See page 122 and Table 8.

**vinorelbine** A cytostatic drug of the vinca alkaloid type. It is used in non-small cell lung cancer and in advanced breast cancer resistant to other drugs.
**Dose:** 25–36 mg/m$^2$ weekly by i.v. infusion. Main side-effect is neutropenia. (Navelbine). See page 122.

**vitamin A** One of the vitamins obtained from fish-liver oils. A deficiency in the diet causes night-blindness, skin changes and a decreased resistance to infection.
**Dose:** 2500–25 000 units daily.

**vitamin B** A group of water soluble vitamins obtained from yeast or rice polishings. The constituents include thiamine, riboflavine, nicotinic acid, pyridoxine, and small amounts of other factors.

**vitamin B$_6$** Pyridoxine.

**vitamin B$_{12}$** Cynacobalamin.

**vitamin C** Ascorbic acid.

**vitamin D** The vitamin essential for the absorption of calcium and phosphorus and subsequent bone formation. Several forms of the vitamin are known, but it is used chiefly as calciferol. Vitamin D is activated in the liver and kidneys to more powerful derivatives such as calcitriol and alfacalcidol.

**vitamin D$_2$** Calciferol.

**vitamin E** The vitamin in the germ of wheat, rice and other grains. Deficiency states are uncommon, but may occur in cystic fibrosis and other conditions where fat absorption is impaired. It has been used empirically in many other conditions, but its therapeutic value is questionable.
**Dose:** 5–15 mg daily. Now largely replaced by the synthetic form tocopherol.

**vitamin K** The vitamin concerned with the formation of prothrombin, and so with blood coagulation. Given as menadiol in haemorrhagic disorders, vitamin K$_1$ or phytomenadione has a similar but more rapid and sustained action. Of no value when the prothrombin level of the blood is adequate.

# W

**warfarin** A synthetic anticoagulant similar to phenindione, but with reduced side-effects and it is now the preferred drug. It is used mainly in deep-vein thrombosis and transient brain ischaemia, in doses based on the prothrombin time as reported by the laboratory in terms of the International Normalized Ratio (INR).
**Dose:** Pending INR report, 10 mg daily initially for up to 3 days. Haemorrhage is the main side-effect, and may require the use of phytomenadione to control the excessive response.

**Whitfield's ointment** Benzoic acid 6%, salicylic acid 3%. Has keratolytic and fungicidal properties, and is used mainly for ringworm.

**wool alcohols** A water-in-oil emulsifying agent obtained from wool fat. It is used in many water-containing ointments, such as ointment of wool alcohols and hydrous ointment.

**wool fat** A pale yellow, waxy substance, also known as lanolin, obtained from sheep's wool. It consists mainly of cholesterol-derivatives, and is a constituent of various water-in-oil emulsifying and emollient ointment bases. It may cause skin sensitization in some susceptible patients.

# X

**xamoterol** A partial $\beta_1$ adrenoceptor agonist with a cardiac stimulant action. It is given only in mild chronic heart failure to control exercise-induced symptoms. **Dose:** 400 mg daily. Side-effects are dizziness, headache and gastrointestinal disturbances. Contraindicated in severe heart failure, and care is necessary in asthmatic conditions. (Corwin). See page 141 and Table 18.

**xipamide** A long-acting diuretic and anti-hypertensive similar to chlorthalidone. **Dose:** in hypertension, 20 mg is given as a morning dose; in oedematous states, 40–80 mg as a single dose, reduced later as necessary. (Diurexan). See page 148 and Table 21.

**xylometazoline** A sympathomimetic agent used as a nasal decongestant, and to relieve allergic conjunctivitis as drops of 0.05–0.1%. Rebound congestion may be a side-effect.

# Z

**zalcitabine**∇ An antiviral agent used in the suppressive treatment of AIDS patients who have become resistant to or have failed to respond to zidovudine therapy. **Dose:** 2.25 mg daily under expert supervision, as the drug has many side-effects including peripheral neuropathy. (Hivid).

**zidovudine** An antiviral agent effective against the human immunodeficiency virus (HIV) associated with the acquired immune deficiency syndrome (AIDS). It inhibits the enzyme reverse transcriptase and, by preventing the formation of viral DNA, it inhibits viral development. **Dose:** 3.5 mg/kg 4-hourly for some months. Side-effects include anaemia, neutropenia, nausea, fever and malaise. Liver-function tests are necessary during treatment. The chronic use of analgesics such as paracetamol may increase the risk of neutropenia. (Retrovir). See page 144 and Table 19.

**zinc oxide** A soft white powder widely used in dusting powders, ointments, pastes, etc., for its mild astringent and antiseptic properties. It is a constituent of Lassar's paste, Unna's paste, Calamine Lotion and similar preparations.

**zinc sulphate** Used as an astringent and stimulating lotion (1%) for indolent ulcers; and in conjunctivitis as eye drops (0.25%).

**zinc undecenoate** A white insoluble powder. Constituent of dusting powders and ointments for mycotic conditions.

**zolmitriptan** A serotonin receptor agonist used only in the treatment of acute migraine. **Dose:** 2.5 mg as soon as possible after onset. A second dose may be given not less than 2 hours later if symptoms persist. (Zomig). See page 154 and Table 23.

**zolpidem** A mild hypnotic that acts by binding with a sub-group of benzodiazepine receptors. It has a rapid action, and is used in the short-term treatment of insomnia. **Dose:** 10 mg. Side-effects are dizziness and gastrointestinal disturbance. (Stilnoct). See page 152 and Table 22.

**zopiclone** A mild hypnotic that binds with a sub-group of benzodiazepine receptors, and may modulate the neurotransmitter GABA. **Dose:** in insomnia and early awakening, 7.5–15 mg with initial doses of 3.75 mg for the elderly. A side-effect is a bitter or metallic after-taste. (Zimovane). See page 152.

**zuclopenthixol** A powerful tranquillizing drug with actions, uses and side-effects similar to those of chlorpromazine. It is of value in schizophrenia with agitation and aggression. **Dose:** 20–30 mg or more up to 150 mg daily. For depot maintenance treatment, 100–200 mg or more by deep i.m. injection at intervals of 2–3 weeks, according to need and response. (Clopixol). See page 168.

# Drugs and their use in some common disorders

**More information about the drugs mentioned in this section is given in the main part of the book, pages 9–107.**

# Allergy

Allergy is a general term applied to certain types of hypersensitivity reactions, some of which such as hayfever are well known, but the factors that cause such reactions vary widely in their nature. In brief, an allergic reaction is immunologically mediated, and originates in an exposure to an excitatory substance referred to as an antigen, which in sensitive individuals is followed by the production of antibodies. Antigens are often protein in nature, and eggs, peanut products, wasp and bee stings, as well as drugs, can function as antigens. Subsequent re-exposure to the antigen may give rise to an antigen-antibody reaction, which is linked with the release of cell-bound histamine and other spasmogens, which in turn act upon various tissues to produce the allergic response. The response may manifest itself in several ways, such as hayfever, rhinitis, bronchoconstriction and rash or urticaria. In severe allergic reactions (anaphylactic shock), an alarming fall in blood pressure may occur with respiratory distress, and requires the immediate i.m. injection of adrenaline solution (0.5–1 ml) together with i.v. hydrocortisone 200 mg and resuscitation measures.

It should be noted that the anaphylactic reactions that occur after the first dose of certain drugs, including contrast media, are more in the nature of an idiosyncratic-toxic reaction than an immunologically mediated response, but may be no less severe, and resuscitation facilities should always be available.

In less severe allergic reactions such as hayfever and allergic rhinitis, antihistamines are widely used for symptomatic relief. They do not interrupt the chain of antigen-antibody-histamine release, but block the access of the released histamine to the sensitized tissues. Their action is palliative and not curative, and the response to treatment is often variable.

They are usually effective in hayfever, urticaria and insect bites, but are of no value in allergic asthma. Some antihistamines also have a sedative action, which may be useful in urticaria, but undesirable in other conditions. This sedative side-effect is less marked with some of the newer antihistamines (see Table 2). In overdose they may cause convulsions in young patients. The extended local application of antihistamines should be avoided, as antihistamines may themselves cause an allergic-type dermatitis. Side-effects include dry mouth, blurred vision and occasional gastrointestinal disturbances. Patients should be warned that drowsiness is a common side-effect that may affect car-driving ability. Attempts have been made to desensitize susceptible patients by injections of specific antigens, such as grass pollens. The method is not without risk, particularly in asthmatic patients, and should be carried out only by experts.

| Approved names | Brand names | Daily dose range |
|---|---|---|
| acrivastine* | Semprex | 24 mg |
| astemizole* | Hismanal, Pollen-Eze | 10 mg |
| azatadine | Optimine | 2–4 mg |
| brompheniramine | Dimotane | 12–32 mg |
| cetrizine* | Zirtek | 10 mg |
| chlorpheniramine | Piriton | 12–24 mg |
| clemastine | Tavegil | 1–2 mg |
| cyproheptadine | Periactin | 8–32 mg |
| loratadine* | Clarityn | 10 mg |
| mezquitazine | Primalan | 5–10 mg |
| phenindamine* | Thephorin | 75–150 mg |
| pheniramine | Daneral SA | 75–150 mg |
| promethazine | Phenergan | 20–75 mg |
| terfenadine* | Triludan | 60–120 mg |
| trimeprazine | Vallergan | 30–100 mg |
| triprolidine | Actidil, Pro-Actidil | 7.5–15 mg |

*Antihistamine with reduced sedative effects

Table 2 Antihistamines.

# Anaemia

Anaemia is essentially a deficiency of red blood cells, and may occur as the result of a lack of certain factors such as iron, folic acid or vitamin $B_{12}$, or from disease in which the rate of breakdown of red cells exceeds the rate of production of new cells. Iron-deficiency anaemia is the most common form, and may occur during pregnancy or as a consequence of restricted diets. Such a deficiency can be dealt with by the oral administration of a suitable iron salt, and ferrous sulphate is widely used. For patients who cannot tolerate ferrous sulphate, other salts are ferrous gluconate and fumarate. Some iron preparations for use during pregnancy also contain folic acid but are too numerous to list here. Slow-release iron products are also available. In all cases of iron-deficiency anaemia, oral treatment should be continued for some months to build up an adequate store of iron.

In a few cases, where oral iron therapy is not possible, iron-deficiency anaemia can be treated with iron-sorbitol solution by deep i.m. injection, using a 'Z' technique to avoid staining the skin. The dose is based on the degree of iron-deficiency. Oral iron should be stopped for at least 24 hours before injection treatment. (Jectofer).

Megaloblastic anaemias are less common, and are due to a deficiency of vitamin $B_{12}$ or of folic acid, or to a defect in the absorption or utilization of those factors, and may be secondary to treatment with cytotoxic agents such as methotrexate. Pernicious anaemia is the most common form of vitamin $B_{12}$ deficiency, and develops insidiously as the normally ample stores of the vitamin in the liver are slowly depleted. Treatment is replacement therapy with hydroxocobalamin, which is the preferred form of vitamin $B_{12}$, as it is excreted more slowly than the older cyanocobalamin, and has a much longer action. Some oral preparations of vitamin $B_{12}$ are available, but in general they are regarded as unsatisfactory for the treatment of vitamin $B_{12}$ deficiency.

Aplastic anaemia is due to a marked reduction in the formation of red blood cell precursors, and is a disease of the bone marrow. It may occur from no known cause, or from exposure to some toxic agents, including cytotoxic drugs. Bone marrow transplants are the only effective treatment, although some androgens such as nandrolone have been used with occasional success. Sideroblastic anaemias are due to a disturbance in the normal utilization of iron, and may respond to large doses of pyridoxine. Haemolytic anaemia is characterized by an excessive breakdown of red blood cells, due to disease or toxic agents. Some of these less common anaemias may respond to corticosteroid therapy. The severe anaemia of end-stage renal disease in dialyzed patients differs from other anaemias in being due to a lack of erythropoietin, the kidney hormone that regulates red blood cell production by the bone marrow. It can now be treated with human erythropoietin obtained by recombinant DNA technology.

| Approved names | Brand names |
|---|---|
| ferrous sulphate | Feospan } <br> Ferrograd } sustained release products <br> Slow-Fe } |
| ferrous fumarate | Fersaday <br> Fersamol <br> Galfer |
| ferrous gluconate | |
| ferrous glycine sulphate | Plesmet <br> Ferrocontin Continus <br>   (sustained release product) |
| ferrous succinate | Ferromyn |
| iron-polysaccharide complex | Niferex |
| sodium iron edetate | Sytron |
| iron-sorbitol injection | Jectofer |
| hydroxocobalamin | Cobalin-H, Neo-Cytamen |
| cyanocobalamin | Cytacon (oral), Cytamen |
| nandrolone | Deca-Durabolin |
| pyridoxine | |
| epoetin (erythropoietin) | Eprex, Recormon |

Table 3  Iron preparations.

# Angina pectoris (angina)

Angina pectoris is a painful cardiac condition that occurs when the work load on the heart and the consequent oxygen demand of the myocardium exceed the ability of the cardiovascular system to meet that demand. The pain may vary from a relatively mild ache to a crushing chest pain which may radiate to the left shoulder and left arm and other areas. It is often triggered off by exertion, and usually subsides rapidly with rest. It is basically a stress response to factors that increase cardiac demand and output, and is often linked with an atheromatous narrowing of the coronary arteries. Treatment of angina is with coronary vasodilator drugs that reduce cardiac drive and lower the myocardial oxygen demand (many of which are also used in the treatment of hypertension – see page 148. They include the time-honoured glyceryl trinitrate (which can be given by several routes), other nitrates, calcium channel blocking agents, beta-adrenergic receptor blocking agents and potassium channel activators. Glyceryl trinitrate is of particular value when a rapid response is required. The following Table gives an indication of the wide range of anti-anginal products currently available.

| Approved names | Brand names | Products |
|---|---|---|
| **nitrates** | | |
| glyceryl trinitrate * | | sublingual tablets 300, 500, 600 mg |
| | **Coro-Nitro Spray*** | spray 400 mg/dose |
| | **Glytrin Spray** | spray 400 mg/dose |
| | **Nitrolingual Spray** | 400 mg/dose |
| | **Nitro-Continus** | long-acting tablets, 6.4 mg |
| | **Suscard** | long-acting tablets, 1 mg, 3 mg, 5 mg |
| | **Sustac** | long-acting tablets, 2.6 mg, 6.4 mg |
| | **Nitrocine injection** | 1 mg |
| | **Nitronal injection** | 1 mg |
| | **Deponit** | patches 5 mg |
| | **Minitran** | patches 5 mg, 10 mg, 15 mg |
| | **Nitro-Dur** | patches 2.5 mg, 5 mg, 10 mg, 15 mg |
| | **Trasiderm-Nitro** | patches 5 mg, 10 mg |
| | **Percutol** | ointment 2% |

Note: Sprays (1–2 doses) are given under the tongue; the mouth should then be closed.

| | | |
|---|---|---|
| sorbide idinitrate | **Isordil** | tablets 5 mg, 10 mg, 30 mg |
| | **Sorbichew** | tablets 5 mg |
| | **Sorbitrate** | tablets 10 mg, 20 mg |
| | | long-acting products |
| | **Cedocard-Retard** | 20 mg, 40 mg |
| | **Isoket Retard** | 20 mg, 40 mg |
| | **Isordil Tembids** | 40 mg |
| | **Sorbid-SA** | 20 mg, 40 mg |
| | **Isoket injection** | 500 mg |
| isosorbide mononitrate | **Elantan** | tablets 10, 20, 40 mg |
| | **Ismo** | tablets 10, 20, 40 mg |
| | **Isotrate** | tablets 20 mg |
| | **Monit** | tablets 10, 20 mg |
| | **Mono-Cedocard** | tablets 10, 20, 40 mg |
| | | long-acting products |
| | **Elantan LA** | capsules 25 mg, 50 mg |
| | **Imdur** | capsules 60 mg |
| | **Ismo Retard** | tablets 40 mg |
| | **MCR-50** | capsules 50 mg |
| | **Monit SR** | tablets 40 mg |
| | **Monomax SR** | capsules 40 mg |

**Table 4  Drugs used in angina.** Continued over.

| Approved names | Brand names | Products |
|---|---|---|
| **nitrates** | | |
| pentaerythritol tetranitrate | **Mycardol** | tablets 30 mg |
| **beta–blockers** | | |
| acebutolol | **Sectral** | capsules 100 mg, 200 mg<br>tablets 400 mg |
| atenolol | **Tenormin** | tablets 25, 50, 100 mg |
| bisoprolol | **Emcor, Monocr** | tablets 5 mg, 10 mg |
| metoprolol | **Betaloc, Lopresor** | tablets 50 mg, 100 mg |
| nadolol | **Corgard** | tablets 40 mg, 80 mg |
| oxprenolol | **Trasicor**<br>**Slow-Trasicor** | tablets 20 mg, 40 mg, 80 mg<br>tablets 160 mg |
| pindolol | **Visken** | tablets 5 mg, 15 mg |
| propranolol | **Inderal**<br>**Inderal–LA** | tablets 10, 40, 80 mg<br>tablets 160 mg |
| **calcium channel blocking agents** | | |
| amlodipine | **Istin** | tablets 5mg, 10 mg |
| diltiazem | **Adizem**<br>**Tildiem** | tablets 60 mg<br>tablets 60 mg |
| (long-acting diltiazem products are:<br>Adizem-XL, Angil SR, Calcicard CR, Diazem SR, Diazem XL, Slozem,<br>Tildiem LA, Tildiem Retard) | | |
| felodipine | **Plendil** | tablets 5 mg, 10 mg |
| nicardipine | **Cardene** | tablets 20 mg, 30 mg |
| nifedipine | **Adalat** | capsules 5 mg, 10 mg |
| (long-acting nifedipine products are:<br>Adalat LA, Adalat Retard, Adipine MR, Angiopine MR, Cardilate MR,<br>Coracten, Hypolar Retard, Nifelease, Nifensar XL, Unipine XL) | | |
| verapamil | **Cordilox**<br>**Securon** | tablets 40, 80, 120, 160 mg<br>tablets 40 mg, 80 mg, 120 mg |
| **Potassium channel activator** | | |
| nicorandil | **Ikorel tablets** | 10 mg, 20 mg |

# Anxiety

Anxiety states may manifest themselves in a variety of ways from a general sense of uneasiness to acute panic attacks. The symptoms may also vary widely, from a minor physical disturbance such as dryness of the mouth and sweating of the hands and 'butterflies in the stomach' to breathlessness, hyperventilation and lightheadedness. Emotional stress often precipitates anxiety, and drug treatment is useful when the cause of the stress is ill-defined or cannot be removed. Such treatment should always be regarded as a short-term measure, as the prolonged use of anxiolytics involves the risks of dependence and the problems of eventual withdrawal. For such short-term treatment of severe anxiety, a benzodiazepine such as diazepam is often the drug of choice, but other drugs such as buspirone are also in use. Some of the potent antipsychotic agents are also given in small doses for the relief of anxiety. The beta-blockers are occasionally useful in controlling some of the symptoms of anxiety, when the possibility of stress can be anticipated, as in public speaking or performance.

117

Anxiety

| Approved name | Brand name | Daily dose range |
|---|---|---|
| alprazolam | Xanax | 750–1500 µg |
| bromazepam | Lexotan | 3–18 mg |
| chlordiazepoxide | Librium | 30–100 mg |
| clorazepate | Tranxene | 7.5–22.5 mg |
| diazepam | Atensine, Valium | 5–30 mg |
| lorazepam | Ativan | 2.5–10 mg |
| oxazepam | | 45–120 mg |

Table 5 Benzodiazepine anxiolytics.

# Asthma

Bronchial asthma is a spasmodic obstructive disease of the airways, and symptoms may vary from wheeziness to severe bronchoconstriction that can be fatal. Attacks may be precipitated by exposure to allergens, which may vary from house dust to pollen, fungal spores and animal hair. In some susceptible patients certain drugs, including aspirin, may initiate a severe asthmatic attack. Treatment is basically with drugs that have a relatively selective bronchodilatory action, and, in the case of those drugs given by aerosol inhalation, patients must be given careful instruction in the use of the inhaler device if the optimum response is to be obtained. Ephedrine and isoprenaline have been used in asthma, but have been virtually replaced by salbutamol and other more selective $\beta_2$-adrenoceptor stimulants. Adrenaline also has a powerful bronchodilator action, but it may cause cardiac arrhythmias, and it is now used mainly in acute anaphylaxis. (See page 10.)

Salbutamol, now widely used, may be given orally by aerosol inhalation, or, in acute conditions, by injection. Ipratropium and oxitropium are anticholinergic agents with a relatively selective bronchodilator action, and are of value in patients who cannot tolerate sympathomimetic agents of the salbutamol type. Other bronchodilators are the xanthines aminophylline and theophylline, but side-effects may limit their use. Some long-acting xanthine products have a sustained action associated with reduced side-effects, but such products are not necessarily bio-equivalent, and a change from one product to another should not be made without good cause. Corticosteroids are also of value in both the prophylaxis and treatment of asthma, and those given by inhalation are beclomethasone, budesonide and fluticasone. The recently introduced salmeterol is a derivative of salbutamol intended for use together with inhaled corticosteroid therapy in the prophylactic treatment of asthma. It has a slow initial action, but twice daily treatment is claimed to give relief over 24 hrs. Other drugs for the prophylaxis of asthma are sodium cromoglycate and nedocromil, given by oral inhalation of a dry powder. Ketotifen is an antihistamine with some of the properties of sodium cromoglycate.

| Approved names | Brand names |
|---|---|
| **selective β2 stimulants** | |
| bambuterol | **Bambec** |
| eformoterol | **Foradil** |
| fenoterol | **Berotec** |
| reproterol | **Bronchodil** |
| salbutamol | **Salbulin,** } **oral**<br>**Ventolin, Volmax** }<br><br>**Aerolin Autohaler,** } **aerosol inhalation**<br>**Salbulin, Ventolin** } **products** |
| salmeterol | **Serevent** |
| terbutaline | **Bricanyl, Monovent** |
| tulobuterol | **Respacal** |
| **other stimulants** | |
| orciprenaline | **Alupent** |
| oxitropium | **Oxivent** |
| **xanthines** | |
| aminophylline | **Pecram, Phyllocontin Continus** |
| theophylline | **Choledyl, Lasma, Nuelin,**<br>**Slo-Phyllin, Theo-Dur, Uniphyllin Continus** |

**Table 6 Anti-asthma drugs.** Continued over.

**Asthma**

| Approved names | Brand names |
| --- | --- |
| **corticosteroids** | |
| beclomethasone | Becotide, Becodisks, Becloforte |
| budesonide | Pulmicort |
| fluticasone | Flixotide |
| **prophylactics** | |
| sodium cromoglycate | Intal |
| ketoprofen | Zaditen |
| nedocromil | Tilade |
| **anticholinergic agents** | |
| ipratropium | Atrovent |
| oxitropium | Oxivent |

# Bell's palsy

Bell's palsy is a unilateral facial paralysis, characterized by sudden onset and pain, usually behind the ear. The cause is unknown, but the symptoms are thought to be due to local swelling and a compression of the facial nerve. Patients should be reassured that the paralysis is unrelated to stroke and spontaneous recovery usually occurs after some weeks. Corticosteroids are effective if the condition is diagnosed early, and prednisolone is given initially in doses of 60–80 mg daily, decreasing by 10 mg every 2 days for about a week. As the palsy may prevent closure of the affected eye, local treatment with artificial tears or liquid paraffin may be required.

| Approved names | Brand names |
| --- | --- |
| hypromellose (artificial tears) | Tears Naturelle Isopto Alkaline & Plain |
| liquid paraffin | Lacri-Lube |
| polyvinyl alcohol | Hypotears |
| prednisolone | Deltacortril, Deltastab, Precortisyl, Prednesol |

Table 7  Drugs given for Bell's palsy.

121

Bell's palsy

# Cancer

The treatment of cancer is difficult because cancer cells are cells that have escaped from the controls that govern normal cell growth and differentiation of function. As a result, uncoordinated growth may develop rapidly, and cancer cells may migrate and invade other tissues. Any anti-cancer drug is therefore likely to damage normal cells, particularly actively growing cells such as those of the bone marrow, and the dose of a cytotoxic agent is often a compromise between that having the desired anti-cancer action and that causing toxicity.

The drugs used in the treatment of cancer can be divided into four main groups, which attack the cells at different points. The alkylating agents interfere with the replication and function of DNA, modify protein synthesis, and have correspondingly wide effects. The antimetabolites interfere with cell metabolism by combining with cell enzymes, or by forming abnormal proteins, or otherwise inhibiting normal development. The cytotoxic antibiotics have an action similar to that of the antimetabolites, but they also have radiomimetic properties, and combined radiotherapy may increase the risks of damage to normal cells. These antibiotics, with the exceptions of dactinomycin and bleomycin, also have undesirable cardiotoxic properties, and dosage requires careful control. Amsacrine is a synthetic cytotoxic agent with some of the properties of the antibiotic group. Some recently introduced drugs include docetaxel, gemcitabine, letrozole, paclitaxel, raltitrexed and topotecan.

The vinca alkaloids are a class apart, as they are plant substances, and act at the metaphase stage of cell division. They are used mainly in acute leukaemias and some lymphomas. Vincristine is almost free from any depressive effects on bone marrow function, vinblastine has some degree of myelosuppressive activity but is less neurotoxic. Vindesine occupies an intermediate position. Etoposide is a synthetic drug with some of the properties of the vinca alkaloids. Other and unclassified cytotoxic agents include the platinum complexes carboplatin and cisplatin, used mainly in ovarian cancer, and the enzyme crisantaspase used in acute lymphoblastic leukaemia. Some cancers are hormone dependent, and the symptoms may be controlled by suitable hormone antagonists. Breast cancer for example may respond to aminoglutethimide, anastrozole, formestane, letrozole and toremifene. Prostatic cancer can be treated with anti-androgens such as fosfesterol, bicalutamide, cyproterone and flutamide. Certain hormone analogues such as buserelin, goserelin, leuprorelin and triptorelin are also used in cancer of the prostate. A distressing side-effect of high-dose cytotoxic chemotherapy was severe and intractable nausea and vomiting, which could be so intense that patients have been known to refuse further anti-cancer treatment. The problem has since been resolved by the introduction of potent antiemetics of the ondansetron type. See page 158.

| Approved names | Brand names |
|---|---|
| **alkylating agents** | |
| busulphan | Myleran |
| carmustine | BiCNU |
| chlorambucil | Leukeran |
| cyclophosphamide | Endoxana |
| estramustine | Estracyt |
| ifosfamide | Mitoxana |
| lomustine | CCNU |
| melphalan | Alkeran |
| mustine | Mustine |
| thiotepa | Thiotepa |
| treosulphan | Treosulfan |
| **antimetabolites** | |
| cladribine | Leustat |
| cytarabine | Alexan, Cytosar |
| fludarabine | Fludara |
| fluorouracil | Fluoro-Uracil, Efudix |
| gemcitabine | Gemzar |
| mercaptopurine | Puri-Nethol |
| methotrexate | Maxtrex |
| raltitrexed | Tomudex |
| thioguanine | Lanvis |

Table 8  Anti-cancer drugs. Continued on pages 124–125.

123

Cancer

| Approved names | Brand names |
|---|---|
| **cytotoxic antibiotics** | |
| **bleomycin** | **Bleomycin** |
| **dactinomycin** | **Cosmegen** |
| **daunorubicin** | **DaunoXome** |
| **doxorubicin** | **Doxorubicin** |
| **epirubicin** | **Pharmarubicin** |
| **idarubicin** | **Zavedos** |
| **mitomycin** | **Mitomycin C** |
| **mitozantrone** | **Novantrone** |
| **vinca alkaloids** | |
| **vinblastine** | **Velbe** |
| **vincristine** | **Oncovin** |
| **vindesine** | **Eldesine** |
| **vinorelbine** | **Navelbine** |
| **other agents** | |
| **aldesleukin** | **Proleukin** |
| **amsacrine** | **Amsidine** |
| **bicalutamide** | **Casodex** |
| **carboplatin** | **Paraplatin** |
| **cisplatin** | **Cisplatin** |
| **dacarbazine** | **DTIC** |
| **docetaxel** | **Taxotere** |

| Approved names | Brand names |
| --- | --- |
| **other agents** | |
| etoposide | Vepesid |
| hydroxyurea | Hydrea |
| iritotecan | Campto |
| letrozole | Femara |
| octreotide | Sandostatin |
| paclitaxel | Taxol |
| pentostatin | Nipent |
| procarbazine | Natulan |
| razoxane | Razoxin |
| topotecan | Hycamptin |
| tretinoin | Vesanoid |
| **hormone antagonists** | |
| aminoglutethimide | Orimeten |
| anastrozole | Armidex |
| bicalutamide | Casodex |
| buserelin | Suprefact |
| cyproterone | Cyprostat |
| flutamide | Drogenil |
| formestane | Lentaron |
| goserelin | Zoladex |
| tamoxifen | Emblon, Noltam, Nolvadex, Tamofen |
| torasemide | Torem |

# Cough

Cough is an explosive expiration of air from the lungs, and is a protective mechanism to expel excessive exudate or foreign bodies from the respiratory tract, but other irritant factors may also stimulate the cough reflex. Productive cough should not be suppressed without good cause, such as when the patient finds cough exhausting or prevents sleep, but suppression may then have the undesirable effect of causing retention of sputum. On the other hand, suppression of the dry, useless or unproductive cough may have corresponding advantages. Many soothing and demulcent preparations represented by simple linctus have been used for the symptomatic relief of cough, and another traditional remedy is steam inhalation, assisted by the addition of Friar's balsam and menthol. Expectorant products such as ammonia and ipecacuanha mixture are also used, even though pharmacological proof of their efficacy may be lacking. Cough suppressants, represented by codeine, have a central depressant action on the cough centre, but effective doses may have the disadvantage of causing constipation. Extended use should be avoided because of the possible risk of habituation. The treatment of severe cough in terminal lung cancer is with more potent cough suppressants such as diamorphine or methadone.

| Approved names | Brand names |
| --- | --- |
| codeine linctus | Galcodine |
| pholcodine linctus | Galenophol, Pavocol D, Pholcomed |

Table 9  Cough suppressants.

# Cystitis

Cystitis is an inflammatory disease of the lower urinary tract, more common in women, with painful urinary frequency and urgency, and often with low back pain. It is usually caused by Gram-negative bacteria, particularly *E. coli*, and first-line treatment is ample fluids. Sodium bicarbonate or sodium/potassium citrate is sometimes given to relieve the dysuria by making the urine alkaline. Uncomplicated cystitis usually responds to a wide-range antibiotic, or to trimethoprim, nitrofurantoin, co-trimoxazole, or a quinolone antibacterial agent such as nalidixic acid. Some of the quinolones are also useful for the long-term suppressive treatment of recurrent infections.

| Approved names | Brand names |
|---|---|
| **antibiotics** | |
| ampicillin | Amifen, Penbritin, Vidopen |
| amoxycillin | Almodan, Amoxil |
| cephalosporins<br>  (see Table 34, page 248) | |
| **quinolones** | |
| ciprofloxacin | Ciproxin |
| cinoxacin | Cinobac |
| nalidixic acid | Mictral, Negram, Uriben |
| norfloxacin | Utinor |
| ofloxacin | Tarivid |
| **other agents** | |
| trimethoprim | Ipral, Monotrim, Trimopan |
| co-trimoxazole<br>  (trimethoprim with sulphamethoxazole) | Bactrim, Septrin |
| fosfomycin | Monuril |
| hexamine | Hiprex |
| nitrofurantoin | Furadantin, Macrodanton |

Table 10  Drugs used to treat cystitis.

# Depression

Depression is a natural reaction to disappointment and grief, but it is normally brief and self-limiting. Excessive or prolonged depression is an illness, sometimes without apparent cause, and it appears to be linked with an imbalance in the brain of certain amine substances, including serotonin, that act as neuroregulators. Drug therapy can assist in restoring a normal balance, but prolonged treatment is usually necessary to evoke a full response. The drugs in most frequent use are the tricyclic antidepressants, so-called from their chemical structure, together with the monoamine oxidase inhibitors (MAOIs). All the tricyclic antidepressants have the same general pattern of activity, but some, such as amitriptyline, are more sedative than others. Some related compounds have a similar antidepressant action, but blood counts are essential with mianserin and convulsions have been reported after maprotiline therapy. The monoamine oxidase inhibitors are phenelzine, isocarboxazid and tranylcypromine. They are now used less often, as they are potent drugs that react with many other therapeutic agents, as well as certain food such as cheese, broad beans, pickled herring, and meat/yeast extracts. A new MAOI is moclobemide, which has a more selective and reversible action on the A-form of MAO. Particular care is necessary with tranylcypromine. Fluvoxamine, fluoxetine, paroxetine and sertraline are newer drugs that have a more selective antidepressant action mediated by inhibiting the re-uptake of serotonin. They are referred to collectively as SSRIs (selective serotonin re-uptake inhibitors).

| Approved names | Brand names | Daily dose range |
|---|---|---|
| **tricyclic and similar antidepressants** | | |
| [a]amitriptyline | Lentizol, Tryptizol | 75–150 mg |
| amoxapine | Asendis | 100–300 mg |
| [a]clomipramine | Anafranil | 30–150 mg |
| [a]dothiepin | Prothiaden | 75–150 mg |
| [a]doxepin | Sinequan | 75–300 mg |
| imipramine | Tofranil | 75–200 mg |
| lofepramine | Gamanil | 140–210 mg |
| [a]maprotiline | Ludiomil | 25–150 mg |
| [a,b]mianserin | Bolvidon, Norval | 30–90 mg |
| nortriptyline | Allegron | 30–100 mg |
| [b]protriptyline | Concordin | 15–60 mg |
| [a]trazodone | Molipaxin | 150–300 mg |
| [a]trimipramine | Surmontil | 50–300 mg |
| viloxazine | Vivalan | 300–400 mg |
| **monoamine oxidase inhibitors** | | |
| isocarboxazid | Marplan | 30–60 mg |
| moclobemide | Manerix | 150–600 mg |
| phenelzine | Nardil | 30–90 mg |
| tranylcypromine | Parnate | 10–30 mg |

[a]These drugs have sedative properties that are of value when depression is complicated by anxiety.
[b]Mianserin is a tetracyclic compound.

**Table 11  Antidepressants. Continued over.**

129

Depression

| Approved names | Brand names | Daily dose range |
|---|---|---|
| **selective serotonin re–uptake inhibitors (SSRIs)** | | |
| citalopram | Cipramil | 20–60 mg |
| fluoxetine | Prozac | 20 mg |
| fluvoxamine | Faverin | 100–300 mg |
| mitazapine | Zispin | 15–45 mg |
| paroxetine | Seroxat | 20–50 mg |
| reboxetine | Edronax | 4–8 mg |
| sertraline | Lustral | 50–200 mg |
| **other antidepressants** | | |
| flupenthixol | Fluanxol | 1–3 mg |
| nefazodone | Dutonin | 200–600 mg |
| tryptophan | Optimax | 3–6 g |
| venlafaxine | Efexor | 75–150 mg |

Depression

# Diabetes

Diabetes mellitus is a deficiency caused by a lack of insulin, a specific hormone secreted by the islet cells of the pancreas, or by a failure of the insulin-release mechanism. As a result of that insulin deficiency, carbohydrates and fats are not fully metabolized. Glucose accumulates in the circulation and causes a diuresis, so that polyuria and thirst are troublesome complications. Insulin-dependent diabetes, which occurs mainly in children and young adults, can be controlled by injections of insulin. Soluble insulin is used for rapid treatment and in emergencies, but stabilized patients can be controlled by one of the longer-acting forms of insulin such as insulin-zinc-suspension. Insulin was once obtained from pigs or cattle, but human types of insulin are now available and used to an increasing extent. (See Table 12.)

In middle age, a non-insulin-dependent type of diabetes may develop. In such patients, the natural secretion of insulin still occurs, but the insulin is not released according to metabolic requirements. Release can, however, be induced by treatment with the orally active hypoglycaemic agents referred to as the sulphonylureas, represented by chlorpropamide (see Table 13). The sulphonylureas are most effective in mature patients who are already stabilized on low doses of insulin, or who do not respond to purely dietary control. Patients receiving less than 20 units of insulin daily can usually be transferred directly to an oral drug, but in other cases the transfer should be carried out over a few days. For those patients who do not respond to the sulphonylureas, an alternative is the biguanide metformin. The mode of action differs, as it functions mainly by increasing the peripheral utilization of glucose. Guar gum has some antidiabetic properties, possibly mediated by interfering with the absorption of carbohydrates, and may be a useful supplementary treatment. Oral therapy with any antidiabetic drug is not suitable for juvenile or unstable diabetics.

Diabetic emergencies may be due to keto-acidosis and/or hyper-osmolar coma, or to hypoglycaemia which may also result in coma. The former requires treatment with i.v. soluble insulin, preferably by an i.v. pump system, failing which the insulin should be given by i.m. injection. Hypoglycaemic coma, which may be due to an overdose of insulin, can be treated with the i.v. infusion of 50% glucose solution, or by the injection of glucagon 1mg by any route. (Diazoxide is used in the control of chronic hypoglycaemia which is due to the overproduction of insulin. It has no place in the emergency treatment of diabetic coma.)

131

**Diabetes**

| Product | Brand or other name | Origin | Approximate duration of action in hrs |
|---|---|---|---|
| **Short-acting** | | | |
| Soluble insulin | Soluble | beef | 5–8 |
| | Human Actrapid | human-pyr | |
| | Human Velosulin | human-emp | |
| | Humulin S | human-prb | |
| | Hypurin Neutral | beef | |
| | Velosulin | pork | |
| | Insulin Lispro* | humalog | |
| **Intermediate-acting** | | | |
| Insulin zinc (IZS) (amorphous) | Semitard MC | pork | 18–24 |
| | Hypurin Isophane | beef | |
| | Pork Insulatard | pork | |
| Isophane insulin (a complex with protamine) | Human Insulatard | human-pyr | |
| | Humulin I | human-prb | |
| | Rapitard MC | beef & pork | |
| | Pork Mixtard | pork | |
| Biphasic insulin | Human Mixtard | human-pyr | |
| | Humulin M1–5 | human-prb | |
| Biphasic isophane insulin (a complex with protamine) | Semitard MC | beef/pork | |
| Insulin zinc (IZS) (amorphous) | | | |

*(recombinant human insulin analogue)

| **Long-acting** | | | |
|---|---|---|---|
| Insulin zinc (IZS) (amorphous + crystalline) | Hypurin Lente | beef | 24–36 |
| | Lentard MC | beef/pork | |
| | Human Monotard | human-pyr | |
| | Humulin Lente | human-prb | |
| Insulin zinc (IZS) (crystalline) | Human Ultratard | human-pyr | 24–36 |
| | Humulin Zn | human-prb | |
| Protamine zinc | Hypurin Protamine Zinc | beef | |

Note: Human type insulins are prepared from enzyme-modified pork insulin (emp), or by pro-insulin recombinant biosynthesis (prb), or via precursor yeast DNA technology (pyr).

**Table 12  Insulin products.**

| Approved names | Brand names |
| --- | --- |
| **sulphonylureas** | |
| chlorpropamide | **Diabinase** |
| glibenclamide | **Daonil, Semi-Daonil, Euglucon** |
| gliclizide | **Diamicron** |
| glimepiride | **Amaryl** |
| glipizide | **Glibenese, Minodiab** |
| gliquidone | **Glurenorm** |
| tolazamide | **Tolanase** |
| tolbutamide | **Rastinon** |
| **biguanide** | |
| metformin | **Glucophage** |
| **others** | |
| acarbose | **Glucobay** |
| guar gum | **Guarem** |
| troglitazone* | **Romozin** |

* Note: This new drug, an insulin enhancer, has recently been withdrawn pending investigations of reports of liver damage.

**Table 13 Anti-diabetic drugs.**

133

Diabetes

# Dysmenorrhoea

The pain of dysmenorrhoea is thought to result from uterine contractions, and mild analgesics may be of some value, as may antispasmodics such as alverine. As the contractions appear to be mediated by prostaglandins, drugs that inhibit the enzymes associated with prostaglandin production may be of more value in spasmodic dysmenorrhoea. Such drugs are represented by naproxen and related compounds used in rheumatoid conditions (see page 165) which are best given before the onset of, and continued during, menstruation. In other cases, suppression of ovulation by progestogens may be effective, as may mixed progestogen/oestrogen contraceptive preparations.

| Approved names | Brand names |
| --- | --- |
| alverine | Spasmonal |
| naproxen | Naprosyn |
| **hormones** | |
| dydrogesterone | Duphaston |
| norethisterone | Primolut N, Utovlan |
| progestogen/oestrogen | Controvlar |

Table 14  Drugs used to treat dysmenorrhoea.

# Epilepsy

Epilepsy, thought to be due to a deficiency of the brain neurotransmitter GABA (gamma-amino-butyric acid), is a condition characterized by convulsions, popularly known as fits, which are the result of excessive stimulation of the brain by a variety of factors. The convulsions may vary from generalized seizures (tonic-clonic/*grand mal*); absence seizures (usually in children) with a transient loss of consciousness that may pass in a fraction of a second almost like a daydream; and localized epilepsy without loss of awareness, that may sometimes appear more like a change of mood (*petit mal*). In *status epilepticus*, seizures follow one another with no intervening period of consciousness.

Although most anti-epileptic drugs function by increasing the activity of GABA which stabilizes neuronal membranes, no single drug is yet available that can control all types of seizures. For many years phenobarbitone was the standard treatment and related drugs such as methyphenobarbitone and primidone appear to owe their action to conversion in the body to phenobarbitone, and they all have sedative side-effects.

For grand mal, phenytoin is often a first choice drug, but careful control of dose is necessary, and carbamazepine has a wider range of safety. Ethosuximide is used mainly in petit mal.

Sodium valproate is effective in most types of epilepsy and some benzodiazepines are also of value as anticonvulsants. A new anti-epileptic drug with a more selective mode of action is vigabatrin. Vigabatrin inhibits the activity of the GABA-metabolizing enzyme, and so permits a rise in the brain level of GABA. At present, vigabatrin is used mainly in the treatment of epilepsy not responding to other drugs. Gabapentin, lamotrigine and topiramate are more recently introduced drugs used mainly as adjunctive therapy in partial seizures, and when control is otherwise difficult.

In all cases, any change in treatment should be carried out slowly to prevent the precipitation of rebound seizures. Those drugs used by injection for the control of status epilepticus are indicated thus* in Table 15.

| Approved names | Brand names |
|---|---|
| **Those effective in petit mal:** | |
| phenobarbitone | Luminal |
| methylphenobarbitone | Prominal |
| clonazepam | Rivotril |
| ethosuximide | Emeside, Zarontin |
| sodium valproate | Epilim |
| **Those effective in grand mal and other types of seizure:** | |
| phenobarbitone | Luminal |
| methylphenobarbitone | Prominal |
| carbamazepine | Tegretol |
| chlormethiazole* | Heminevrin |
| clonazepam* | Rivotril |
| diazepam* | Diazemuls, Valium |
| gabapentin | Neurontin |
| lamotrigine | Lamictal |
| lorazepam* | Almazine, Ativan |
| phenytoin* | Epanutin |
| primidone | Mysoline |
| sodium valproate | Epilim |
| topiramate | Topamax |
| vigabatrin | Sabril |

*Indicates those drugs used in status epilepticus.

**Table 15** Anticonvulsants.

# Glaucoma

Glaucoma is an insidious ophthalmic disorder of the elderly, and is characterized by an increase in the intraocular pressure. That rise, if not treated, may lead to damage of the optic nerve and eventual blindness.

The condition is basically due to a reduction in the normal outflow of the aqueous humour through the trabecular network and Schlemm's canal. Treatment is aimed at reducing the formation of the aqueous humour, usually with eye drops containing a beta-blocker. When such treatment is not tolerated or contraindicated, eye drops containing an alpha$_2$-adrenergic receptor agonist such as brimonidine may be useful, either as monotherapy or as adjunctive treatment.

Another approach is the local use of a prostaglandin analogue (latanoprost) which acts by increasing aqueous humour outflow.

Other alternative or supplementary therapy is oral treatment with a carbonic anhydrase inhibitor, which has an indirect action by reducing the amount of sodium bicarbonate in the aqueous humour. Older drugs are represented by the miotics, although they have the disadvantage of causing some blurring of vision.

It must also be remembered that with eye drops of the beta-blocker type, some systemic absorption may occur, so care is necessary when using such eye drops in patients with a history of obstructive disease of the airways such as asthma.

| Approved names | Proprietary names | Product |
|---|---|---|
| **beta-blockers** | | |
| betaxolol | **Beoptic** | eye drops 0.5% |
| carteolol | **Teoptic** | eye drops 1% |
| levobunolol | **Betagan** | eye drops 0.5% |
| mitopranolol | | eye drops 0.1% |
| timolol | **Timoptol** **Glaucol** | eye drops 0.25% |
| **alpha$_2$-agonist** | | |
| brimonidine | **Alphagan** | eye drops 0.13% |
| **prostaglandin** | | |
| latanoprost | **Xalatan** | eye drops 0.01% |
| **carbonic anhydrase inhibitors** | | |
| acetazolamide | **Diamox** | 0.15–1 g daily |
| dorzolamide | **Trusopt** | eye drops 2% |
| **others** | | |
| adrenaline | **Eppy, Simplene** | eye drops 1% |
| dipivefrine | **Propine** | eye drops 0.1% |
| guanethidine | **Ganda** | eye drops 1–3% |
| carbachol | | eye drops 3% |
| pilocarpine | **Carpine, Sno-Pilo** | eye drops 0.5–4% |

Note: Corticosteroids should not be used as eye drops as they may disguise a viral infection, and with extended use both locally and orally may cause a steroid glaucoma.

**Table 16 Drugs used in glaucoma.**

# Gout

Gout is an arthritic inflammation occurring mainly in the joints of the fingers and toes, and predominantly in males. It is due to the local deposition of sodium urate crystals from body fluids saturated with urates. An acute attack of gout may occur without warning and is an inflammatory reaction to the crystals, but the continued deposit of such crystals leads to the slow erosion of the affected joints and the development of gouty accretions known as tophi that are characteristic of chronic gout.

The treatment of acute gout is with high doses of one of the many non-steroidal anti-inflammatory agents now available (NSAIDs). An older but no less effective treatment is the alkaloid colchicine, but its side-effects are often dose-limiting. On the other hand, it has the advantage of being suitable for use in heart failure complicated by gout, as it does not cause fluid retention. Colchicine is also useful in preventing the attacks of acute gout that may occur during the initial stages of treatment of chronic gout with other drugs.

In chronic gout the aim of treatment is the reduction of uric acid formation or the increase of its urinary excretion. Uric acid is formed in the body from purines, a process mediated in part by the enzyme xanthine-oxidase. Inhibition of xanthine-oxidase activity brings about a slow reduction of serum urate levels, and an inhibitory drug of that type is allopurinol. Extended treatment is required to evoke a full response. Allopurinol should not be given during an attack of acute gout, as it may exacerbate the symptoms. Paradoxically the initial use of allopurinol in the treatment of chronic gout may provoke an attack of acute gout, and it is usual to give a course of colchicine or a NSAID prophylactically before allopurinol therapy is commenced. An alternative treatment of chronic gout is the use of drugs that promote the excretion of uric acid, and such uricosuric drugs are represented by probenicid and sulphinpyrazone.

It should be noted that although NSAIDs are used in acute gout, aspirin should not be used as it impairs uric acid excretion, and azapropazone should be used only after other NSAIDs have proved ineffective.

| Approved names | Brand names | Daily dose range |
|---|---|---|
| allopurinol | Zyloric | 100–600 mg |
| colchicine | | 1 mg |
| probenicid | Benemid | 500 mg–2 g |
| sulphinpyrazone | Anturan | 100–600 mg |
| NSAIDs with the exception of aspirin and azapropazone | | |

Table 17 Drugs used to treat gout.

# Heart failure

Heart failure is an inability of the heart to meet all the normal physiological demands of the body. In the early stages heart failure may be noted only on exercise, when the reduction in cardiac efficiency causes shortness of breath. As the condition progresses the heart fails to empty completely, so blood accumulates in the heart, and the back-pressure thus set up leads to further breathlessness, with congestion of the lungs and fluid accumulation which leads to ankle oedema. Basically, treatment is aimed at breaking the vicious circle of heart failure-congestion-oedema-increasing heart weakness.

For mild heart failure, without marked pulmonary oedema, first-line treatment is with a thiazide diuretic, such as bendrofluazide, which by reducing the volume of fluid in the circulation relieves the cardiac work-load and improves the cardiac efficiency (see Table 18). Some of the vasodilatory drugs used in the treatment of hypertension (see page 148) are also of value in heart failure, as the vasodilation they produce lowers the peripheral resistance and so improves the cardiac output.

In more severe heart failure, digoxin, the glycoside of the foxglove, remains the drug of choice. It has a selective stimulatory action on the myocardium, resulting in more powerful and efficient contractions of the heart muscle, and improves the general circulation.

Digoxin also acts on the vagus nerve and reduces the heart rate, and with increased cardiac efficiency the myocardial oxygen demand is reduced. The improvement in the circulation also promotes renal efficiency and relieves the oedema. Digitoxin has a similar action.

Another type of cardiac drug widely used in the treatment of heart failure is the angiotensin-converting enzyme inhibitors (ACE-inhibitors). They prevent the conversion of the inert angiotensin I into angiotensin II, which has a potent pressor action on the arterial vascular system. They are used in conjunction with diuretics and digoxin. Enoximone and milrinone are enzyme inhibitors that have a digoxin-like action on the myocardium, and are used in congestive heart failure not responding to other drugs. Xamoterol is a sympathomimetic agent used only in exercise-induced mild heart failure. It should be withdrawn if the condition deteriorates.

| Approved names | Brand names |
| --- | --- |
| **diuretics** | |
| bendrofluazide | Aprinox, Neo-Naclex |
| See also page 149 | |
| **cardiac glycosides** | |
| digoxin | Lanoxin, Lanoxin-PG |
| digitoxin | |
| **ACE inhibitors** | |
| captopril | Capoten |
| cilazapril | Vascace |
| enalapril | Innovace |
| fosinopril | Staril |
| lisinopril | Carace, Zestril |
| moexipril | Perdix |
| perindopril | Coversyl |
| quinapril | Accupro |
| ramipril | Tritace |
| trandolapril | Gopten, Odrik |

Table 18 Drugs used to treat heart failure. Continued over.

| Approved names | Brand names |
|---|---|
| **others** | |
| enoximone | Perfan |
| milrinone | Primacor |
| prazocin | Hypovase |
| xamoterol | Corwin |
| See also page 141 | |

**mixed products**

Accuretic (contains quinapril and hydrochlorothiazide)

Acezide (contains captopril and hydrochlorothiazide)

Capozide (contains captopril and hydrochlorothiazide)

Carace Plus (contains lisinopril and hydrochlorothiazide)

Innozide (contains enalapril and hydrochlorothiazide)

Zestoretic (contains lisinopril and hydrochlorothiazide)

**cardiac (inotropic) stimulants**

| | |
|---|---|
| dobutamine | Dobutrex, Posiject |
| dopamine | |
| dopexamine | Dopacard |

143

**Heart failure**

# Herpes simplex and other viral infections

Herpes simplex or cold sore is a recurrent viral infection, which appears as a small cluster of vesicles, filled with clear fluid in an inflamed area. It usually appears on the lips and mucosa, but genital herpes can also occur. (Herpes simplex keratitis is a viral infection of the eye.) Herpes zoster is a related but more severe skin condition. Treatment is with antiviral drugs such as idoxuridine, acyclovir and penciclovir applied locally; acyclovir, famciclovir and valaciclovir are also given orally. In severe and systemic infections, acyclovir is given by i.v. infusion. In immunocompromised patients, acyclovir is also given orally for long-term prophylaxis. Inosine pranobex is also used in the treatment of superficial herpes, and as auxiliary therapy in genital warts. Didanosine, lamivudine, stavudine, zalcatabine and zidovudine are reversed transcriptase inhibitors, used in the treatment of AIDS; ganciclovir and foscarnet are of value in AIDS-associated cytomegalovirus (CMV) infections, particularly CMV retinitis.

| Approved names | Brand names |
| --- | --- |
| acyclovir | Zovirax |
| famciclovir | Famvir |
| penciclovir | Vectavir |
| tribavarin | Virazid |
| valciclovir | Valtrex |
| **Drugs used in AIDS and CMV infections** | |
| cidovir | Vistide |
| didanosine | Videx |
| foscarnet | Foscavir |
| ganciclivir | Cymevene |
| lamivudine | Epivir |
| ritonavir | Norvir |
| saquinavir | Invirase |
| stavudine | Zerit |
| zalcatabine | Hivid |
| zidovudine | Retrovir |

Table 19 Drugs used to treat herpes simplex.

145

Herpes simplex and
other viral infections

# Hyperlipidaemia

Coronary atherosclerosis and associated conditions are linked with a high plasma level of cholesterol and triglycerides. Those plasma lipids are not present as such, as they are protein bound, and circulate as macromolecular complexes termed lipoproteins. They can be divided into very low-density lipoproteins (VLDL), low-density lipoproteins (LDL) and a very high-density fraction (VHDL). Most of the plasma cholesterol is transported by LDL, and a high level of LDL is associated with increased cardiovascular risks. High levels of LDL can be reduced to some extent by a low-fat diet, but therapy by the use of plasma lipid-lowering drugs is often required.

Nicotinic acid reduces the formation of LDL in the liver, but the high doses necessary, up to 3 g daily, cause marked peripheral vasodilation, a side-effect that makes the drug unacceptable by many patients. Nicofuranose and acipimox, which are derivatives of nicotinic acid, have a similar but less intense vasodilatory action. Probucol, an unrelated compound, appears to act at an early stage of cholesterol synthesis, and to promote the clearance of LDL. Fish oil lowers triglyceride levels, but reliance is largely placed on the use of ion-exchange resins, represented by cholestyramine, and on drugs of the clofibrate group. The exchange resins bind bile acids in the intestines, and interrupt the enterohepatic circulation of bile acids by preventing their re-absorption. The metabolic synthesis of cholesterol from bile acids is thus indirectly inhibited. That inhibition leads to a mobilization of cholesterol from stores in the liver, or withdrawal from cholesterol-containing LDL. The result is a slow lowering of both cholesterol and LDL plasma levels, but prolonged treatment is necessary.

Clofibrate and similar drugs reduce plasma triglyceride levels by stimulating the enzyme lipoprotein lipase. They also reduce cholesterol levels, but to a lesser extent. The side-effects of the clofibrate group include nausea and abdominal discomfort and care is necessary in renal impairment. Clofibrate increases biliary excretion of cholesterol, and accelerates gall stone formation. With gemfibrozil, blood and liver function tests should be carried out before and during treatment. A new approach to the problem of hyperlipidaemia is the use of selective enzyme inhibitors.

Cholesterol is synthesized to a great extent in the liver, and one of the enzymes concerned in that complex process is referred to as HMG-CoA reductase. Simvastatin, fluvastatin, atorvastatin and pravastatin are inhibitors of that enzyme, and so prevent further cholesterol synthesis. Plasma levels of cholesterol are maintained by drawing on reserves of the liver, and as those reserves dwindle the plasma levels of cholesterol gradually fall. These drugs are used in hyperlipidaemia not responding to other therapy, and, as extended treatment is necessary, liver function tests should be carried out at intervals of 4–6 weeks. Side-effects are constipation, nausea, abdominal pain, rash and diarrhoea.

| Approved names | Brand names | Daily dose |
|---|---|---|
| **nicotinic acid and derivatives** | | |
| nicotinic acid | | 1–6 g |
| acipimox | Olbetam | 500–750 mg |
| **exchange resins** | | |
| cholestyramine | Questran | 12–24 g |
| colestipol | Colestid | 10–30 g |
| **clofibrate and similar drugs** | | |
| bezafibrate | Bezalip | 600 mg |
| ciprofibrate | Modalim | 100 mg |
| clofibrate | Atromid-S | 2 g |
| fenofibrate | Lipantil | 300 mg |
| gemfibrozil | Lopid | 1–2 g |
| **enzyme inhibitors** | | |
| atorvastatin | Lipitor | 10 mg |
| fluvastatin | Lescol | 20–40 mg |
| pravastatin | Lipostat | 10–40 mg |
| simvastatin | Zocor | 10–40 mg |
| **others** | | |
| fish oil | Maxepa | 10 g |

Table 20 Antihyperlipidaemic drugs.

**Hyperlipidaemia**

# Hypertension

Hypertension is a state of continued high blood pressure (diastolic pressure over 95 mmHg). Essential hypertension is of no known or obvious cause, and is often linked with age. Secondary hypertension may be caused by renal disease, pregnancy or rarely by an adrenaline-producing tumour (phaeochromocytoma). Treatment is aimed at reducing the elevated blood pressure to a level consistent with the age and condition of the patient, and not to an artificially low level that might reduce the blood supply to essential organs such as the kidneys. The range of drugs used in hypertension is extensive and combined therapy with drugs that act at different points may give the best overall control.

Beta-adrenoceptor blocking agents (beta-blockers) of which propanolol is one of many, are in wide use (see Table 21), and are often given in association with thiazide diuretics (see bendrofluazide). The calcium channel blocking agents used in angina are also effective in hypertension, but are indicated mainly in patients not responding to other therapy. Another approach to the treatment of hypertension is the use of angiotensin-converting enzyme inhibitors (ACE inhibitors). These drugs act by inhibiting the formation of angiotensin II, the most powerful natural pressor substance, and are highly effective as blood pressure lowering agents. They also have applications in the treatment of heart failure. In general they are well tolerated, but initial therapy requires care, as they bring about a marked first-dose fall in blood pressure, and a first dose should be taken at night with the patient in bed. Losartan and valsartan act at a later stage, as they function as angiotensin II antagonists.

Other hypertensive drugs act by blocking alpha-adrenoceptors, and may also cause a first-dose hypotension. Other drugs in less frequent use are represented by bethanidine, debrisoquine, guanethidine, hydralazine and methyldopa. Minoxidil is given in severe hypertension resistant to other drugs; clonidine, diazoxide and sodium nitroprusside are given by i.v. in the control of hypertensive crisis.

| Approved names | Brand names |
|---|---|
| **beta-adrenoceptor blocking agents (beta-blockers)** | |
| acebutolol | Sectral |
| atenolol | Tenormin |
| betaxolol | Kerlone |
| bisoprolol | Emcor, Monocor |
| carvedilol | Eucardic |
| celiprolol | Celectol |
| esmolol | Brevibloc |
| labetalol | Trandate |
| metoprolol | Betaloc, Lopressor, Betaloc SA*, Lopresor SR* |
| nadolol | Corgard |
| oxprenolol | Trasicor, Slow-Trasicor* |
| pindodol | Visken |
| sotalol | Beta-Cardone, Sotacor |
| timolol | Betim, Blocadren |

* Long-acting products

| thiazide and other diuretics | |
|---|---|
| amiloride** | Midamor |
| bendrofluazide | Aprinox, Berkozide, Centyl, Neo-Naclex |
| bumetanide* | Burinex |
| carenoate*** | Spiroctan-M |
| chorothiazide | Saluric |
| chlorthalidone | Hygroton |
| cyclopenthiazide | Navidrex |
| ethacrynic acid* | Edecrin |

**Table 21 Antihypertensive drugs.** Continued on pages 150–152.

| Approved names | Brand names |
|---|---|
| **thiazide and other diuretics** | |
| frusemide* | Lasix |
| hydrochlorothiazide | HydroSaluric |
| hydroflumethiazide | Hydrenox |
| indapamide | Natrilix |
| mefruside | Baycaron |
| metolazone | Netinex S |
| piretanide* | Arelix |
| polythiazide | Nephril |
| spironolactone*** | Aldactone, Spiroctan |
| toresamide* | Torem |
| triamterene** | Dytac |
| xipamide | Diurexan |

\* loop  \*\* potassium-sparing  \*\*\* aldosterone antagonists

| | |
|---|---|
| **calcium channel blocking agents** | |
| amlodipine | Istin |
| diltiazem | Britiazem, Tildiem |
| felodipine | Plendil |
| isradipine | Prescal |
| lacidipine | Motens |
| nicardipine | Cardone |
| nifedipine | Adalat, Adipine, Coracten |
| nimodipine | Nimotop |
| verapamil | Berkatens, Cordilox, Securon, Securon SR*, Univer* |

*Sustained release

| Approved names | Brand names |
|---|---|
| **ACE inhibitors** | |
| captopril | Acepril, Capoten |
| cilazapril | Vascace |
| enalapril | Innovace |
| fosinopril | Staril |
| lisinopril | Carace, Zestril |
| meoxipril | Perdix |
| perindopril | Coversyl |
| quinapril | Accupro |
| ramipril | Tritace |
| trandolapril | Gopten, Odrik |

* Acezide and Capozide contain captopril and hydrochlorthiazide

| angiotensin II receptor antagonists | |
|---|---|
| losartan | Cozaar |
| valsartan | Diovan |

| others | |
|---|---|
| bethanidine | Bendogen |
| clonidine | Catapres |
| debrisoquine | Declinax |
| diazoxide | Eudemine |
| doxazocin | Cardura |
| guanethidine | Ismelin |
| hydralazine | Apresoline |
| indoramin | Baratol |
| methyldopa | Aldomet |
| minoxodil | Loniten |

151

**Hypertension**

| Approved names | Brand names |
| --- | --- |
| others | |
| phenoxybenzamine | Dibenyline |
| phentolamine | Rogitine |
| prazocin | Hypovase |
| sodium nitroprousside | Nipride |
| terazocin | Hytrin |

# Insomnia

Insomnia is a common condition, and with advancing age the total sleep period tends to shorten, and become more interrupted. It is sometimes more apparent than real, as although insomniacs may have a disturbed sleep pattern, they may in fact sleep more than they realize. Initial insomnia, or difficulty in falling asleep, may be due to anxiety, whereas early morning awakening, after which the individual finds difficulty in falling asleep again, may be associated with depression, or be merely part of the ageing process. In all cases, before any treatment is instituted, any underlying cause of the insomnia such as cough or pain should be dealt with, and any stimulants should be avoided.

The drugs used to treat insomnia include sedatives and hypnotics. Sedatives reduce mental activity and predispose to sleep, whereas hypnotics are sleep-inducing drugs, but there is no sharp distinction, as small doses of hypnotics may have a useful sedative effect. Barbiturates were once widely used as hypnotics, but as tolerance and dependence may easily occur, their use has declined sharply since the introduction of the hypnotic benzodiazepines represented by nitrazepam. These drugs are suitable for the short-term treatment of insomnia, and are best given about 30 minutes before bedtime. Some have a longer action than others, and may have hangover effects, and with extended treatment may have a cumulative action. Chloral is a time-honoured hypnotic which is also suitable in small doses for children; triclofos is a chloral derivative. Promethazine is an antihistamine that is also used as a mild hypnotic. Chlormethiazole is more suitable for elderly patients as it has few after-effects. Zolpidem and zopiclone are new and unrelated hypnotics. Any treatment with a hypnotic should be withdrawn slowly to reduce any rebound insomnia.

| Approved names | Brand names | Daily dose range |
| --- | --- | --- |
| **benzodiazepines** | | |
| flunitrazepam | Rohypnol | 0.5–2 mg |
| flurazepam | Dalmane | 15–30 mg |
| loprazolam | | 1–2 mg |
| lormetazepam | | 0.5–1.5 mg |
| nitrazepam | Mogadon, Somnite | 5–10 mg |
| temazepam[a] | Normisan | 10–40 mg |
| **other hypnotics** | | |
| chloral hydrate | Notec | 0.5–2 g |
| chloral betaine | Welldorm | 0.5–2 g |
| chlormethiazole | Heminevrin | 192–384 mg |
| promethazine | Phenergan, Sominex | 25–50 mg |
| triclofos | | 1–2 g . |
| zolpidem | Stilnoct | 5–10 mg |
| zopiclone | Zimovane | 7.5–15 mg |

[a]short-acting hypnotic

**Table 22 Hypnotics.**

153

Insomnia

# Migraine

Migraine is an episodic condition characterized by severe headache, visual disturbances, nausea and vomiting. The flashes of light that occur may be due to cerebral vasoconstriction, but the headache is thought to be linked with vasodilation of the cranial arteries. The cause is unknown, but some apparently innocuous dietary products such as chocolate or cheese may initiate an attack, and oral contraceptives may both precipitate migraine and increase the severity of an established attack. Some cases of migraine may respond to simple analgesics like aspirin and paracetamol, but more potent treatment is usually required. Ergotamine is often the first choice, as it constricts the cranial arteries, but it has little effect on the visual disturbances, and may even increase the nausea and vomiting, and require antiemetic therapy (see page 158). When vomiting is a problem, ergotamine can be given by aerosol inhalation or by suppository. Isometheptene is a sympathomimetic agent and has vasoconstrictor properties that are also useful in the treatment of migraine.

For the prophylactic treatment of migraine reliance is often placed on pizotifen, which has some antiserotonin and anti-histaminic properties, but it may bring about an increase in weight. Cyproheptadine has similar properties and uses. Beta-blockers and some tricyclic antidepressants such as propanolol are also used in the prophylaxis of migraine, and the use of a long-acting product may permit a single daily dose (see page 66). Methysergide is used in the prophylaxis of very severe migraine not responding to other drugs, but it may cause fibrotic reactions, and is used only under hospital supervision.

More recently, it has become clear that serotonin ($5–HT_1$-) has a more specific action in bringing about cranial vasoconstriction, an effect mediated via the $5–HT_1$-like receptors. A serotonin analogue with a selective action on those receptors is sumatriptan. It is given in doses of 6 mg by s.c. injection via an auto-injection device as soon as possible after an attack of migraine has begun, when it gives rapid relief of migraine and cluster headache. A second dose if required may be given after 1 hour up to a maximum dose of 12 mg in 24 hours. Like ergotamine, sumatriptan is not suitable for prophylaxis. Naratriptan and zolmitriptan are newer $5–HT_1$ agonists for the treatment of acute migraine. Recently aspirin in doses of 75 mg daily has been used in the prophylaxis of migraine, particularly during pregnancy, where other drugs may have adverse effects on the fetus.

| Approved names | Brand names |
| --- | --- |
| ergotamine | Cafergot*, Lingraine, Migril*, Medihaler-Ergotamine |
| clonidine | Dixarit |
| cyproheptadine | Periactin |
| isometheptene | Midrid* |
| methysergide | Deseril |
| naratriptan | Naramig |
| pizotifen | Sanomigran |
| sumatriptan | Imigran |
| zolmitriptan | Zomig |

* These are mixed products with supplementary drugs such as caffeine or
paracetamol. Migraleve, Migraves and Faramax are antiemetic products containing
metoclopramide with a mild analgesic.

**Table 23 Drugs used to treat migraine.**

# Myocardial infarction

Myocardial infarction, often referred to as coronary thrombosis or a heart attack, is a sudden reduction in the flow of blood to part of the myocardium (but mainly the left ventricle), and is associated with the presence of a blood clot. It is characterized by a severe and prolonged angina-like pain and cardiac arrhythmias. The pain is seldom relieved by glyceryl trinitrate (unlike angina pectoris), and injections of morphine, buprenorphine or a similar powerful analgesic may be required, but remedial treatment is with a fibrinolytic agent, given as soon as possible by i.v. injection. Other treatment is with drugs of the lignocaine type to control the cardiac arrhythmias, together with digoxin and diuretics for the heart failure. Subsequent long-term control involves the use of beta-blockers, specific anti-arrhythmic agents, lipid-lowering drugs, exchange resins, enzyme inhibitors, platelet stabilizers and anticoagulants. See Hyperlipidaemia (page 146).

| Approved names | Brand names |
|---|---|
| **fibrinolytic/thrombolytic agents** | |
| alteplase | Actilase |
| anistreplase | Eminase |
| reteplase | Rapilysin |
| streptokinase | Kabikinase, Streptase |
| urokinase | Ukidan |
| **anti-arrhythmics** | |
| disopyramide | Rythmodan |
| flecainide | Tambocor |
| lignocaine | Xylocard |
| **beta-blockers** | |
| atenolol | Tenormin |
| metoprolol | Betaloc, Lopresor |
| propranolol | Inderal, Apsolol, Berkolol, Cardinol |
| timolol | Betim, Blocadren |
| **platelet stabilizers** | |
| aspirin | Angettes, Platet |
| dipyridamole | Persantin |

Note: Many of the auxiliary drugs used in the management of post-myocardial infarction conditions are also those used in the treatment of hypertension, and are referred to on page 148, Table 21.

**Table 24 Drugs used in myocardial infarction.**

# Nausea and vomiting

Nausea and vomiting can be triggered off by a number of factors, ranging from gastric irritation, including that caused by drugs, disturbances of balance such as vertigo, or by pregnancy and travelling. The condition is ultimately linked with a stimulation of the vomiting centre of the brain, and most antiemetics function by an action on that centre. The alkaloid hyoscine is widely used in travel sickness, as are the antihistamines, and for the best results should be taken prophylactically before a journey. As an alternative to oral therapy, a skin patch containing hyoscine may be used to obtain an extended action. Many of these antiemetics have sedative side-effects, and they should not be used routinely in the vomiting of pregnancy. Some antipsychotic agents of the chlorpromazine type have a more selective action, as they are dopamine antagonists and have a blocking action on the chemoreceptor trigger zone of the vomiting centre. Domperidone and nabilone are other powerful antiemetics with similar uses.

It has long been known that the vomiting reflex is stimulated by the release of serotonin in the gut, and metoclopramide has an antiemetic action, mediated in part at least by serotonin blockade. It has been given in high doses in the severe nausea and vomiting caused by chemotherapeutic agents in the treatment of cancer where the nausea could be so intense that patients have refused further treatment. Recently it has been shown that a sub-group of serotonin receptors (the 5–HT$_3$ receptors) is linked with the initiation of the vomiting reflex. Specific drugs for the blockade of 5–HT$_3$ receptors are now available (Table 25), and their introduction has opened a new approach to the problem of controlling the severe nausea and vomiting in patients receiving high doses of cyclophosphamide and similar drugs in bone marrow transplants and other conditions associated with severe nausea and vomiting.

| Approved names | Brand names |
| --- | --- |
| hyoscine | Scopoderm TTS (skin patch) |
| **antihistamines** | |
| cinnarizine | Stugeron |
| cyclizine | Valoid |
| dimenhydrinate | Dramamine |
| promethazine | Phenergan |
| promethazine theoclate | Avomine |
| **chlorpromazine group** | |
| chlorpromazine | Largactil |
| perphenazine | Fentazin |
| prochlorperazine | Buccastem, Stemetil, Vertigon |
| thiethylperazine | Torecan |
| **5–HT$_3$ antagonists** | |
| granisetron | Kytril |
| ondansetron | Zofran |
| tropisetron | Navoban |
| **others** | |
| metoclopramide | Gastromax, Maxolon |
| nabilone | Cesamet |

Table 25 Antiemetics.

# Parkinsonism

Parkinsonism is a degenerative disease associated with a progressive reduction in the amount of dopamine, a neurotransmitter substance formed in the substantia nigra of the brain. As a result, the normal balance between the brain levels of dopamine and acetylcholine is disturbed, and is the basic cause of the tremor, muscular rigidity and slowness characteristic of parkinsonism. For many years the only treatment was the anticholinergic agents, and they remain of value in controlling the rigidity and tremor of mild forms of the illness. Amantadine is an unrelated drug with reduced side-effects, but some patients may fail to respond, and tolerance may limit its value.

Although parkinsonism is due to a dopamine deficiency, dopamine cannot be given directly as replacement therapy as it is poorly absorbed, and does not cross the blood-brain barrier, and its amino acid precursor, levodopa, although better absorbed, is inactivated to some extent by liver enzymes, and so fails to reach the brain in a fully effective concentration. The problem can be partly overcome by giving levodopa together with a specific inhibitor such as benserazide or carbidopa. The combination permits a larger amount of levodopa to reach the brain where it is converted to active dopamine. Additional therapy with an anticholinergic agent may improve the response, and in some cases permit a reduction in the 'end-of-dose' loss of symptomatic control. Selegiline acts upon another enzyme, and is given together with levodopa in severe parkinsonism. Bromocriptine is a secondary drug that appears to act by stimulating any surviving dopamine receptors in the brain, but side-effects may limit its value. Lysuride is a new drug with a similar stimulatory action.

Pergolide is another new dopamine agonist that acts on both $D_1$ and $D_2$ receptors. Combined treatment with these auxiliary drugs, and careful adjustment of doses, including those of levodopa, may improve the overall response, reduce the severity of side-effects, and possibly delay further deterioration of the patient's condition.

| Approved names | Brand names |
|---|---|
| **anticholinergic/antimuscarinic agents** | |
| **benzhexol** | **Artane, Broflex** |
| **benztropine** | **Cogentin** |
| **biperidon** | **Akineton** |
| **orphenadrine** | **Biorphen, Disipal** |
| **procyclidine** | **Arpicolin, Kemadrin** |
| **levodopa and mixed products** | |
| **levodopa** | **Larodopa** |
| **co-beneldopa** (levodopa with benserazide) | **Madopar** |
| **co-careldopa** (levodopa with carbidopa) | **Sinemet** |
| **others** | |
| **amantadine** | **Symmetrel** |
| **bromocriptine** | **Parlodel** |
| **lysuride** | **Revanil** |
| **pergolide** | **Celance** |
| **ropinirole** | **Requip** |
| **selegiline** | **Eldepryl** |
| **tolcapone** | **Tasmar** |

Note: Apomorphine is sometimes used in refractory and fluctuating Parkinson's disease. Treatment is commenced in hospital, as the drug must be given initially by subcutaneous infusion, together with an antiemetic to control the side-effects of apomorphine. Only well-motivated patients are likely to accept such treatment.

**Table 26  Anti-parkinsonism drugs.**

161

Parkinsonism

# Peptic ulcer

The term peptic ulcer includes gastric ulcer, duodenal ulcer and the less common oesophageal ulcers. It is a medical axiom that 'no acid – no ulcer', and for many years gastric ulcers were treated with antacids such as magnesium trisilicate. Bismuth chelate has a protective action by coating the ulcerated areas, whereas sucralfate appears to act by protecting the gastric mucosa from acid-pepsin attack.

Acid secretion can be suppressed by anti-cholinergic agents and misoprostol is a prostaglandin analogue which also inhibits gastric acid secretion, and it is of value in the prophylaxis of peptic ulcers induced by non-steroidal anti-inflammatory drugs (NSAIDs).

In recent years, reliance has been placed to an increasing extent on the histamine $H_2$-receptor blocking agents, which have a selective inhibitory action on gastric acid secretion, and so promote the healing of peptic ulcers by a more direct attack on the initial cause. Extended treatment with intermittent rest periods is necessary to avoid relapse.

Another approach to the treatment of gastric ulcer is the inhibition of the release of acid from the gastric parietal cells, a process mediated by the enzyme hydrogen/potassium adenosine triphosphatase, the so-called 'proton pump' system. Omeprazole and lansoprazole act as proton pump inhibitors, and are effective in the control of peptic ulcers resistant to other drugs. They are also preferred for the treatment of erosive oesophagitis, and in combination with antibiotics, such as amoxycillin and clarithromycin, are effective in ulcer relapse associated with the presence of *Helicobacter pylori*.

| Approved names | Brand names |
| --- | --- |
| bismuth chelate | De-Noltab |
| carbenoxolone | Pyrogastrone* |
| misoprostol | Cytotec |
| sucralfate | Antepsin |
| H$_2$-receptor blocking agents | |
| cimetidine | Dyspamet, Tagamet, Algitec |
| famotidine | Pepcid |
| nizatidine | Axid |
| ranitidine | Zantac |
| ranitidine bismuth citrate | Pylorid |
| enzyme inhibitors | |
| lansoprazole | Zoton |
| omeprazole | Losec |
| pantoprazole | Protium |

*Also contains antacids.

Table 27  Anti-ulcer drugs.

Peptic ulcer

# Prostatic hyperplasia

Benign prostatic hyperplasia (BPH) is common in men over 50 years of age, and is associated with a varying degree of bladder obstruction and consequent incomplete emptying of the bladder. Such symptoms facilitate infection and may lead to inflammation of the bladder and urinary tract, and cause progressive urinary frequency. Although surgery offers the prospect of radical cure, it is often possible to stabilize the condition in mild cases by medical treatment, and, in those patients awaiting surgery, symptomatic relief may be obtained by drug therapy.

Alpha-adrenergic receptors are present in prostatic tissue, and stimulation of those receptors causes contraction of the smooth muscle of the bladder, and on that basis some alpha-adrenoceptor antagonists have been used for the symptomatic treatment of BPH. Some drugs of that type are also used in hypertension, and a side-effect in BPH is a marked first-dose hypotension.

Androgens are also necessary for prostatic development, so another approach to the treatment of BPH is with anti-androgen therapy. Testosterone is the principal male hormone, but the development of the prostate gland is dependent on the conversion of that hormone to dihydrotestosterone (DHT) within the gland. That conversion is mediated by the enzyme 5-alpha reductase. A selective inhibitor of that enzyme, now available for the treatment of BPH, is finasteride. It is given in daily doses of 5 mg, but prolonged administration is necessary to obtain an adequate shrinking in size of the prostate gland and the corresponding symptomatic relief.

| Approved names | Brand names | Daily dose range |
|---|---|---|
| **alpha–adrenoceptor antagonists** | | |
| **alfusocin** | **Xatral** | **5–10 mg** |
| **doxazocin** | **Cardura** | **1–4 mg** |
| **indoramin** | **Doralese** | **40–100 mg** |
| **prazocin** | **Hypovase** | **1–4 mg** |
| **tamsulosin** | **Flomax** | **400 mg** |
| **tetrazocin** | **Hytrin** | **1–10 mg** |
| **anti–androgen** | | |
| **finasteride** | **Proscar** | **5 mg** |

Note: Some of these alpha-adrenoceptor antagonists are also used in the treatment of hypertension (page 148), and may cause a marked first-dose postural hypertension and collapse. Care is also necessary when giving such a drug to a patient already being treated for hypertension.

**Table 28  Drugs used in benign prostatic hyperplasia.**

# Rheumatoid and osteoarthritis

Rheumatoid arthritis is a chronic inflammatory disease of the joints with local swelling and pain. The cause is unknown and, although partial remission and exacerbations occur, the disease is a progressive one, and in severe conditions bedrest may be necessary. In osteoarthritis, degeneration of the joints also occurs. Treatment is largely symptomatic, and is based on the non-steroidal anti-inflammatory drugs (NSAIDs) of which aspirin is the oldest and one of the most widely used. The NSAIDs have analgesic as well as anti-inflammatory properties, and act by suppressing the production of inflammatory prostaglandins. The choice of a NSAID depends much upon individual response, as they are potential gastric irritants, and are best taken after food. Patients vary widely in their tolerance to any particular NSAID, and the drugs have many side-effects. To obtain prolonged relief at night, and to reduce morning stiffness, some NSAIDs are available as suppositories.

Corticosteroids are used mainly in conditions not responding to NSAIDs, and are sometimes given by direct injection into a joint. In some cases of rheumatoid arthritis, the progression of the disease can be halted for a time by drugs that modify the underlying degenerative process, as with gold salts, penicillamine, and less frequently chloroquine and salazypyrine. Sodium aurothiomalate is a gold compound given by injection, but auranofin is an orally active gold preparation. Some immunosuppressive drugs such as azothioprine have a action similar to that of the gold compounds. The use of all these disease-modifying drugs requires great care. The treatment of gout is referred to on page 140.

| Approved names | Brand names |
|---|---|
| **non-steroidal anti-inflammatory drugs (NSAIDs)** | |
| aceclofenac | **Preservex** |
| acemetacin | **Emflex** |
| azapropazone | **Rheumox** |
| benorylate | **Benoral** |
| *diclofenac | **Diclomax, Motifene, Voltarol** |
| diflunisal | **Dolobid** |
| etodolac | **Lodine** |
| fenbrufen | **Lederfen** |
| fenoprofen | **Fenopron, Progesic** |
| flurbiprofen | **Froben** |
| ibuprofen | **Apsifen, Brufen, Fenbid, Ibular, Lidofen, Motrin, Paxofen** |
| *indomethacin | **Flexin, Imbrilon, Indocid, Indolar, Indomed, Mobilan, Rheumacin, Slo-Indo** |
| *ketoprofen | **Alrheumat, Orudis, Orivail** |
| mefenamic acid | **Ponstan** |
| nabumetone | **Relifex** |
| *naproxen | **Laraflex, Naprosyn, Synflex** |
| *piroxicam | **Feldene, Larapam** |

**Table 29  Drugs used to treat rheumatoid arthritis. Continued over.**

| Approved names | Brand names |
| --- | --- |
| sulindac | Clinoril |
| tenoxicam | Mobilflex |
| tiaprofenic acid | Surgam |
| tolmetin | Tolectin |
| **gold compounds** | |
| auranofin | Ridura |
| sodium aurothiomalate | Myocrisin |
| **others** | |
| chloroquine | Avloclor, Nivaquine |
| penicillamine | Distamine, Pendramine |
| salazopyrine | Salazopyrin |
| **immunosuppressants** | |
| azathioprine | Azamune, Berkaprine, Imuran |
| chlorambucil | Leukeran |
| cyclophosphamide | Endoxana |
| cyclosporin | Sandimmun Neoral |
| methotrexate | Maxtrex |

* also available as suppositories

Rheumatoid
and osteoarthritis

# Schizophrenia

Schizophrenia is a serious mental disorder, with hallucinations and delusions, a deterioration in thought patterns and reasoning ability, and an increasing disability to distinguish between the imaginary and the real. It may develop slowly, or be a rapid response to stress. In some patients a condition of apathy and withdrawal may be the most prominent symptom. The range of antipsychotic drugs used in the treatment of schizophrenia is wide and extending, as new types of drugs are introduced. The drugs in most frequent use are phenothiazines of the chlorpromazine type referred to as either antipsychotic drugs or major tranquillizers. The different members of the group exhibit certain differences in action, as some may be more effective in controlling the most marked symptoms of schizophrenia, and others may be of more value in apathetic patients, but the distinction is not sharp. In all cases, prolonged treatment is essential, as improvement may be slow, and drug withdrawal should be correspondingly slow, as relapse may occur.

Schizophrenia is considered to be due to an imbalance of certain factors in the brain, and many antipsychotic drugs act by blocking dopamine receptors, thus permitting a rise in the brain level of dopamine. That rise may be associated with some of the side-effects of the chlorpromazine group of drugs. In some cases, improvement once achieved can be maintained by the use of long-acting depot injections of the drug concerned, which reduce to some extent the problems of patient compliance with therapy.

Many other antipsychotic drugs unrelated to chlorpromazine have a basically similar action. Sulpiride is exceptional, as in high doses it can control the more severe forms of schizophrenia, whereas in small doses it has a modifying effect on withdrawn patients.

| Approved names | Brand names |
|---|---|
| **sedative phenothiazines** | |
| chlorpromazine | Largactil |
| methotrimeprazine | Nozinan |
| promazine | Sparine |
| **less sedative phenothiazines** | |
| pericyazine | Neulactil |
| pipothiazine | Piportil |
| thioridazine | Melleril |
| **phenothiazines with increased extra-pyramidal side-effects** | |
| fluphenazine | Moditen |
| perphenazine | Fentazin |
| prochlorperazine | Stemetil, Buccastem |
| trifluoperazine | Stelazine |
| **other antischizophrenics** | |
| clozapine | Clozaril |
| flupenthixol | Depixol |
| haloperidol | Dozic, Serenace |
| loxapine | Loxapac |
| olanzapine | Zyprexa |
| oxypertine | Integrin |
| pimozide | Orap |
| quetiapine | Seroquel |
| risperidone | Risperdal |
| sulpiride | Dolmatil, Sulpitil, Sulparex |
| trifluoperidol | Triperidol |
| zuclopenthixol | Clopixol |

Table 30 Drugs used to treat schizophrenia.

# Tuberculosis

Tuberculosis was once a dreaded and lingering lung infection for which no treatment was known. The incidence of the disease declined with the general improvement in living standards, and at one time was thought to be under control, but the incidence has risen again with the marked changes in migrant populations. Immunocompromised patients may also develop tuberculosis, and the disease was recently described as a 'global emergency'.

The primary infection, due to *Mycobacterium tuberculosis*, is usually mild and asymptomatic, but later the classical symptoms of cough, purulent sputum, haemoptysis and loss of weight develop, as may the risk of spread to other tissues such as the bones and joints. The causative organism is slow-growing, and its waxy coating hinders drug penetration, and the aim of treatment is to reduce the population of the invading organism as soon as possible, and to prevent the emergence of drug-resistant strains of *M. tuberculosis*.

As a rule, antitubercular therapy is commenced with three drugs, isoniazid, rifampicin and pyrazinamide, and continued for 2 months. Further treatment for at least 4 months is with a two-drug dose scheme, usually with isoniazid and rifampicin. Alternative drugs for use when resistance is known or suspected include ethambutol, streptomycin, capreomycin, cycloserine and rifambutin. Pyrazinamide is used for initial treatment only, as it acts mainly on the intracellular and dividing forms of the bacterium. The successful treatment of tuberculosis is essentially long-term, and requires considerable patient compliance.

Most antitubercular drugs have toxic effects on the liver, and hepatic function tests should be carried out before and during treatment, together with tests for renal efficiency. Peripheral neuropathy is an occasional side-effect of isoniazid, and patients should be advised to report any tingling sensation. Pyridoxine 10 mg daily may be given daily for prophylaxis and treatment. A typical dosage scheme is as follows, but others are also in use:

| | |
|---|---|
| isoniazid | 300 mg daily for 6 months; |
| rifampicin | 450–600 mg daily for 6 months; |
| pyrazinamide | 1.5–2 g daily for the first 2 months only. |

For the prophylactic treatment of those in close contact with tuberculous patients, isoniazid may be given alone in doses of 300 mg daily, or together with rifampicin in doses of 600 mg daily for 6 months.

| Approved names | Brand names | Dose |
|---|---|---|
| capreomycin | Capastat | 1 g daily by deep i.m. injection |
| cycloserine | | 500 mg daily for 2 weeks |
| ethambutol | Myambutol | 25 mg/kg daily |
| isoniazid | | 300 mg daily |
| pyrazinamide | Zinamide | 2 g three times a week |
| rifabutin | Mycobutin | 150–400 mg daily |
| rifampicin | Rifadin, Rimactane | 600–900 mg three times a week |
| streptomycin | Rimactane | 1 g daily by deep i.m. injection |

Table 31 Antitubercular drugs.

Tuberculosis

# Ulcerative colitis

Ulcerative colitis is an abnormal condition of the lower intestinal tract, particularly the colon, and is characterized by a breakdown of the mucosal layer with inflammation and ulceration, and attacks of bloody diarrhoea, abdominal pain and dehydration. Remission and recurrence may occur without apparent cause. As the disease progresses, the muscular coat of the intestines may be involved, with further ulceration. Crohn's disease is very similar, but may affect other parts of the intestinal tract. Mild conditions may respond to codeine, but more specific treatment is with sulphasalazine and prednisolone, which may be given orally or as retention enemas, and less frequently azathiaprine is given. Sulphasalazine has certain side-effects associated with the 'sulpha' part of the drug, and the derivatives mesalazine and olsalazine may be better tolerated.

| Approved names | Brand names |
| --- | --- |
| azathioprine | Azamune, Berkaprine, Imuran |
| balsalazide | Colazide |
| mesalazine | Asocol, Pentasa, Salofalk |
| olsalazine | Dipentum |
| prednisolone | Deltacortril Enteric<br>Deltastab<br>Precortisyl<br>Prednesol<br>*Predenema<br>*Predfoam<br>*Predsol |
| sulphasalazine | Salazopyrin |

\* Rectal products

Table 32 Drugs used to treat ulcerative colitis.

Ulcerative colitis

# Urinary incontinence and frequency

Normal urinary control is the result of a complex process involving many factors, including the interaction of both smooth and voluntary muscle. Loss of that control may arise from a variety of causes, including a disturbance of the local nerve supply to the bladder, when the term neurogenic bladder is sometimes used, or it may arise from trauma or infection. Urinary incontinence is characterized by an involuntary passing of urine, which is preceded by an urgent desire to void. Stress incontinence is an uncontrollable loss of urine as a result of coughing, straining or any other activity that brings about a sudden increase in the intra-abdominal pressure. It is more common in women than in men.

Overflow incontinence usually occurs as the result of an obstruction, or of impaired detrusor muscle contraction. The bladder fills until the urinary pressure overcomes the sphincter resistance, and the urine then dribbles from the urethra, whereas frequency may be due to trauma, infection or inflammation. Nocturnal enuresis is the involuntary and periodic urination that occurs during sleep in children, and is more common in boys than in girls.

For symptomatic treatment, reliance is based largely on the anticholinergic agents represented by propantheline. Such agents inhibit the effects of acetycholine on smooth muscle, reduce erratic detrusor muscle contractions and increase stability. The use of certain tricyclic antidepressants in the treatment of frequency and urinary incontinence is also based on their anticholinergic action. Ephedrine is used mainly in enuresis, as it relaxes the detrusor muscle. A few drugs, such as flavoxate, have a direct antispasmodic action. Desmopressin, an analogue of the pressor principle of the posterior pituitary gland, has also been used for the treatment of enuresis. In some cases of cystitis where the urine is acid, the urinary discomfort can be relieved by the alkalinization of the urine by the oral administration of sodium bicarbonate, sodium citrate or potassium citrate. See also page 127.

| Approved names | Brand names |
| --- | --- |
| **anticholinergic/antimuscarinic agents** | |
| oxybutynin | Cystrin, Ditropan |
| propantheline | Pro-Banthine |
| **tricyclic antidepressants** | |
| amitriptyline | Domical, Lentizol, Tryptizol |
| imipramine | Tofranil |
| nortriptyline | Concordin |
| **others** | |
| desmopressin | DDAVP, Desmospray |
| ephedrine | |
| flavoxate | Urispas |

**Table 33 Drugs used in incontinence.**

| Approved name | Proprietary name | Main action or indication |
| --- | --- | --- |
| abciximab | ReoPro | heparin adjunct |
| acamprosate | Campral | alcoholism |
| acarbose | Glucobay | diabetes |
| acebutolol | Sectral | hypertension |
| aceclofenac | Preservex | arthritis |
| acemetacin | Emflex | arthritis |
| acetazolamide | Diamox | glaucoma |
| acetylcysteine | Parvolex | mucolytic; paracetamol overdose |
| aciclovir | Zovirax | antiviral |
| acipimox | Olbetam | hyperlipidaemia |
| acitretin | Neotigason | psoriasis |
| aclarubicin | Aclacin | cytotoxic |
| acrivastine | Semprex | antihistamine |
| actinomycin D | Cosmegen | cytotoxic |
| adapalene | Differin gel | acne |
| adenosine | Adenocor | paroxysmal tachycardia |
| albendazole | Eskazole | anthelmintic |
| alclometasone | Modrasone | topical corticosteroid |
| aldesleukin | Proleukin | cytotoxic |
| alendronic acid | Fosamax | osteoporosis |
| alfacalcidol | One-Alpha | vitamin D deficiency |
| alfentanil | Rapifen | narcotic analgesic |
| alfuzosin | Xatral | prostatic hypertrophy |
| alimemazine | Vallergan | antihistamine |
| allopurinol | Zyloric | gout |

Approved and proprietary names of drugs

| Approved name | Proprietary name | Main action or indication |
|---|---|---|
| alprazolam | Xanax | anxiety |
| alprostadil | Prostin VR | maintenance of ductus arteriosus in neonates |
| alteplase | Actilyse | fibrinolytic |
| altretamine | Hexalen | cytotoxic |
| alverine | Spasmonal | antispasmodic |
| amantadine | Symmetrel | parkinsonism |
| amifostine | Ethylol | cytoprotectant |
| amikacin | Amikin | antibiotic |
| amiloride | Midamor | diuretic |
| aminoglutethimide | Orimeten | cytotoxic |
| aminophylline | Pecram; Phyllocontin | asthma |
| amiodarone | Cordarone | anti-arrhythmic |
| amitriptyline | Lentizol; Tryptizol | antidepressant |
| amlodipine | Istin | calcium antagonist |
| amorolfine | Loceryl | topical antifungal |
| amoxapine | Asendis | antidepressant |
| amoxycillin | Almodan; Amoxil | antibiotic |
| amphotericin B | Fungilin; Fungizone | antifungal |
| ampicillin | Penbritin; Vidopen | antibiotic |
| amsacrine | Amsidine | cytotoxic |
| amylobarbitone | Amytal | hypnotic |
| anastrozole | Arimidex | cytotoxic |
| anistreplase | Eminase | fibrinolytic |
| apomorphine | Britaject | parkinsonism |
| apraclonidine | Iopidine | glaucoma |

177

Approved and proprietary
names of drugs

| Approved name | Proprietary name | Main action or indication |
|---|---|---|
| aprotinin | Trasylol | haemostatic |
| astemizole | Hismanal | antihistamine |
| atenolol | Tenormin | beta-blocker |
| atorvastatin | Lipitor | hyperlipidaemia |
| atovaquone | Malarone<br>Wellvone | antimalarial<br>AIDS |
| atracurium | Tracrium | muscle relaxant |
| auranofin | Ridaura | rheumatoid arthritis |
| azapropazone | Rheumox | antirheumatic |
| azatadine | Optimine | antihistamine |
| azathioprine | Azamune; Imuran | immunosuppressive |
| azelaic acid | Skinoren | acne |
| azelastine | Rhinolast | topical antihistamine |
| azithromycin | Zithromax | antibiotic |
| azlocillin | Securopen | antibiotic |
| aztreonam | Azactam | antibiotic |
| baclofen | Lioresal | muscle relaxant |
| balsalazide | Colazide | ulcerative colitis |
| bambuterol | Bambec | asthma |
| beclomethasone | Becotide;<br>Propaderm | corticosteroid;<br>topical corticosteroid |
| bendrofluazide | Aprinox; Neo-Naclex | diuretic |
| benorylate | Benoral | analgesic |
| benperidol | Anquil | tranquillizer |
| benzhexol | Artane; Broflex | parkinsonism |
| benztropine | Cogentin | parkinsonism |
| benzylpenicillin | Crystapen | antibiotic |

| Approved name | Proprietary name | Main action or indication |
|---|---|---|
| beractant | Survanta | lung surfactant |
| betahistine | Serc | Ménière's syndrome |
| betamethasone | Betnelan; Betnesol; Betnovate | corticosteroid; topical corticosteroid |
| betaxolol | Betopic; Kerlone | beta-blocker; glaucoma |
| bethanechol | Myotonine | smooth muscle stimulant |
| bethanidine | Bendogen | hypertension |
| bezafibrate | Bezalip | hyperlipidaemia |
| bicalutamide | Casodex | cytotoxic |
| biperiden | Akineton | parkinsonism |
| bisacodyl | Ducolax | laxative |
| bisoprolol | Emcor; Monocor | beta-blocker |
| botulinum toxin | Botox; Dysport | blepharospasm |
| bretylium tosylate | Bretylate | cardiac arrhythmias |
| brimonidine | Alphagan | glaucoma |
| bromazepam | Lexcotan | anxiolytic |
| bromocriptine | Parlodel | dopamine agonist |
| bromopheniramine | Dimotane | antihistamine |
| budesonide | Pulmicort; Rhinocort | asthma; rhinitis |
| bumetanide | Burinex | diuretic |
| bupivacaine | Marcaine | anaesthetic |
| buprenorphine | Temgesic | analgesic |
| buserelin | Suprefact | prostatic carcinoma |
| buspirone | Buspar | anxiolytic |

| Approved name | Proprietary name | Main action or indication |
| --- | --- | --- |
| busulphan | Myleran | cytotoxic |
| butobarbitone | Soneryl | hypnotic |
| cabergoline | Cabaser; Dostinex | dopamine agonist |
| cadexomer iodine | Iodosorb | leg ulcers |
| calcipotriol | Dovonex | psoriasis |
| calcitonin | Calcitare | hypercalaemia |
| calcitriol | Rocatrol | vitamin D deficiency |
| canrenoate | Spiroctan-N | diuretic |
| capreomycin | Capastat | antibiotic |
| captopril | Acepril; Capoten | ACE inhibitor |
| carbamazepine | Tegretol | epilepsy |
| cabaryl | Carylderm; Derbac | parasiticide |
| carbenoxolone | Bioplex; Bioral | mouth ulcers |
| carbimazole | Neo-Mercazole | thyrotoxicosis |
| carbocisteine | Mucodyne | mucolytic |
| carboplatin | Paraplatin | cytotoxic |
| carboprost | Hemabate | post-partum haemorrhage |
| carisoprodol | Carisoma | muscle relaxant |
| carmustine | BiCNU | cytotoxic |
| carteolol | Teoptic | glaucoma |
| carvedilol | Eucardic | beta-blocker |
| cefaclor | Distaclor | antibiotic |
| cefadroxil | Baxan | antibiotic |
| cefamandole | Kefadol | antibiotic |
| cefixime | Suprax | antibiotic |
| cefodizime | Timecef | antibiotic |

| Approved name | Proprietary name | Main action or indication |
| --- | --- | --- |
| cefotaxime | Claforan | antibiotic |
| cefoxitin | Mefoxin | antibiotic |
| cefpirome | Cefrom | antibiotic |
| cefpodoxime | Orelox | antibiotic |
| ceftazidime | Fortum | antibiotic |
| ceftibuten | Cedax | antibiotic |
| ceftizoxime | Cefizox | antibiotic |
| ceftriaxone | Rocephin | antibiotic |
| cefuroxime | Zinacef; Zinnat | antibiotic |
| celiprolol | Celectol | hypertension |
| cephalexin | Ceporex; Keflex | antibiotic |
| cephamandole | Kefadol | antibiotic |
| cephazolin | Kefzol | antibiotic |
| cephradine | Velosef | antibiotic |
| cerivastatin | Lipobay | hyperlipidaemia |
| certoparin | Alphaparin | anticoagulant |
| cetirizine | Zirtek | antihistamine |
| chenodeoxycholic acid | Chendol; Chenofalk | gall stones |
| chloral betaine | Welldorm | hypnotic |
| chloral hydrate | Noctec | hypnotic |
| chlorambucil | Leukeran | cytotoxic |
| chloramphenicol | Chloromycetin; Kemicetine | antibiotic |
| chlordiazepoxide | Librium | anxiolytic |
| chlorhexidine | Hibitane | antiseptic |
| chlormethiazole | Heminevrin | hypnotic; anticonvulsant |

Approved and proprietary names of drugs

| Approved name | Proprietary name | Main action or indication |
|---|---|---|
| chloroquine | Avloclor; Nivaquine | antimalarial |
| chlorothiazide | Saluric | diuretic |
| chlorpheniramine | Piriton | antihistamine |
| chlorpromazine | Largactil | tranquillizer |
| chlorpropamide | Diabinese | hypoglycaemic |
| chlortetracycline | Aureomycin | antibiotic |
| chlorthalidone | Hygroton | diuretic |
| cholestyramine | Questran | bile acid binder |
| choline theophyllinate | Choledyl | bronchodilator |
| cidofovir | Vistide | antiviral |
| cilazapril | Vascase | ACE inhibitor |
| cimetidine | Dyspamet; Tagamet | $H_2$-blocker |
| cinchocaine | Nupercainal | local anaesthetic |
| cinnarizine | Stugeron | antiemetic |
| cinoxacin | Cinobac | antibiotic |
| ciprofibrate | Modalim | hyperlipidaemia |
| ciprofloxacin | Ciproxin | antibacterial |
| cisapride | Prepulsid | oesophageal reflux |
| cisatracurium | Nimbex | muscle relaxant |
| citalopram | Cipramil | antidepressant |
| cladribine | Leustat | cytotoxic |
| clarithromycin | Klaricid | antibiotic |
| clemastine | Tavegil | antihistamine |
| clindamycin | Dalacin C | antibiotic |
| clobazam | Frisium | tranquillizer |
| clobetasol | Dermovate | topical corticosteroid |

| Approved name | Proprietary name | Main action or indication |
|---|---|---|
| clobetasone | Eumovate | topical corticosteroid |
| clofazimine | Lamprene | antileprotic |
| clofibrate | Atromid S | hyperlipidaemia |
| clomiphene | Clomid; Serophene | infertility |
| clomipramine | Anafranil | antidepressant |
| clonazepam | Rivotril | epilepsy |
| clonidine | Catapres; Dixarit | hypertension; migraine |
| clorazepate | Tranxene | anxiolytic |
| clotrimazole | Canestan | antifungal |
| cloxacillin | Orbenin | antibiotic |
| clozapine | Clozaril | antipsychotic |
| co-amilofruse | Frumil; Lasoride | diuretic |
| co-amilozide | Amil-co; Moduretic | diuretic |
| co-amoxiclav | Augmentin | antibiotic |
| co-beneldopa | Madopar | parkinsonism |
| co-careldopa | Sinemet | parkinsonism |
| co-codamol | Panadeine; Paracodol; Parake | analgesic |
| co-codaprin | Codis | analgesic |
| co-dergocrine | Hydergine | dementia |
| co-dydramol | Paramol | analgesic |
| co-fluampicil | Magnapen | antibiotic |
| co-flumactone | Aldactide | diuretic |
| colestipol | Colestid | exchange resin |
| colfosceril | Exosurf | neonatal respiratory distress |
| colistin | Colomycin | antibiotic |

Approved and proprietary names of drugs

| Approved name | Proprietary name | Main action or indication |
|---|---|---|
| co-phenotrope | Lomotil | diarrhoea |
| co-prenozide | Trasidrex | hypertension |
| co-proxamol | Cosalgesic; Distalgesic | analgesic |
| cortisone | Cortisyl | corticosteroid |
| co-tenidone | Tenoret 50; Tenoretic | hypertension |
| co-triamterzide | Dyazide | diuretic |
| co-trimoxazole | Bactrim; Laratrim; Septrin | antibacterial |
| crisantapase | Erwinase | leukaemia |
| crotamiton | Eurax | antipruritic |
| cyanocobalamin | Cytacon; Cytamen | anti-anaemic |
| cyclizine | Marzine; Valoid | antiemetic |
| cyclopenthiazide | Navidrex | diuretic |
| cyclopentolate | Mydrilate | mydriatic |
| cyclophosphamide | Endoxana | cytotoxic |
| cyclosporin | Neoral | immunosuppressant |
| cyproheptadine | Periactin | antihistamine |
| cyproterone | Androcur; Cyprostat | anti-androgen |
| cytarabine | Cytosar | cytotoxic |
| dacarbazine | DTIC | cytotoxic |
| dactinoycin | Cosmogen | cytotoxic |
| dalteparin | Fragmin | anticoagulant |
| danazol | Danol | endometriosis |
| dantrolene | Dantrium | muscle relaxant |
| daunorubicin | DaunoXome | cytotoxic |
| deflazocort | Calcort | corticosteroid |

| Approved name | Proprietary name | Main action or indication |
|---|---|---|
| demeclocycline | Ledermycin | antibiotic |
| desferrioxamine | Desferal | iron poisoning |
| desflurane | Suprane | inhalation anaesthetic |
| desmopressin | DDAVP | diabetes insipidus |
| desoxymethasone | Stiedex | topical corticosteroid |
| dexamethasone | Decadron | corticosteroid |
| dexamphetamine | Dexedrine | appetite suppressant |
| dextran | Gentran; Rheomacrodex | plasma substitute |
| dextromoramide | Palfium | analgesic |
| dextropropoxyphene | Doloxene | analgesic |
| diazepam | Diazemuls; Stesolid; Valium | anxiety; epilepsy |
| diazoxide | Eudemine | hypertension; hypoglycaemia |
| diclofenac | Voltarol | antirheumatic |
| dicobalt edetate | Kelocyanor | cyanide poisoning |
| dicyclomine | Merbentyl | antispasmodic |
| didanosine | Videx | antiviral |
| diethylcarbamazine | Banocide | filariasis |
| diflucortolone | Nerison | topical corticosteroid |
| diflunisal | Dolobid | analgesic |
| digoxin | Lanoxin | heart failure |
| digoxin antibody | Digibind | digoxin overdose |
| dihydrocodeine | D.F.118 | analgesic |
| dihydrotachysterol | A.T.10 | hypocalcaemia |
| diloxanide furoate | Furamide | amoebiasis |

Approved and proprietary
names of drugs

| Approved name | Proprietary name | Main action or indication |
| --- | --- | --- |
| diltiazem | Adizem; Tildiem | calcium antagonist |
| dimenhydrinate | Dramamine | antihistamine |
| dinoprost | Prostin F2 | uterine stimulant |
| dinoprostone | Prostin E2 | uterine stimulant |
| diphenoxylate | Lomotil | diarrhoea |
| dipivefrine | Propine | glaucoma |
| dipyridamole | Persantin | vasodilator |
| disodium etidronate | Didronel | Paget's disease |
| disodium pamidronate | Aredia | Paget's disease |
| disopyramide | Dirythmin-SA; Rythmoden | cardiac arrhythmias |
| distigmine | Ubretid | urinary retention |
| disulfiram | Antabuse | alcoholism |
| dobutamine | Dobutrex | cardiac support |
| docetaxel | Taxotere | cytotoxic |
| docusate sodium | Dioctyl | laxative |
| domperidone | Motilium | antiemetic |
| donepezil | Aricept | Alzheimer's disease |
| dopamine | Intropin | cardiac stimulant |
| dopexamine | Dopacard | cardiac support |
| dornase alfa | Pulmozyme | cystic fibrosis |
| dorzolamide | Trusopt | glaucoma |
| dothiepin | Prothiaden | antidepressant |
| doxapram | Dopram | respiratory stimulant |
| doxazosin | Cardura | hypertension |
| doxepin | Sinequan | antidepressant |

| Approved name | Proprietary name | Main action or indication |
|---|---|---|
| doxorubicin | Caelyx | cytotoxic |
| doxycycline | Vibramycin | antibiotic |
| droperidol | Droleptan | neuroleptic |
| dydrogesterone | Duphaston | progestogen |
| econazole | Ecostatin; Pevaryl | antifungal |
| eformoterol | Foradil | bronchodilator |
| enalapril | Innovace | ACE inhibitor |
| enflurane | Enthrane | inhalation anaesthetic |
| enoxaparin | Clexane | thrombosis |
| enoximone | Perfan | heart failure |
| epirubicin | Pharmorubicin | cytotoxic |
| epoetin alfa beta | Eprex; Recormon | anaemia in chronic renal failure |
| epoprostenol | Flolan | bypass surgery |
| ergotamine | Lingraine | migraine |
| erythromycin | Erythrocin; Ilotycin | antibiotic |
| esmolol | Brevibloc | beta-blocker |
| estramustine | Estracyt | cytotoxic |
| estropipate | Harmogen | oestrogen |
| ethacrynic acid | Edecrin | diuretic |
| ethambutol | Myambutol | tuberculosis |
| ethamsylate | Dicynene | haemostatic |
| ethosuximide | Emeside; Zarontin | anticonvulsant |
| etidronate | Didronel | Paget's disease |
| etodolac | Lodine | arthritis |
| etomidate | Hypnomidate | i.v. anaesthetic |

Approved and proprietary
names of drugs

| Approved name | Proprietary name | Main action or indication |
| --- | --- | --- |
| etoposide | Vepesid | cytotoxic |
| etretinate | Tigason | psoriasis |
| Factor VIIa | NovoSeven | haemophilia A |
| Factor VIII | Kogenate; Monoclate-P | haemophilia B |
| Factor IX | Mononine; Replenine | haemophilia B |
| famciclovir | Famvir | antiviral |
| famotidine | Pepcid-PM | $H_2$-blocker |
| felodipine | Plendil | calcium antagonist |
| fenbufen | Lederfen | antirheumatic |
| fenofibrate | Lipantil | hyperlipidaemia |
| fenoprofen | Fenopron | arthritis |
| fenoterol | Berotec | asthma |
| fentanyl | Sublimaze | analgesic |
| fenticonazole | Lomexin | antifungal |
| fexofenadine | Telfast | antihistamine |
| filgrastim | Neupogen | neutropenia |
| finasteride | Proscar | prostatic hypertrophy |
| flavoxate | Urispas | antispasmodic |
| flecainide | Tambocor | cardiac arrhythmias |
| flucloxacillin | Floxapen | antibiotic |
| fluconazole | Diflucan | antifungal |
| flucytosine | Alcobon | antifungal |
| fludarabine | Fludara | cytotoxic |
| fludrocortisone | Florinef | Addison's disease |
| flumazenil | Anexate | benzodiazepine antagonist |

| Approved name | Proprietary name | Main action or indication |
|---|---|---|
| flunisolide | Syntaris | allergic rhinitis |
| flunitrazepam | Rohypnol | hypnotic |
| fluocinolone | Synalar | topical corticosteroid |
| fluocinonide | Metosyn | topical corticosteroid |
| fluocortolone | Ultralanum | topical corticosteroid |
| fluorometholone | FML | topical corticosteroid |
| fluoxetine | Prozac | antidepressant |
| flupenthixol | Depixol | schizophrenia |
| fluphenazine | Modecate; Moditen | schizophrenia |
| flurandrenolone | Haelan | topical corticosteroid |
| flurazepam | Dalmane | hypnotic |
| flurbiprofen | Froben | arthritis |
| flutamide | Drogenil | prostatic carcinoma |
| fluticasone | Flixonase | topical corticosteroid |
| fluvastatin | Lescol | hyperlipidaemia |
| fluvoxamine | Faverin | antidepressant |
| folinic acid | Refolinon | methotrexate antidote |
| formestane | Lentaron | cytotoxic |
| foscarnet | Foscavir | antiviral |
| fosfestrol | Honvan | cytotoxic |
| fosfomycin | Monuril | antibacterial |
| fosinopril | Staril | ACE inhibitor |
| framycetin | Soframycin | topical antibiotic |
| frusemide | Lasix | diuretic |
| fusafungine | Locabiotal | antibiotic |
| gabapentin | Neurontin | epilepsy |

189

Approved and proprietary
names of drugs

190
Approved and proprietary
names of drugs

| Approved name | Proprietary name | Main action or indication |
| --- | --- | --- |
| gallamine | Flaxedil | muscle relaxant |
| gamolenic acid | Epogam | eczema |
| ganciclovir | Cymevene | antiviral |
| gemcitabine | Gemzar | cytotoxic |
| gemfibrozil | Lopid | hyperlipidaemia |
| gentamicin | Cidomycin; Genticin | antibiotic |
| gestrinone | Dimetriose | endometriosis |
| gestronol | Depostat | endometrial carcinoma |
| glibenclamide | Daonil; Euglucon | hypoglycaemic |
| gliclazide | Diamicron | hypoglycaemic |
| glimepiride | Amaryl | hypoglycaemic |
| glipizide | Glibenese; Minodiab | hypoglycaemic |
| gliquidone | Glurenorm | hypoglycaemic |
| glucagon | GlucaGen | hypoglycaemic |
| glutaraldehyde | Glutarol | warts |
| gonadorelin | Fertiral | infertility |
| goserelin | Zoladex | prostatic carcinoma |
| granisetron | Kytril | migraine |
| griseofulvin | Fulcin; Grisovin | antifungal |
| guanethidine | Ismelin | hypertension |
| halcinonide | Halciderm | topical corticosteroid |
| haloperidol | Dozic; Haldol; Serenace | schizophrenia |
| halofantrine | Halfan | antimalarial |
| halothane | Fluothane | anaesthetic |
| hetastarch | Hespan | plasma substitute |

| Approved name | Proprietary name | Main action or indication |
|---|---|---|
| hexamine hippurate | Hiprex | urinary antiseptic |
| hyaluronidase | Hyalase | enzyme |
| hydralazine | Apresoline | hypertension |
| hydrochlorothiazide | HydroSaluric | diuretic |
| hydrocortisone | Corlan; Efcortesol; Solu-Cortef | corticosteroid |
| hydroflumethiazide | Hydrenox | diuretic |
| hydromorphone | Palladone | narcotic analgesic |
| hydroxocobalamin | Cobalin-H; Neo-Cytamen | anti-anaemic |
| hydroxychloroquine | Plaquenil | antimalarial |
| hydroxyprogesterone | Proluton-Depot | progestogen |
| hydroxyurea | Hydrea | cytotoxic |
| hydroxyzine | Atarax | tranquillizer |
| hyoscine butyl bromide | Buscopan | antispasmodic |
| ibuprofen | Brufen; Fenbid | arthritis |
| idarubicin | Zavedos | cytotoxic |
| idoxuridine | Herpid; Iduridin; Virudox | antiviral |
| ifosfamide | Mitoxana | cytotoxic |
| imipenem | Primaxin | antibiotic |
| imipramine | Tofranil | antidepressant |
| indapamide | Natrilix | hypertension |
| indinavir | Crixivan | antiviral |
| indomethacin | Indocid; Indomax | arthritis |
| indoramin | Baratol | beta-blocker |
| indoramin | Doralese | prostatic hypertrophy |

Approved and proprietary names of drugs

| Approved name | Proprietary name | Main action or indication |
| --- | --- | --- |
| inosine pranobex | Imunovir | antiviral |
| inositol nicotinate | Hexopal | vasodilator |
| interferon | Intron; Roferon; Wellferon | leukaemia |
| ipratropium | Atrovent | bronchodilator |
| irbisartan | Aprovel | hypertension |
| irinotecan | Campto | cytotoxic |
| iron-sorbitol | Jectofer | anaemia |
| isocarboxazid | Marplan | antidepressant |
| isoconazole | Travogyn | candidiasis |
| isoprenaline | Saventrine | heart block |
| isosorbide dinitrate | Isoket; Isordil; Sorbitrate | angina |
| isosorbide mononitrate | Elantan; Ismo; Monit | angina |
| isotretinoin | Roaccutane | severe acne |
| isradipine | Prescal | calcium antagonist |
| itraconazole | Sporanox | antifungal |
| ivermectin | Mectizan | filariasis |
| kanamycin | Kannasyn | antibiotic |
| ketamine | Ketalar | anaesthetic |
| ketoconazole | Nizoral | antifungal |
| ketoprofen | Alrheumat; Orudis | arthritis |
| ketorolac | Toradol | analgesic |
| ketotifen | Zaditen | anti-asthmatic |
| labetalol | Trandate | beta-blocker |
| lacidipine | Motens | calcium antagonist |

| Approved name | Proprietary name | Main action or indication |
|---|---|---|
| lactulose | Duphalac | laxative |
| lamivudine | Epivir | antiviral |
| lamotrigine | Lamictal | epilepsy |
| lansoprazole | Zoton | peptic ulcer |
| latanoprost | Xalantan | glaucoma |
| lenograstim | Granocyte | neutropenia |
| letrozole | Femara | cytotoxic |
| leuprorelin | Prostap | prostatic carcinoma |
| levobunolol | Betagan | glaucoma |
| levocabastine | Livostin | allergic conjunctivitis |
| lignocaine | Xylocaine | local anaesthetic |
| liothyronine | Tertroxin | thyroid deficiency |
| lisinopril | Carace; Zestril | ACE inhibitor |
| lithium carbonate | Camcolit; Phasal | mania |
| lodoxamide | Alomide | allergic conjunctivitis |
| lofepramine | Gamanil | antidepressant |
| lofexidine | BritLofex | anti-opioid |
| lomustine | CCNU | cytotoxic |
| loperamide | Arret; Imodium | diarrhoea |
| loratadine | Clarityn | antihistamine |
| lorazepam | Ativan | tranquillizer |
| losartan | Cozaar | hypertension |
| loxapine | Loxapac | antipsychotic |
| lymecycline | Tetralysal | antibiotic |
| lypressin | Syntopressin | diabetes insipidus |
| lysuride | Revanil | parkinsonism |

Approved and proprietary names of drugs

| Approved name | Proprietary name | Main action or indication |
|---|---|---|
| malathion | Derbac; Prioderm | parasiticide |
| maprotiline | Ludiomil | antidepressant |
| mebendazole | Vermox | anthelmintic |
| mebeverine | Colofac | antispasmodic |
| medroxyprogesterone | Provera | progestogen |
| mefenamic acid | Ponstan | arthritis |
| mefloquine | Larium | malaria |
| mefruside | Baycaron | diuretic |
| megestrol | Megace | cytotoxic |
| meloxicam | Mobic | osteoarthritis |
| melphalan | Alkeran | cytotoxic |
| meprobamate | Equanil | tranquillizer |
| meptazinol | Meptid | analgesic |
| mepyramine | Anthisan | topical antihistamine |
| mequitazine | Primalan | antihistamine |
| mercaptopurine | Puri-Nethol | cytotoxic |
| meropenem | Meropen | antibiotic |
| mesalazine | Asacol; Pentasa | ulcerative colitis |
| mesna | Utomitexan | urotoxicity due to cyclophosphamide |
| mesterolone | Pro-Viron | androgen |
| metaraminol | Aramine | hypotension |
| metformin | Glucophage | hypoglycaemic |
| methadone | Physeptone | analgesic |
| methocarbamol | Robaxin | muscle relaxant |
| methohexitone | Brietal | anaesthetic |

| Approved name | Proprietary name | Main action or indication |
|---|---|---|
| methotrexate | Maxtrex | cytotoxic |
| methotrimeprazine | Nozinan | pain in terminal cancer |
| methoxamine | Vasoxine | vasoconstrictor |
| methylcellulose | Celevac | laxative |
| methylcysteine | Visclair | mucolytic |
| methyldopa | Aldomet; Dopamet | hypertension |
| methylphenidate | Ritalin | hyperactivity |
| methylphenobarbitone | Prominal | epilepsy |
| methylprednisolone | Medrone | corticosteroid |
| methysergide | Deseril | migraine |
| metirosine | Demser | phaeochromocytoma |
| metoclopramide | Maxolon; Gastromax | antiemetic |
| metolazone | Metenix | diuretic |
| metoprolol | Betaloc; Lopressor | beta-blocker |
| metronidazole | Flagyl; Zadstat | trichomoniasis |
| metyrapone | Metopirone | resistant oedema |
| mexiletine | Mexitil | cardiac arrhythmias |
| miconazole | Dakterin | antifungal |
| midazolam | Hypnovel | i.v. sedative |
| mifepristone | Mifegyne | antiprogestogen |
| milrinone | Primacor | severe heart failure |
| minocycline | Minocin | antibiotic |
| minoxidil | Loniten | hypertension |
| mirtazapine | Zispin | antidepressant |
| misoprostol | Cytotec | peptic ulcer |
| mitozantrone | Novantrone | cytotoxic |

| Approved name | Proprietary name | Main action or indication |
|---------------|------------------|---------------------------|
| mivacurium | Mivacron | muscle relaxant |
| moclobemide | Manerix | antidepressant |
| moexipril | Perdix | hypertension |
| molgramostim | Leucomax | neutropenia |
| mometasone | Elocon | topical corticosteroid |
| moracizine | Ethmozine | anti-arrhythmic |
| morphine | MST Continus; Sevredol | analgesic |
| moxisylyte | Erecnos | induction of erection |
| moxonidine | Physiotens | hypertension |
| mupirocin | Bactroban | topical antibiotic |
| mycophenylate | CellCept | immunosuppressant |
| nabumetone | Relifex | arthritis |
| nadolol | Corgard | beta-blocker |
| nafarelin | Synarel | endometriosis |
| naftidrofuryl | Praxilene | vasodilator |
| nalbuphine | Nubain | analgesic |
| nalidixic acid | Negram | urinary antiseptic |
| naloxone | Narcan | narcotic antagonist |
| naltrexone | Nalorex | opioid dependence |
| nandrolone | Deca-Durabolin | anabolic steroid |
| naproxen | Naprosyn; Synflex | arthritis |
| naratriptan | Naramig | migraine |
| nedocromil | Tilade | anti-asthmatic |
| nefazodone | Dutonin | antidepressant |
| nefopam | Acupan | analgesic |

| Approved name | Proprietary name | Main action or indication |
| --- | --- | --- |
| neostigmine | Prostigmin | myasthenia |
| netilmicin | Netillin | antibiotic |
| nicardipine | Cardene | calcium antagonist |
| niclosamide | Yomesan | anthelmintic |
| nicorandil | Ikorel | angina |
| nicotinyl alcohol | Ronicol | vasodilator |
| nicoumalone | Sinthrome | anticoagulant |
| nifedipine | Adalat; Coracten | calcium antagonist |
| nimodipine | Nimotop | calcium antagonist |
| nisoldipine | Syscor | angina; hypertension |
| nitrazepam | Mogadon, Somnite | hypnotic |
| nitrofurantoin | Furadantin; Macrodantin | urinary antiseptic |
| nizatidine | Axid, Zinga | $H_2$-blocker |
| noradrenaline | Levophed | hypotension |
| norethisterone | Menzol; Primolut N | progestogen |
| norfloxacin | Utinor | urinary tract infections |
| nortriptyline | Allegron | antidepressant |
| nystatin | Nystan | antifungal |
| octreotide | Sandostatin | carcinoid syndrome |
| ofloxacin | Exocin; Tarivid | urinary tract infection |
| olanzapine | Zyprexa | schizophrenia |
| olsalazine | Dipentum | ulcerative colitis |
| omeprazole | Losec | peptic ulcer |
| ondansetron | Zofran | antinauseant |
| orciprenaline | Alupent | bronchospasm |

Approved and proprietary names of drugs

| Approved name | Proprietary name | Main action or indication |
|---|---|---|
| orphenadrine | Biorphen; Disipal | parkinsonism |
| oxazepan | Oxanid | tranquillizer |
| oxitropium | Oxivent | bronchodilator |
| oxpentifylline | Trental | vasodilator |
| oxprenolol | Trasicor | beta-blocker |
| oxybutynin | Cystrin; Ditropan | urinary incontinence |
| oxypertine | Integrin | tranquillizer |
| oxytetracycline | Terramycin | antibiotic |
| oxytocin | Syntocinon | induction of labour |
| paclitaxel | Taxol | cytotoxic |
| pamidronate | Aredia | osteoporosis |
| pancuronium | Pavulon | muscle relaxant |
| pantoprazole | Protium | peptic ulcer |
| paroxetine | Seroxat | antidepressant |
| penciclovir | Vectavir | antiviral |
| penicillamine | Distamine; Pendramine | Wilson's disease |
| pentaerythritol tetranitrate | Mycardol | angina |
| pentamididine | Pentacarinat | leishmaniasis |
| pentazocine | Fortral | analgesic |
| pentostatin | Nipent | cytotoxic |
| pergolide | Celance | parkinsonism |
| pericyazine | Neulactil | schizophrenia |
| perindopril | Coversyl | ACE inhibitor |
| permethrin | Lyclear | pediculocide |
| perphenazine | Fentazin | schizophrenia |

| Approved name | Proprietary name | Main action or indication |
| --- | --- | --- |
| phenazocine | Narphen | analgesic |
| phenelzine | Nardil | antidepressant |
| phenindamine | Thephorin | antihistamine |
| phenindione | Dindevan | anticoagulant |
| pheniramine | Daneral | antihistamine |
| phenoperidine | Operidine | analgesic |
| phenoxybenzamine | Dibenyline | vasodilator |
| phentolamine | Rogitine | phaeochromocytoma |
| phenylbutazone | Butacote | ankylosing spondylitis |
| phenytoin | Epanutin | epilepsy |
| phytomenadione | Konakion | hypoprothrombinaemia |
| pimozide | Orap | schizophrenia |
| pindolol | Visken | beta-blocker |
| piperacillin | Pipril | antibiotic |
| pipothiazine | Piportil | antipsychotic |
| piracetam | Nootropil | myoclonus |
| pirbuterol | Exirel | bronchodilator |
| piretanide | Arelix | diuretic |
| piroxicam | Feldene | antirheumatic |
| pivampicillin | Pondocillin | antibiotic |
| pizotifen | Sanomigran | migraine |
| podophyllotixin | Condyline | penile warts |
| polyestradiol | Estradurin | prostatic carcinoma |
| polygeline | Haemaccel | blood volume expander |
| polystyrene resin | Resonium | hyperkalaemia |
| polythiazide | Nephril | diuretic |

Approved and proprietary
names of drugs

| Approved name | Proprietary name | Main action or indication |
|---|---|---|
| poractant | Curosurf | lung surfactant |
| pravastatin | Lipostat | hyperlipidaemia |
| prazosin | Hypovase | hypertension |
| prednisolone | Deltacortril; Precortisyl; Prednesol | corticosteroid |
| prilocaine | Citanest | anaesthetic |
| primidone | Mysoline | epilepsy |
| probenecid | Benemid | gout |
| procainamide | Pronestyl | cardiac arrhythmias |
| procarbazine | Natulan | cytotoxic |
| prochlorperazine | Stemetil | antiemetic; vertigo |
| procyclidine | Kemadrin | parkinsonism |
| proguanil | Paludrine | antimalarial |
| promazine | Sparine | tranquillizer |
| promethazine | Phenergan | antihistamine |
| promethazine theoclate | Avomine | antiemetic |
| propafenone | Arythmol | cardiac arrhythmias |
| propantheline | Pro-Banthine | spasmolytic |
| propofol | Diprivan | anaesthetic |
| propranolol | Inderal | beta-blocker |
| protriptyline | Concordin | antidepressant |
| proxymetacaine | Ophthaine | corneal anaesthetic |
| pumactant | Alec | lung surfactant |
| pyrazinamide | Zinamide | tuberculosis |
| pyridostigmine | Mestinon | myasthenia |
| pyridoxine | Benadon | vitamin B deficiency |

| Approved name | Proprietary name | Main action or indication |
|---|---|---|
| pyrimethamine | Daraprim | antimalarial |
| quetiapine | Seroquel | schizophrenia |
| quinagolide | Norprolac | hyperprolactinaemia |
| quinalbarbitone | Seconal | hypnotic |
| quinapril | Accupro | ACE inhibitor |
| raltitrexed | Tomudex | cytotoxic |
| ramipril | Tritace | ACE inhibitor |
| ranitidine | Zantac | $H_2$-blocker |
| razoxane | Razoxin | cytotoxic |
| reboxetine | Edronax | antidepressant |
| remifentanil | Ultiva | analgesic |
| reproterol | Bronchodil | bronchodilator |
| reteplase | Rapilysin | myocardial infarction |
| rifabutin | Myocobutin | tuberculosis |
| rifampicin | Rifacin; Rimactane | tuberculosis |
| riluzole | Rilutek | motor neurone disease |
| risperidone | Risperdal | schizophrenia |
| ritodrine | Yutopar | premature labour |
| ritonavir | Norvir | antiviral |
| roboxetine | Edronax | antidepressant |
| rocuronium | Esmeron | muscle relaxant |
| roprinirole | Requip | parkinsonism |
| ropivacaine | Naropin | local anaesthetic |
| salbutamol | Ventolin | bronchospasm |
| salcatonin | Calsynar; Miacalcic | Paget's disease |
| salmeterol | Serevent | bronchospasm |

Approved and proprietary names of drugs

| Approved name | Proprietary name | Main action or indication |
|---|---|---|
| saquinavir | Invirase | antiviral |
| selegiline | Eldepryl | parkinsonism |
| sermorelin | Geref | growth hormone |
| sertindole | Serdolect | schizophrenia |
| sertraline | Lustral | antidepressant |
| silver sulphadiazine | Flamazine | antibacterial |
| simvastatin | Zocor | hyperlipidaemia |
| sodium atendronate | Fosomax | osteoporosis |
| sodium aurothiomalate | Myocrisin | rheumatoid arthritis |
| sodium clodronate | Loron; Bonefos | hypercalcaemia of malignancy |
| sodium cromoglycate | Intal; Rynacrom | anti-allergic |
| sodium fusidate | Fucidin | antibiotic |
| sodium iron edetate | Sytron | anti-anaemic |
| sodium stibogluconate | Pentostam | leishmaniasis |
| sodium valproate | Epilim | epilepsy |
| somatropin | Zomacton | growth hormone |
| sotalol | Beta-Cardone; Sotacor | beta-blocker |
| spectinomycin | Trobicin | antibiotic |
| spironolactone | Aldactone; Spiroctan | diuretic |
| stanozolol | Stromba | anabolic steroid |
| stavudine | Zerit | antiviral |
| streptokinase | Kabikinase; Streptase | fibrinolytic |
| sucralfate | Antepsin | peptic ulcer |
| sulconazole | Exelderm | antifungal |
| sulfametopyrazine | Kelfizine | sulphonamide |

| Approved name | Proprietary name | Main action or indication |
|---|---|---|
| sulindac | Clinoril | arthritis |
| sulphasalazine | Salazopyrin | ulcerative colitis |
| sulphinpyrazone | Anturan | gout |
| sulpiride | Dolmatil; Sulpitil | schizophrenia |
| sumatriptan | Imigran | migraine |
| suxamethonium | Anectine; Scoline | muscle relaxant |
| tacalcitol | Curaderm | psoriasis |
| tacrolimus | Prograf | immunosuppressant |
| tamoxifen | Nolvadex | cytotoxic |
| tamsulosin | Flomax | prostatic hypertrophy |
| tazarotene | Zorac | psoriasis |
| tazobactam | Tazocin | antibiotic |
| teicoplanin | Targocid | antibiotic |
| temazepam | Normison | hypnotic |
| temocillin | Temopen | antibiotic |
| tenoxicam | Mobiflex | arthritis |
| terazosin | Hytrin | hypertension |
| terbinafine | Lamisil | antifungal |
| terbutaline | Bricanyl | bronchospasm |
| terfenadine | Triludan | antihistamine |
| testosterone | Virormone | hypogonadism |
| tetracosactrin | Synacthen | corticotrophin |
| tetracycline | Achromycin | antibiotic |
| thiabendazole | Mintezol | anthelmintic |
| thiambutosine | Ciba 1906 | anthelmintic |

Approved and proprietary names of drugs

| Approved name | Proprietary name | Main action or indication |
| --- | --- | --- |
| thiamine | Benerva | vitamin B$_1$ deficiency |
| thioguanine | Lanvin | cytotoxic |
| thiopentone | Intraval | i.v. anaesthetic |
| thioridazine | Melleril | tranquillizer |
| thymoxamine | Opilon | vasodilator |
| thyroxine | Eltroxin | thyroid deficiency |
| tiaprofenic acid | Surgam | antirheumatic |
| tibolone | Livial | menopause |
| ticarcillin | Timentin | antibiotic |
| tiludronic acid | Skelid | Paget's disease |
| timolol | Betim; Blocadren | beta-blocker |
| tinidazole | Fasigyn | anaerobic infections |
| tinzaparin | Innohep | anticoagulant |
| tioconazole | Trosyl | antifungal |
| tizanidine | Zanaflex | spasticity |
| tobramycin | Nebcin; Tobralex | antibiotic |
| tolazamide | Tolanase | hypoglycaemic |
| tolbutamide | Rastinon | hypoglycaemic |
| tolcapone | Tasmar | parkinsonism |
| tolfenamic acid | Clotam | migraine |
| tolmetin | Tolectin | antirheumatic |
| topiramate | Topamax | epilepsy |
| topotecan | Hycamtin | cytotoxic |
| torasemide | Torem | diuretic |
| toremifene | Fareston | cytotoxic |
| tramadol | Zydol | analgesic |

| Approved name | Proprietary name | Main action or indication |
|---|---|---|
| trandolapril | Gopten; Odrik | ACE inhibitor |
| tranexamic acid | Cyklokapron | antifibrinolytic |
| tranylcypromine | Parnate | antidepressant |
| trazodone | Molipaxin | antidepressant |
| tretinoin | Retin-A; Retinova; Vesaniod | acne; photodamage; leukaemia |
| triamcinolone | Adcortyl; Ledercort | corticosteroid |
| triameterene | Dytac | diuretic |
| tribavirin | Virazid | antiviral |
| trifluoperazine | Stelazine | tranquillizer |
| trilostane | Modrenal | aldosteronism |
| trimeprazine | Vallergan | antihistamine |
| trimethoprim | Ipral; Monotrim; Trimopan | antibacterial |
| trimetrexate | Neutrexin | AIDS |
| trimipramine | Surmontil | antidepressant |
| triptorelin | Decapeptyl | cytotoxic |
| troglitazone | Romozin | insulin enhancer |
| tropicamide | Mydriacyl | mydriatic |
| tropisetron | Navoban | antinauseant |
| tryptophan | Optimax | antidepressant |
| tulobuterol | Respacal | bronchodilator |
| urea hydrogen peroxide | Otex | ear drops |
| urofollitrophin | Orgafol | infertility |
| urokinase | Ukidan | hyphaemia; embolism |
| ursodeoycholic acid | Destolit; Ursofalk | gallstones |
| valaciclovir | Valtrex | antiviral |

205

Approved and proprietary
names of drugs

| Approved name | Proprietary name | Main action or indication |
|---|---|---|
| valproic acid | Convulex | epilepsy |
| valsartan | Diovan | hypertension |
| vancomycin | Vancocin | antibiotic |
| vecuronium | Norcuron | muscle relaxant |
| venlafaxine | Efexor | antidepressant |
| verapamil | Cordilox; Univer | angina; hypertension |
| vigabatrin | Sabril | anticonvulsant |
| viloxazine | Vivalan | antidepressant |
| vinblastine | Velbe | cytotoxic |
| vincristine | Oncovin | cytotoxic |
| vindesine | Eldisine | cytotoxic |
| vinorelbine | Navelbine | cytotoxic |
| warfarin | Marevan | anticoagulant |
| xamoterol | Corwin | mild heart failure |
| xipamide | Diurexan | diuretic |
| xylometazoline | Otrivine | nasal decongestant |
| zalcitabine | Hivid | HIV infections |
| zidovudine | Retrovir | antiviral |
| zolmitriptan | Zomig | migraine |
| zolpidem | Stilnoct | insomnia |
| zopiclone | Zimovane | hypnotic |
| zuclopenthixol | Clopixol | schizophrenia |

206
Approved and proprietary
names of drugs

| Proprietary name | Approved name | Main action or indication |
|---|---|---|
| Accupro | quinapril | ACE inhibitor |
| Acepril | captopril | ACE inhibitor |
| Achromycin | tetracycline | antibiotic |
| Aclacin | aclarubicin | cytotoxic |
| Actilyse | alteplase | fibrinolytic |
| Acupan | nefopam | analgesic |
| Adalat | nifedipine | calcium antagonist |
| Adcortyl | triamcinolone | topical corticosteroid |
| Adenocor | adenosine | paroxysmal tachycardia |
| Adipine | nifedipine | angina |
| Adizem | diltiazem | angina |
| Akineton | biperiden | parkinsonism |
| Alcobon | flucytosine | antifungal |
| Aldactide | co-flumactone | diuretic |
| Aldactone | spironolactone | resistant oedema |
| Aldomet | methyldopa | hypertension |
| Alec | pumactant | lung surfactant |
| AlfaD | alfacalcidol | vitamin D deficiency |
| Alimix | cisapride | oesophageal reflux |
| Alkeran | melphalan | cytotoxic |
| Allegron | nortriptyline | antidepressant |
| Aller-eeze | clemastine | antihistamine |
| Almodan | amoxycillin | antibiotic |
| Alomide | lodoxamide | allergic conjunctivitis |
| Alphagan | brimonidine | glaucoma |
| Alphaparin | certoparin | anticoagulant |

Approved and proprietary
names of drugs

| Proprietary name | Approved name | Main action or indication |
| --- | --- | --- |
| Alupent | orciprenaline | bronchodilator |
| Amaryl | glimepiride | antidiabetic |
| AmBisome | amphotericin | antifungal |
| Amikin | amikacin | antibiotic |
| Amil-co | co-amilozide | diuretic |
| Amoxil | amoxycillin | antibiotic |
| Amphocil | amphotericin | antifungal |
| Amsidine | amacrine | cytotoxic |
| Amytal | amylobarbitone | hypnotic |
| Anaflex | polynoxylin | antiseptic |
| Androcur | cyproterone | anti-androgen |
| Anectine | suxamethonium | muscle relaxant |
| Anexate | flumazenil | benzodiazepine antagonist |
| Angilol | propanolol | beta-blocker |
| Angiozem | diltiazem | angina |
| Anquil | benperidol | tranquillizer |
| Antabuse | disulfiram | alcoholism |
| Antepsin | sulcralfate | peptic ulcer |
| Anthisan | mepyramine | topical antihistamine |
| Anturan | sulphinpyrazone | gout |
| Apresoline | hydralazine | hypertension |
| Aprinox | bendrofluazide | diuretic |
| Aprovel | irbisartan | hypertension |
| Apsifen | ibuprofen | arthritis |
| Aquadrate | urea | ichthyosis |
| Aramine | metaraminol | vasoconstrictor |

| Proprietary name | Approved name | Main action or indication |
| --- | --- | --- |
| Aredia | disodium pamidronate | hypercalcaemia of malignancy |
| Arfonad | trimetaphan | hypotensive surgery |
| Aricept | donepezil | Alzheimer's disease |
| Arimidex | anastrozole | breast cancer |
| Arpicolin | procyclidine | parkinsonism |
| Arpimycin | erythromycin | antibiotic |
| Arret | loperamide | diarrhoea |
| Artane | benzhexol | parkinsonism |
| Arythmol | propafenone | cardiac arrhythmias |
| Asacol | mesalazine | ulcerative colitis |
| Ascabiol | benzyl benzoate | scabies |
| Asendis | amoxapine | antidepressant |
| A.T.10 | dihydrotachysterol | hypocalcaemia |
| Atarax | hydroxyzine | tranquillizer |
| Ativan | lorazepam | tranquillizer |
| Atromid-S | clofibrate | hypercholesterolaemia |
| Atrovent | ipratropium | bronchodilator |
| Aureomycin | chlortetracycline | antibiotic |
| Augmentin | co-amoxiclav | antibiotic |
| Avloclor | chloroquine | antimalarial |
| Avomine | promethazine | antiemetic |
| Axid | nizatidine | $H_2$-blocker |
| Azactam | aztreonam | antibiotic |
| Azamune | azathioprine | cytotoxic |
| Bactrim | co-trimoxazole | antibacterial |

| Proprietary name | Approved name | Main action or indication |
|---|---|---|
| Bactroban | mupirocin | topical antibiotic |
| Bambec | bambuterol | asthma |
| Banocide | diethylcarbamazine | filariasis |
| Baratol | indoramin | beta-blocker |
| Baxan | cefadroxil | antibiotic |
| Baycaron | mefruside | diuretic |
| Becloforte | beclomethasone | corticosteroid |
| Beconase | beclomethasone | rhinitis |
| Becotide | beclomethasone | corticosteroid |
| Bedranol SR | propranolol | beta-blocker |
| Benadon | pyridoxine | vitamin $B_6$ deficiency |
| Bendogen | bethanidine | hypertension |
| Benemid | probenecid | gout |
| Benerva | thiamine | vitamin $B_1$ deficiency |
| Benoral | benorylate | analgesic |
| Benoxyl | benzyl peroxide | acne |
| Berkatens | verapamil | angina; hypertension |
| Berkmycen | oxytetracycline | antibiotic |
| Berkolol | propranolol | beta-blocker |
| Berkozide | bendrofluazide | diuretic |
| Berotec | fenoterol | bronchitis |
| Beta-Cardone | sotalol | beta-blocker |
| Betadine | povidone-iodine | antiseptic |
| Betagan | levobunolol | glaucoma |
| Betaloc | metoprolol | beta-blocker |
| Betim | timolol | beta-blocker |

| Proprietary name | Approved name | Main action or indication |
| --- | --- | --- |
| Betnelan | betamethasone | corticosteroid |
| Betnesol | betamethasone | corticosteroid |
| Betnovate | betamethasone | topical corticosteroid |
| Betoptic | betaxolol | glaucoma |
| Bezalip | bezafibrate | hyperlipidaemia |
| BiCNU | carmustine | cytotoxic |
| Biltricide | praziquantel | anthelmintic |
| Bioplex | carbenoxolone | mouth ulcers |
| Biorphen | orphenadrine | parkinsonism |
| Blocadren | timolol | beta-blocker |
| Bonefos | sodium clodronate | hypercalcaemia of malignancy |
| Botox | botulinum toxin | blepharospasm |
| Bretylate | bretylium | cardiac arrhythmias |
| Brevibloc | esmolol | beta-blocker |
| Bricanyl | terbutaline | bronchospasm |
| Brietal | methohexitone | anaesthetic |
| Britaject | apomorphine | parkinsonism |
| Britiazim | diltiazem | angina |
| BritLofex | lofexidine | anti-opioid |
| Broflex | benzhexol | parkinsonism |
| Brolene | propamidine | conjunctivitis |
| Bronchodil | reproterol | bronchodilator |
| Brufen | ibuprofen | arthritis |
| Buccastem | prochlorperazine | vertigo |
| Burinex | bumetanide | diuretic |

| Proprietary name | Approved name | Main action or indication |
| --- | --- | --- |
| Buscopan | hyoscine butyl bromide | antispasmodic |
| Buspar | buspirone | anxiolytic |
| Butacote | phenylbutazone | ankylosing spondylitis |
| Cabaser | cabergoline | dopamine agonist |
| Cacit | calcium carbonate | osteoporosis |
| Caelyx | doxorubicin | cytotoxic |
| Calabren | glibenclamide | hypoglycaemic |
| Calciparine | calcium heparin | anticoagulant |
| Calcisorb | sodium cellulose phosphate | hypercalciuria |
| Calcitare | calcitonin | Paget's disease |
| Calcium Resonium | exchange resin | hyperkalaemia |
| Calpol | paracetamol | analgesic |
| Calsynar | salcatonin | Paget's disease |
| Camcolit | lithium carbonate | mania |
| Campral | acamprosate | opioid antagonist |
| Campto | irinotecan | cytotoxic |
| Canestan | clotrimazole | antifungal |
| Capastat | capreomycin | tuberculosis |
| Caplenal | allopurinol | gout |
| Capoten | captopril | ACE inhibitor |
| Caprin | aspirin | arthritis |
| Carace | lisinopril | ACE inhibitor |
| Cardilate | nifedipine | angina |
| Cardinol | propranolol | beta-blocker |
| Cardura | doxazosin | hypertension |

| Proprietary name | Approved name | Main action or indication |
|---|---|---|
| Carisoma | carisprodol | muscle relaxant |
| Carylderm | carbaryl | parasiticide |
| Casodex | bicalutamide | cytotoxic |
| Catapres | clonidine | hypertension |
| CCNU | lomustine | cytotoxic |
| Cedax | ceftibuten | antibiotic |
| Cedocard | isosorbide dinitrate | angina |
| Cefrom | cefpirome | antibiotic |
| Celance | pergolide | parkinsonism |
| Celectol | celiprolol | hypertension |
| Celevac | methylcellulose | laxative |
| CellCept | mycophenylate | immunosuppressant |
| Ceporex | cephalexin | antibiotic |
| Cesamet | nabilone | antiemetic |
| Chendol | chenodeoxycholic acid | gall stones |
| Chenofalk | chenodeoxycholic acid | gall stones |
| Chloromycectin | chloramphenicol | antibiotic |
| Choledyl | choline theophyllinate | bronchodilator |
| Ciba 1906 | thiambutosine | leprosy |
| Cidomycin | gentamicin | antibiotic |
| Ciloxan | ciprafloxacin | corneal ulcer |
| Cinobac | cinoxacin | antibiotic |
| Cipramil | citalopram | antidepressant |
| Ciproxin | ciprofloxacin | antibacterial |
| Citanest | prilocaine | anaesthetic |
| Claforan | cefotaxime | antibiotic |

| Proprietary name | Approved name | Main action or indication |
|---|---|---|
| Clarityn | loratadine | antihistamine |
| Clexane | enoxaparin | thrombosis |
| Clinoril | sulindac | arthritis |
| Cloburate | clobetasone | eye drops |
| Clomid | clomiphene | gonadotrophin inhibitor |
| Clopixol | zuclopenthixol | schizophrenia |
| Clotam | tolfenamic acid | migraine |
| Clozaril | clozapine | antipsychotic |
| Cobalin H | hydroxocobalamin | antianaemic |
| Codis | co-codamol | analgesic |
| Cogentin | benztropine | parkinsonism |
| Colazide | balsalazide | ulcerative colitis |
| Colestid | colestipol | exchange resin |
| Colofac | mebeverine | antispasmodic |
| Colomycin | colistin | antibiotic |
| Colpermin | peppermint oil | antispasmodic |
| Comox | co-trimoxazole | antibacterial |
| Concordin | protriptyline | antidepressant |
| Condyline | podophyllotoxin | penile warts |
| Convulex | valproic acid | epilepsy |
| Coracten | nifedipine | calcium antagonist |
| Cordarone X | amiodarone | cardiac arrhythmias |
| Cordilox | verapamil | angina |
| Corgard | nadolol | beta-blocker |
| Corlan | hydrocortisone | local corticosteroid |
| Coro-Nitro | glyceryl trinitrate | angina |

| Proprietary name | Approved name | Main action or indication |
|---|---|---|
| Cortisyl | cortisone | corticosteroid |
| Corwin | xamoterol | mild heart failure |
| Cosmegen | actinomycin D | cytotoxic |
| Coversyl | perindopril | ACE inhibitor |
| Cozaar | losartan | hypertension |
| Creon | pancreatin | cystic fibrosis |
| Crixivan | indinavir | antiviral |
| Crystapen | benzylpenicillin | antibiotic |
| Curatoderm | tacalcitol | psoriasis |
| Curosurf | poractant | lung surfactant |
| Cyclogest | progesterone | premenstrual syndrome |
| Cyklokapron | tranexamic acid | antifibrinolytic |
| Cymevene | ganciclovir | antiviral |
| Cyprostat | cyproterone | prostatic carcinoma |
| Cytacon | cyanocobalamin | anti-anaemic |
| Cytamen | cyanocobalamin | anti-anaemic |
| Cytosar | cytarabine | cytotoxic |
| Cytotec | misoprostol | peptic ulcer |
| Daktarin | miconazole | antifungal |
| Dalacin C | clindamycin | antibiotic |
| Dalmane | flurazepam | hypnotic |
| Daneral SA | pheniramine | antihistamine |
| Danol | danazol | endometriosis |
| Dantrium | dantrolene | muscle relaxant |
| Daonil | glibenclamide | hypoglycaemia |
| Daraprim | pyrimethamine | antimalarial |

| Proprietary name | Approved name | Main action or indication |
|---|---|---|
| DaunoXome | daunorubicin | cytotoxic |
| DDAVP | desmopressin | diabetes insipidus |
| Decadron | dexamethasone | corticosteroid |
| Deca-Durabolin | nandrolone | cytotoxic |
| Decapeptyl | triptorelin | cytotoxic |
| Declinax | debrisoquine | hypertension |
| Deltacortril | prednisolone | corticosteroid |
| Deltastab | prednisolone | corticosteroid |
| Demser | metirosine | phaeochromocytoma |
| De-Nol | bismuth chelate | peptic ulcer |
| Depixol | flupenthixol | schizophrenia |
| Deponit | glyceryl trinitrate | angina |
| Depostat | gestronol | endometrial carcinoma |
| Derbac | carbaryl | parasiticide |
| Dermovate | clobetasol | topical corticosteroid |
| Deseril | methysergide | migraine |
| Desferal | desferrioxamine | iron poisoning |
| Destolit | ursodeoxycholic acid | gall stones |
| Dexedrine | dexamphetamine | appetite suppressant |
| D.F.118 | dihydrocodeine | analgesic |
| Diabinese | chlorpropamide | hypoglycaemic |
| Diamicron | gliclazide | hypoglycaemic |
| Diamox | acetazolamide | glaucoma |
| Diazemuls | diazepam | anxiolytic |
| Dibenyline | phenoxybenzamine | vasodilator |
| Dicynene | ethamsylate | haemostatic |

| Proprietary name | Approved name | Main action or indication |
| --- | --- | --- |
| Didronel | disodium etidronate | Paget's disease |
| Differin gel | adapalene | acne |
| Diflucan | fluconazole | antifungal |
| Digibind | digoxin antibody | digoxin overdose |
| Dilzem | diltiazem | angina; hypertension |
| Dimetriose | gestrinone | endometriosis |
| Dimotane | brompheniramine | antihistamine |
| Dindevan | phenindione | anticoagulant |
| Dioctyl | docusate sodium | laxative |
| Diovan | valsartan | hypertension |
| Dipentum | olsalazine | ulcerative colitis |
| Diprivan | propofol | i.v. anaesthetic |
| Dirythmin-SA | disopyramide | cardiac arrhythmias |
| Disipal | orphenadrine | parkinsonism |
| Distaclor | cefaclor | antibiotic |
| Distamine | penicillamine | Wilson's disease |
| Ditropan | oxybutynin | urinary incontinence |
| Diurexan | xipamide | diuretic |
| Dixarit | clonidine | migraine |
| Dobutrex | dobutamine | cardiac stimulant |
| Dolmatil | sulpiride | schizophrenia |
| Dolobid | diflunisal | analgesic |
| Doloxene | dextropropoxyphene | analgesic |
| Domical | amitriptyline | antidepressant |
| Dopacard | dopexamine | cardiac surgery |
| Dopamet | methyldopa | hypertension |

| Proprietary name | Approved name | Main action or indication |
| --- | --- | --- |
| Dopram | doxopram | respiratory stimulant |
| Doralese | indoramin | hypertension |
| Dostinex | cabergoline | dopamine agonist |
| Dovonex | calcipotriol | psoriasis |
| Dozic | haloperidol | antipsychotic |
| Dramamine | dimenhydrinate | antihistamine |
| Drogenil | flutamide | prostatic carcinoma |
| Droleptan | droperidol | analgesic |
| Dryptal | frusemide | diuretic |
| DTIC | dacarbazine | cytotoxic |
| Dulcolax | bisacodyl | laxative |
| Duphalac | lactulose | laxative |
| Duphaston | dydrogestone | progestogen |
| Durogesic | fentanyl-patch | analgesic |
| Duromine | phentermine | appetite suppressant |
| Dutonin | nefazodone | antidepressant |
| Dyazide | co-triamterzide | diuretic |
| Dyspamet | cimetidine | H$_2$-blocker |
| Dysport | botulinum toxin | blepharospasm |
| Dytac | triamterine | diuretic |
| Ebufac | ibuprofen | arthritis |
| Ecostatin | econazole | antifungal |
| Edecrin | ethacrynic acid | diuretic |
| Edronax | roboxetine | antidepressant |
| Efalith | lithium succinate | seborrhoea |
| Efcortesol | hydrocortisone | topical corticosteroid |

| Proprietary name | Approved name | Main action or indication |
|---|---|---|
| Efexor | venlafaxine | antidepressant |
| Efudix | fluorouracil | cytotoxic |
| Elantan | isosorbide mononitrate | angina |
| Eldepryl | selegiline | parkinsonism |
| Eldisine | vindesine | cytotoxic |
| Eltroxin | thyroxine | thyroid deficiency |
| Elyzol | metronidazole | anaerobic infections |
| Emblon | tamoxifen | cytotoxic |
| Emcor | bisoprolol | beta-blocker |
| Emflex | acemetacin | arthritis |
| Eminase | anistreplase | fibrinolytic |
| Endoxana | cyclophosphamide | cytotoxic |
| Epanutin | phenytoin | anticonvulsant |
| Ephynal | tocopherol | vitamin E deficiency |
| Epilim | sodium valproate | anticonvulsant |
| Epivir | lamivudine | antiviral |
| Epogam | gamolenic acid | eczema |
| Eppy | adrenaline | glaucoma |
| Eprex | eryhthropoietin | anaemia in chronic renal failure |
| Equanil | meprobamate | tranquillizer |
| Erecnos | moxisylyte | erection stimulant |
| Erwinase | crisantaspase | leukaemia |
| Erycen | erythromycin | antibiotic |
| Erymax | erythromycin | antibiotic |
| Erythrocin | erythromycin | antibiotic |

Approved and proprietary names of drugs

| Proprietary name | Approved name | Main action or indication |
| --- | --- | --- |
| Erythroped | erythromycin | antibiotic |
| Eskazole | albendazole | hydatid disease |
| Esmeron | rocuronium | muscle relaxant |
| Estracyt | estramustine | cytotoxic |
| Estradurin | polyestradiol | prostatic carcinoma |
| Ethmozine | moracizine | anti-arrhythmic |
| Ethyol | amifostine | cytoprotectant |
| Eucardic | carvedilol | hypertension |
| Eudemine | diazoxide | hypertension; hypoglycaemia |
| Euglucon | glibenclamide | hypoglycaemia |
| Eumovate | clobetasone | topical corticosteroid |
| Eurax | crotamiton | antipruritic |
| Exelderm | sulconazole | antifungal |
| Exosurf | colfosceril | neonatal respiratory distress |
| Famvir | famciclovir | antiviral |
| Fareston | toremifene | cytotoxic |
| Farlutal | medroxyprogesterone | progestogen |
| Fasigyn | tinidazole | anaerobic infections |
| Faverin | fluvoxamine | antidepressant |
| Feldene | piroxicam | arthritis |
| Femara | letrozole | cytotoxic |
| Femulen | ethynodiol | oral contraceptive |
| Fenbid | ibuprofen | arthritis |
| Fenopron | fenoprofen | arthritis |
| Fentazin | perphenazine | tranquillizer |

| Proprietary name | Approved name | Main action or indication |
|---|---|---|
| Fertiral | gonadorelin | infertility |
| Flagyl | metronidazole | trichomoniasis |
| Flamazine | silver sulphadiazine | antibacterial |
| Flaxedil | gallamine | muscle relaxant |
| Flixonase | fluticasone | topical corticosteroid |
| Flolan | epoprostenol | preserving platelet function in by-pass surgery |
| Flomax | tamsulosin | prostatic hypertrophy |
| Florinef | fludrocortisone | corticosteroid |
| Floxapen | flucloxacillin | antibiotic |
| Flu-Amp | co-fluampicil | antibiotic |
| Fluanoxol | flupenthixol | antidepressant |
| Fludara | fludarabine | cytotoxic |
| Fluothane | halothane | inhalation anaesthetic |
| FML | fluoromethalone | topical corticosteroid |
| Foradil | eformoterol | bronchodilator |
| Forane | isoflurane | inhalation anaesthetic |
| Fortral | pentazocine | analgesic |
| Fortum | ceftazidime | antibiotic |
| Fosamax | alendronic acid | osteoporosis |
| Foscavir | foscarnet | antiviral |
| Fragmin | deltaparin | anticoagulant |
| Frisium | clobazam | anxiolytic |
| Froben | flurbiprofen | antirheumatic |
| Frumil | co-amilofruse | diuretic |
| Fucidin | sodium fusidate | antibiotic |

Approved and proprietary
names of drugs

| Proprietary name | Approved name | Main action or indication |
|---|---|---|
| Fulcin | griseofulvin | antifungal |
| Fungilin | amphotericin B | antifungal |
| Fungizone | amphotericin B | antifungal |
| Furadantin | nitrofurantoin | urinary antiseptic |
| Furamide | diloxanide furoate | amoebiasis |
| Galenamox | amoxycillin | antibiotic |
| Galenphol | pholcodine | antitussive |
| Gamanil | lofepramine | antidepressant |
| Garamycin | gentamicin | antibiotic |
| Gastromax | metoclopramide | antiemetic |
| Gelofusine | gelatin | blood volume expander |
| Gemzar | gemcitabine | cytotoxic |
| Genotropin | somatropin | growth hormone |
| Genticin | gentamicin | antibiotic |
| Gentran | dextran | plasma substitute |
| Geref | sermorelin | growth hormone |
| Glibenese | glipizide | hypoglycaemic |
| Glucobay | acarbose | diabetes |
| Glucophage | metformin | hypoglycaemic |
| Glurenorm | gliquidone | hypoglycaemic |
| Glypressin | terlipressin | oesophageal varices |
| Gopten | trandolapril | ACE inhibitor |
| Granocyte | lenograstim | neutropenia |
| Grisovin | griseofulvin | antifungal |
| Guarem | guar gum | hypoglycaemic |
| Haelan | fluandrenolone | topical corticosteroid |

| Proprietary name | Approved name | Main action or indication |
| --- | --- | --- |
| Halciderm | halcinonide | topical corticosteroid |
| Haldol | haloperidol | schizophrenia |
| Halfan | halofantrine | antimalarial |
| Harmogen | oestrone | menopause |
| Hebamate | carboprost | post-partum haemorrhage |
| Heminevrin | chlormethiazole | psychosis; hypnotic |
| Hep-Flush | heparin | anticoagulant |
| Heplok | heparin | anticoagulant |
| Hepsal | heparin | anticoagulant |
| Herpid | idoxuridine | antiviral |
| Hespan | hetastarch | plasma substitute |
| Hetrazan | diethylcarbamazine | filariasis |
| Hexalen | altretamine | cytotoxic |
| Hexopal | inositol nicotinate | vasodilator |
| Hibitane | chlorhexidine | antiseptic |
| Hiprex | hexamine hippurate | urinary antiseptic |
| Hismanal | astemizole | antihistamine |
| Hivid | zalcatabine | antiviral |
| Honvan | fosfestrol | cytotoxic |
| Humatrope | somatropin | growth hormone |
| Humegon | gonadotrophin | infertility |
| Hyalase | hyaluronidase | enzyme |
| Hycamtin | topotecan | cytotoxic |
| Hydergine | co-dergocrine | dementia |
| Hydrea | hydroxyurea | cytotoxic |
| Hydrenox | hydroflumethiazide | diuretic |

223

Approved and proprietary
names of drugs

| Proprietary name | Approved name | Main action or indication |
| --- | --- | --- |
| Hydrocortistab | hydrocortisone | corticosteroid |
| Hydrocortisyl | hydrocortisone | corticosteroid |
| Hydrocortone | hydrocortisone | corticosteroid |
| HydroSaluric | hydrochlorothiazide | diuretic |
| Hygroton | chlorthalidone | diuretic |
| Hypnomidate | etomidate | i.v. anaesthetic |
| Hypnovel | midazolam | hypnotic |
| Hypovase | prazosin | hypertension |
| Hytrin | terazocin | hypertension |
| Ibular | ibuprofen | arthritis |
| Iduridin | idoxuridine | antiviral |
| Ikorel | nicorandil | angina |
| Ilosone | erythromycin | antibiotic |
| Imbrilon | indomethacin | arthritis |
| Imdur | isosorbide mononitrate | angina |
| Imigran | sumatriptan | migraine |
| Imtack | isosorbide dinitrate | angina |
| Immunoprin | azathioprine | immunosuppressant |
| Imodium | loperamide | diarrhoea |
| Imunovir | inosine pranobex | antiviral |
| Imuran | azathioprine | immunosuppressant |
| Inderal | propranolol | beta-blocker |
| Indocid | indomethacin | arthritis |
| Indolar SR | indomethacin | arthritis |
| Indomod | indomethacin | arthritis |
| Innohep | tinzaparin | anticoagulant |

| Proprietary name | Approved name | Main action or indication |
|---|---|---|
| Innovace | enalapril | ACE inhibitor |
| Inoven | ibuprofen | analgesic |
| Intal | sodium cromoglycate | asthma |
| Integrin | oxypertine | antipsychotic |
| Intraval | thiopentone | i.v. anaesthetic |
| Intron A | interferon | leukaemia |
| Invirase | saquinavir | antiviral |
| Iodosorb | cadexomer iodine | leg ulcers |
| Ionamin | phentamine | appetite suppressant |
| Iopidine | apraclonidine | glaucoma |
| Ipral | trimethoprim | antibacterial |
| Ismelin | guanethidine | hypertension |
| Ismo | isosorbide mononitrate | angina |
| Isordil | isosorbide dinitrate | angina |
| Isotrate | isosorbide mononitrate | angina |
| Isotrex | isotretinoin | acne |
| Istin | amlodipine | calcium antagonist |
| Jectofer | iron-sorbitol | iron deficiency anaemia |
| Kabikinase | streptokinase | fibrinolytic |
| Kannasyn | kanamycin | antibiotic |
| Kefadol | cephamandole | antibiotic |
| Keflex | cephalexin | antibiotic |
| Kefzol | cephamandole | antibiotic |
| Kelfizine | sulfametopyrazine | sulphonamide |
| Kelocyanor | dicolbalt edetate | cyanide poisoning |
| Kemadrin | procyclidine | parkinsonism |

Approved and proprietary
names of drugs

| Proprietary name | Approved name | Main action or indication |
| --- | --- | --- |
| Kemicetine | chloromycetin | antibiotic |
| Kenalog | triamcinolone | corticosteroid |
| Kerlone | betaxolol | beta-blocker |
| Ketalar | ketamine | i.v. anaesthetic |
| Kinidin | quinidine | cardiac arrhythmias |
| Klaricid | clarithromycin | antibiotic |
| Kogenate | factor VIII | haemophilia |
| Konakion | phytomenadione | hypoprothrombinaemia |
| Kytril | granisetron | antiemetic |
| Ladropen | flucloxacillin | antibiotic |
| Lamictal | lamotrigine | epilepsy |
| Lamisil | terbinafine | antifungal agent |
| Lamprene | clofazimine | leprosy |
| Lanoxin | digoxin | heart failure |
| Lanvis | thioguanine | cytotoxic |
| Laractone | spironolactone | diuretic |
| Laraflex | naproxen | arthritis |
| Larapam | piroxicam | arthritis |
| Laratrim | co-trimoxazole | antibacterial |
| Largactil | chlorpromazine | antipsychotic |
| Larium | mefloquine | malaria |
| Larodopa | levodopa | parkinsonism |
| Lasix | frusemide | diuretic |
| Lasma | theophylline | bronchodilator |
| Lasoride | co-amilofruse | diuretic |
| Laxoberal | sodium picosulphate | laxative |

| Proprietary name | Approved name | Main action or indication |
|---|---|---|
| Lederfen | fenbufen | antirheumatic |
| Ledermycin | demeclocycline | antibiotic |
| Lederspan | triamcinolone | corticosteroid |
| Lentaron | formestane | cytotoxic |
| Lentizol | amitriptyline | antidepressant |
| Lescol | fluvastatin | hyperlipidaemia |
| Leucomax | molgramostim | neutropenia |
| Leukeran | chlorambucil | cytotoxic |
| Leustat | cladribine | cytotoxic |
| Levophed | noradrenaline | vasoconstrictor |
| Lexotan | bromazepam | anxiolytic |
| Libanil | glibenclamide | hypoglycaemic |
| Librium | chlordiazepoxide | antipsychotic |
| Lidifen | ibuprofen | arthritis |
| Limclair | trisodium edetate | ocular lime burns |
| Lingraine | ergotamine | migraine |
| Lioresal | baclofen | muscle relaxant |
| Lipantil | fenofibrate | hyperlipidaemia |
| Lipitor | atorvastatin | hyperlipidaemia |
| Lipobay | cerivastatin | hyperlipidaemia |
| Lipostat | pravastatin | hyperlipidaemia |
| Liskonum | lithium carbonate | mania |
| Litarex | lithium citrate | mania |
| Livial | tibolone | menopausal symptoms |
| Livostin | levocabastine | allergic conjunctivitis |
| Locabiotal | fusafungine | antibiotic |

227

Approved and proprietary
names of drugs

| Proprietary name | Approved name | Main action or indication |
|---|---|---|
| Loceryl | amorolfine | topical antifungal |
| Lodine | etodolac | arthritis |
| Lomexin | fenticonazole | antifungal |
| Lomotil | co-phenotrope | diarrhoea |
| Loniten | minoxidil | hypertension |
| Lopid | gemfibrozil | hyperlipidaemia |
| Lopressor | metoprolol | beta-blocker |
| Loron | sodium clodronate | hypercalcaemia of malignancy |
| Losec | omeprazole | peptic ulcer |
| Loxapac | loxapine | antipsychotic |
| Ludiomil | maprotiline | antidepressant |
| Lustral | sertraline | antidepressant |
| Lyclear | permethrin | pediculocide |
| Macrodantin | nitrofurantoin | urinary infections |
| Macrodox | dextran | plasma substitute |
| Madopar | co-beneldopa | parkinsonism |
| Magnapen | co-fluampicil | antibiotic |
| Malarone | atoraquone | antimalarial |
| Manerix | moclobemide | antidepressant |
| Marcain | bupivacaine | anaesthetic |
| Marevan | warfarin | anticoagulant |
| Marplan | isocarboxazid | antidepressant |
| Maxolon | metoclopramide | antiemetic |
| Maxtrex | methotrexate | cytotoxic |
| Mectizan | ivermectin | filariasis |

| Proprietary name | Approved name | Main action or indication |
|---|---|---|
| Medrone | methylprednisolone | corticosteroid |
| Mefoxin | cefoxitin | antibiotic |
| Megace | megestrol | cytotoxic |
| Melleril | thioridazine | tranquillizer |
| Menzol | norethisterone | menorrhagia |
| Meptid | meptazinol | analgesic |
| Merbentyl | dicyclomine | antispasmodic |
| Meronem | meropenem | antibiotic |
| Mestinon | pyridostigmine | myasthenia |
| Metenix | metolazone | diuretic |
| Metopirone | metyrapone | resistant oedema |
| Metosyn | fluocinonide | corticosteroid |
| Metrodin | urofollitrophin | infertility |
| Metrolyl | metronidazole | amoebicide |
| Metrotop | metronidazole | topical deodorant |
| Mexitil | mexilitene | cardiac arrhythmias |
| Miacalcic | salcatonin | Paget's disease |
| Mifegyne | mifepristone | antiprogestogen |
| Minocin | minocycline | antibiotic |
| Minodiab | glipizide | hypoglycaemic |
| Mintec | peppermint oil | antispasmodic |
| Mintezol | thiabendazole | anthelmintic |
| Mitoxana | ifosfamide | cytotoxic |
| Mivacron | mivacurium | muscle relaxant |
| Mobic | meloxicam | osteoarthritis |
| Mobiflex | tenoxicam | arthritis |

229

Approved and proprietary
names of drugs

| Proprietary name | Approved name | Main action or indication |
|---|---|---|
| Modalim | ciprofibrate | hyperlipidaemia |
| Modecate | fluphenazine | antipsychotic |
| Moditen | fluphenazine | schizophrenia |
| Modrasone | alclometasone | topical corticosteroid |
| Modrenal | trilostane | adrenal cortex inhibitor |
| Moduret 25 | co-amilozide | diuretic |
| Moduretic | co-amilozide | diuretic |
| Mogadon | nitrazepam | hypnotic |
| Molipaxin | trazodone | antidepressant |
| Monit | isosorbide mononitrate | angina |
| Mono Cedocard | isosorbide mononitrate | angina |
| Monoclate-P | Factor VIII | haemophilia |
| Monocor | bisoprolol | beta-blocker |
| Mononine | Factor IX | haemophilia |
| Monoparin | heparin | anticoagulant |
| Monotrim | trimethaprim | antibacterial |
| Monovent | terbutaline | bronchospasm |
| Monuril | fosfomycin | antibacterial |
| Motens | lacidipine | hypertension |
| Motilium | domperidone | antiemetic |
| Motrin | ibuprofen | arthritis |
| MST Continus | morphine | analgesic |
| Mucodyne | carbocisteine | mucolytic |
| Multiparin | heparin | anticoagulant |
| Myambutol | ethambutol | tuberculosis |

| Proprietary name | Approved name | Main action or indication |
| --- | --- | --- |
| Mycardol | pentaerythritol | coronary dilator |
| Mycifradin | neomycin | antibiotic |
| Mycobutin | rifabutin | tuberculosis |
| Mydriacyl | tropicamide | mydriatic |
| Mydrilate | cyclopentolate | mydriatic |
| Myleran | busulphan | cytotoxic |
| Myocrisin | sodium aurothiomalate | rheumatoid arthritis |
| Myotonine | bethanechol | cholinergic |
| Mysoline | primidone | epilepsy |
| Nalcrom | sodium cromoglycate | anti-allergic |
| Nalorex | naltrexone | opioid dependence |
| Naprosyn | naproxen | arthritis |
| Naramig | naratriptan | migraine |
| Narcan | naloxone | narcotic antagonist |
| Nardil | phenelzine | antidepressant |
| Naropin | ropivacaine | local anaesthetic |
| Narphen | phenazocine | analgesic |
| Natrilix | indapamide | hypertension |
| Natulan | procarbazine | cytotoxic |
| Navelbine | vinorelbine | cytotoxic |
| Navidrex | cyclopenthiazide | diuretic |
| Navoban | tropisetron | antiemetic |
| Nebcin | tobramycin | antibiotic |
| Negram | nalidixic acid | urinary antiseptic |
| Neo-Cytamen | hydroxocobalamin | anti-anaemic |

| Proprietary name | Approved name | Main action or indication |
| --- | --- | --- |
| Neo-Mercazole | carbimazole | thyrotoxicosis |
| Neo-Naclex | bendrofluazide | diuretic |
| Neoral | cyclosporin | immunosuppressant |
| Neotigason | acitretin | psoriasis |
| Nephril | polythiazide | diuretic |
| Nerisone | diflucortolone | corticosteroid |
| Netillin | netilmicin | antibiotic |
| Neulactil | pericyazine | schizophrenia |
| Neupogen | filgrastim | neutropenia |
| Neurontin | gabapentin | epilepsy |
| Neutrexin | trimetrexate | AIDS |
| Nimbex | cisatracurium | muscle relaxant |
| Nimotop | nimodipine | subarachnoid haemorrhage |
| Nipent | pentostatin | cytotoxic |
| Nitoman | tetrabenazine | chorea |
| Nitrocine | glyceryl trinitrate | angina |
| Nitrolingual | glyceryl trinitrate | angina |
| Nitronal | glyceryl trinitrate | angina |
| Nivaquine | chloroquine | antimalarial |
| Nivemycin | neomycin | antibiotic |
| Nizoral | ketoconazole | antifungal |
| Nolvadex | tamoxifen | cytotoxic |
| Nootropil | piracetam | myoclonus |
| Norcuron | vecuronium | muscle relaxant |
| Norditropin | somatropin | growth hormone |

Approved and proprietary
names of drugs

| Proprietary name | Approved name | Main action or indication |
| --- | --- | --- |
| Norprolac | quinagolide | hyperprolactinaemia |
| Norvir | ritonavir | antiviral |
| Novantrone | mitozantrone | cytotoxic |
| NovoSeven | Factor VIIa | haemophilia A |
| Nozinan | methotrimeprazine | pain in terminal cancer |
| Nubain | nalbuphine | analgesic |
| Nupercainal | cinchocaine | local anaesthetic |
| Nycopren | naproxen | arthritis |
| Nystan | nystatin | antifungal |
| Ocusert Pilo | pilocarpine | glaucoma |
| Odrik | trandolapril | ACE inhibitor |
| Olbetam | acipimox | hyperlipidaemia |
| Omnopon | papaveretum | analgesic |
| Oncovin | vincristine | cytotoxic |
| One-Alpha | alfacalcidol | vitamin D deficiency |
| Ophthaine | proxymetacaine | corneal anaesthetic |
| Opilon | thymoxamine | vasodilator |
| Opticrom | sodium cromoglycate | allergic conjunctivitis |
| Optimax | tryptophan | antidepressant |
| Optimine | azatadine | antihistamine |
| Orap | pimozide | schizophrenia |
| Orbenin | cloxacillin | antibiotic |
| Orgaron | danaparoid | anticoagulant |
| Orelox | cefpodoxime | antibiotic |
| Orgafol | urofillitrophin | infertility |
| Orimeten | aminoglutethimide | cytotoxic |

Approved and proprietary
names of drugs

| Proprietary name | Approved name | Main action or indication |
| --- | --- | --- |
| Orudis | ketoprofen | arthritis |
| Oruvail | ketoprofen | arthritis |
| Otrivine | xylometazoline | nasal congestion |
| Ovex | mebendazole | anthelmintic |
| Oxivent | oxitropium | bronchodilator |
| Palfium | dextromoramide | analgesic |
| Palladone | hydromorphone | analgesic |
| Paludrine | proguanil | antimalarial |
| Panadeine | co-codamol | analgesic |
| Panadol | paracetamol | analgesic |
| Paracodol | co-codamol | analgesic |
| Parake | co-codamol | analgesic |
| Paramol | co-dydramol | analgesic |
| Paraplatin | carboplatin | cytotoxic |
| Parlodel | bromocriptine | lactation suppressant |
| Parmid | metoclopramide | antiemetic |
| Parnate | tranylcypromine | antidepressant |
| Paroven | oxyrutins | varicose states |
| Parvolex | acetylcysteine | paracetamol overdose |
| Pavulon | pancuronium | muscle relaxant |
| Pecram | aminophylline | bronchodilator |
| Penbritin | ampicillin | antibiotic |
| Pendramine | penicillamine | Wilson's disease |
| Pentacarinat | pentamidine | leishmaniasis |
| Pentasa | mesalazine | ulcerative colitis |
| Pentostam | sodium stibogluconate | leishmaniasis |

| Proprietary name | Approved name | Main action or indication |
|---|---|---|
| Pepcid | famotidine | $H_2$-blocker |
| Percutol | glyceryl trinitrate | angina |
| Perdix | moexipril | hypertension |
| Perfan | enoximone | heart failure |
| Pergonal | menotrophin | hypogonadism |
| Periactin | cyproheptadine | antihistamine |
| Persantin | dipyridamole | angina |
| Pevaryl | econazole | antifungal |
| Pharmorubicin | epirubicin | cytotoxic |
| Phenergan | promethazine | antihistamine |
| Phyllocontin | aminophylline | bronchodilator |
| Physeptone | methadone | analgesic |
| Physiotens | moxonidine | hypertension |
| Picolax | sodium picosulphate | laxative |
| Piportil | pipothiazine | antipsychotic |
| Pipril | piperacillin | antibiotic |
| Piriton | chlorpheniramine | antihistamine |
| Plaquenil | hydroxychloroquine | antimalarial |
| Plendil | felodipine | calcium antagonist |
| Pondocillin | pivampicillin | antibiotic |
| Ponstan | mefenamic acid | arthritis |
| Posiject | dobutamine | cardiac support |
| Potaba | potassium p-aminobenzoate | scleroderma |
| Praxilene | naftidrofuryl | vasodilator |
| Precortisyl | prednisolone | corticosteroid |

Approved and proprietary names of drugs

| Proprietary name | Approved name | Main action or indication |
|---|---|---|
| Predsol | prednisolone | corticosteroid |
| Premarin | oestrogen | menopause |
| Prepidil | dinoprostone | cervical ripening |
| Prepulsid | cisapride | oesophageal reflux |
| Prescal | isradipine | calcium antagonist |
| Preservex | aceclofenac | arthritis |
| Priadel | lithium carbonate | mania |
| Primacor | milrinone | severe heart failure |
| Primalan | mequitazine | antihistamine |
| Primaxin | imipenem | antibiotic |
| Primolut N | norethisterone | progestogen |
| Primperan | metoclopramide | antiemetic |
| Pro-Banthine | propantheline | spasmolytic |
| Profasi | gonadotrophin | infertility |
| Prograf | tacrolimus | immunosuppressant |
| Proleukin | aldesleukin | cytotoxic |
| Proluton-Depot | hydroxyprogesterone | progestogen |
| Prominal | methylphenobarbitone | epilepsy |
| Pronestyl | procainamide | cardiac arrhythmias |
| Propaderm | beclomethasone | topical corticosteroid |
| Propine | dipivefrin | glaucoma |
| Proscar | finasteride | prostatic hypertrophy |
| Prostap | leuprorelin | prostatic carcinoma |
| Prostin F2 | dinoprost | uterine stimulant |
| Prostin VR | aprostadil | maintenance of ductus arteriosus in neonates |

| Proprietary name | Approved name | Main action or indication |
|---|---|---|
| Prothiaden | dothiepin | antidepressant |
| Protium | pantoprazole | peptic ulcer |
| Provera | medroxyprogesterone | progestogen |
| Pro-Viron | mesterolone | androgen deficiency |
| Prozac | fluoxetine | antidepressant |
| Pulmicort | budesonide | rhinitis |
| Pulmozyme | dornase alfa | pulmonary surfactant |
| Puri-Nethol | mercaptopurine | cytotoxic |
| Pylorid | ranitidine bismuth citrate | peptic ulcer |
| Quellada | lindane | pediculosis |
| Questran | cholestyramine | bile acid binder |
| Rapifen | alfentanyl | narcotic analgesic |
| Rapitil | nedocromil | ocular allergy |
| Rapilysin | reteplase | fibrinolytic |
| Rastinon | tolbutamide | hypoglycaemic |
| Razoxin | razoxane | cytotoxic |
| Recormon | epoetin beta | anaemia in chronic renal railure |
| Redoxon | ascorbic acid | vitamin C deficiency |
| Refolinon | folinic acid | methotrexate antidote |
| Regaine | minoxidil | baldness |
| Relefact | gonadorelin | test of pituitary function |
| Relifex | nabumetone | arthritis |
| Remnos | nitrazepam | hypnotic |
| Reo-Pro | abciximab | antiplatelet |
| Replenine | Factor IX | haemophilia B |

| Proprietary name | Approved name | Main action or indication |
| --- | --- | --- |
| Requip | ropinirole | parkinsonism |
| Respacal | tulobuterol | bronchodilator |
| Resonium-A | exchange resin | hyperkalaemia |
| Restandol | testosterone | androgen deficiency |
| Retin A | tretinoin | acne |
| Retrovir | zidovudine | antiviral |
| Revanil | lysuride | parkinsonism |
| Rheomacrodex | dextran | blood volume expander |
| Rheumox | azapropazone | arthritis |
| Rhinocort | budesonide | rhinitis |
| Rhinolast | azelastine | topical antihistamine |
| Ridaura | auranofin | rheumatoid arthritis |
| Rifadin | rifampicin | tuberculosis |
| Rilutek | riluzole | motor neurone disease |
| Rimactane | rifampicin | tuberculosis |
| Rinatec | ipratropium | rhinorrhoea |
| Risperdal | risperidone | schizophrenia |
| Ritalin | methylphenidate | hyperactivity |
| Rivotril | clonazepam | anticonvulsant |
| Roaccutane | isotretinoin | severe acne |
| Robaxin | methocarbamol | muscle relaxant |
| Rocaltrol | calcitriol | vitamin D deficiency |
| Rocephin | ceftriaxone | antibiotic |
| Roferon-A | interferon | leukaemia |
| Rogitine | phentolamine | phaeochromocytoma |
| Rohypnol | flunitrazepam | hypnotic |

Approved and proprietary
names of drugs

| Proprietary name | Approved name | Main action or indication |
|---|---|---|
| Romozin | troglitazone | insulin enhancer |
| Ronicol | nicotinyl alcohol | vasodilator |
| Rosex | metronidazole | acne |
| Rynacrom | sodium cromoglycate | allergic rhinitis |
| Rythmodan | disopyramide | cardiac arrhythmias |
| Sabril | vigabatrin | anticonvulsant |
| Saizen | somatropin | growth hormone |
| Salamol | salbutamol | asthma |
| Salazopyrin | sulphasalazine | ulcerative colitis |
| Salbulin | salbutamol | bronchodilator |
| Salofalk | mesalazine | ulcerative colitis |
| Saluric | chlorothiazide | diuretic |
| Sandimmun | cyclosporin | immunosuppressant |
| Sandoglobulin | immunoglobulin | hepatitis |
| Sandostatin | octreotide | carcinoid syndrome |
| Sanomigran | pizotifen | migraine |
| Saventrine | isoprenaline | heart block |
| Scoline | suxamethonium | muscle relaxant |
| Scopoderm TTS | hyoscine | motion sickness |
| Seconal | quinalbarbitone | hypnotic |
| Sectral | acebutolol | beta-blocker |
| Securon | verapamil | angina |
| Securopen | azlocillin | antibiotic |
| Selsun | selenium sulphide | dandruff |
| Semprex | acrivastine | antihistamine |
| Septrin | co-trimoxazole | antibacterial |

| Proprietary name | Approved name | Main action or indication |
|---|---|---|
| Serc | betahistine | Ménière's syndrome |
| Serdolect | sertindole | schizophrenia |
| Serenace | haloperidol | schizophrenia |
| Serevent | salmeterol | bronchospasm |
| Serophene | clomiphene | infertility |
| Seroquel | quetiapine | schizophrenia |
| Seroxat | paroxetine | antidepressant |
| Sevredol | morphine | analgesic |
| Simplene | adrenaline | glaucoma |
| Sinemet | co-careldopa | parkinsonism |
| Sinequan | doxepin | antidepressant |
| Sinthrome | nicoumalone | anticoagulant |
| Sintisone | prednisolone | corticosteroid |
| Skelid | tiludronic acid | Paget's disease |
| Skinoren | azelaic acid | acne |
| Slo-Phyllin | theophylline | bronchodilator |
| Slow-Trasicor | oxprenolol | beta-blocker |
| Soframycin | framycetin | antibiotic |
| Solu-Cortef | hydrocortisone | corticosteroid |
| Solu-Medrone | methylprednisolone | corticosteroid |
| Sominex | promethazine | mild hypnotic |
| Somnite | nitrazepam | hypnotic |
| Soneryl | butobarbitone | hypnotic |
| Sorbid SA | isosorbide dinitrate | angina |
| Sorbitrate | isosorbide dinitrate | angina |
| Sotacor | sotalol | beta-blocker |

| Proprietary name | Approved name | Main action or indication |
|---|---|---|
| Sparine | promazine | antipsychotic |
| Spasmonal | alverine | antispasmodic |
| Spiroctan-M | canrenoate | diuretic |
| Spirolone | spironolactone | diuretic |
| Sporanox | itraconazole | antifungal |
| Stafoxil | flucloxacillin | antibiotic |
| Staril | fosfinopril | ACE inhibitor |
| Stelazine | trifluoperazine | antipsychotic |
| Stemetil | prochlorperazine | antiemetic |
| Stesolid | diazepam | anxiolytic |
| Stiedex | desoxymethasone | topical corticosteroid |
| Stiemycin | erythromycin | acne |
| Stilnoct | zolpidem | insomnia |
| Streptase | streptokinase | fibrinolytic |
| Stromba | stanozolol | anabolic steroid |
| Stugeron | cinnarizine | antiemetic |
| Sublimaze | fentanyl | analgesic |
| Sulpitil | sulpiride | schizophrenia |
| Suprane | desflurane | inhalation anaesthetic |
| Suprax | cefixime | antibiotic |
| Suprecur | buserelin | endometriosis |
| Suprefact | buserelin | prostatic carcinoma |
| Surgam | tiaprofenic acid | arthritis |
| Surmontil | trimipramine | antidepressant |
| Survanta | beractant | lung surfactant |
| Suscard | glyceryl trinitrate | angina |

| Proprietary name | Approved name | Main action or indication |
|---|---|---|
| Sustac | glyceryl trinitrate | angina |
| Sustamycin | tetracycline | antibiotic |
| Sustanon | testosterone | androgen deficiency |
| Symmetrel | amantadine | parkinsonism |
| Synacthen | tetracosactrin | corticotrophin |
| Synalar | fluocinolone | topical corticosteroid |
| Synarel | nafarelin | endometriosis |
| Synflex | naproxen | arthritis |
| Syntaris | flunisolide | local corticosteroid |
| Syntocinon | oxytocin | post-partum haemorrhage |
| Syntopressin | lypressin | diabetes insipidus |
| Syscor | nisoldipine | angina |
| Sytron | sodium iron edetate | anti-anaemic |
| Tagamet | cimetidine | peptic ulcer |
| Tambocor | flecainide | cardiac arrhythmias |
| Tamofen | tamoxifen | cytotoxic |
| Targocid | teicoplanin | antibiotic |
| Tarivid | ofloxacin | urinary tract infections |
| Tasmar | tolcapone | parkinsonism |
| Tavegil | clemastine | antihistamine |
| Taxol | paclitaxel | cytotoxic |
| Taxotere | docetaxel | cytotoxic |
| Tazocin | tazobactam | antibiotic |
| Tegretol | carbamazepine | anticonvulsant |
| Telfast | fexofenodine | antihistamine |
| Temgesic | buprenorphine | analgesic |

| Proprietary name | Approved name | Main action or indication |
|---|---|---|
| Temopen | temocillin | antibiotic |
| Ternormin | atenolol | beta-blocker |
| Teoptic | carteolol | glaucoma |
| Terramycin | oxytetracycline | antibiotic |
| Tertroxin | liothyronine | thyroid deficiency |
| Tetralysal | lymecylycline | antibiotic |
| Theo-Dur | theophylline | bronchospasm |
| Thephorin | phenindamine | antihistamine |
| Tilade | neocromil | asthma |
| Tilarin | nedocromil | allergic conjunctivitis |
| Tildiem | diltiazem | calcium antagonist |
| Timentin | ticarcillin | antibiotic |
| Timecef | cefodizime | antibiotic |
| Timoptol | timolol | glaucoma |
| Tobralex | tobramycin | eye infections |
| Tofranil | imipramine | antidepressant |
| Tolanase | tolazamide | hypoglycaemic |
| Tolectin | tolmetin | antirheumatic |
| Tomudex | raltitrexed | cytotoxic |
| Topamax | topiramate | epilepsy |
| Topicycline | tetracycline | acne |
| Toradol | ketorolac | analgesic |
| Torem | torasemide | diuretic |
| Tracrium | atracurium | muscle relaxant |
| Tramake | tramadol | analgesic |
| Trandate | labetalol | beta-blocker |

Approved and proprietary
names of drugs

| Proprietary name | Approved name | Main action or indication |
|---|---|---|
| Transiderm-Nitro | glyceryl trinitrate | angina |
| Tranxene | clorazepate | anxiolytic |
| Trasicor | oxprenolol | beta-blocker |
| Trasidrex | co-prenozide | hypertension |
| Trasylol | aprotinin | pancreatitis |
| Travogyn | isoconazole | candidiasis |
| Traxam gel | felbinac | sprains |
| Trental | oxpentifylline | vasodilator |
| Triludan | terfenadine | antihistamine |
| Trimogal | trimethoprim | antibacterial |
| Trimopan | trimethoprim | antibacterial |
| Tritace | ramipril | ACE inhibitor |
| Trobicin | spectinomycin | antibiotic |
| Tropium | chlordiazepoxide | anxiety |
| Trosyl | tioconazole | antifungal |
| Trusopt | dorzolamide | glaucoma |
| Tryptizol | amitriptyline | antidepressant |
| Ubretid | distigmine | urinary retention |
| Ukidan | urokinase | hyphaema; embolism |
| Ultralanum | fluocortolone | topical corticosteroid |
| Ultiva | remifentanil | analgesic |
| Uniparin | heparin | anticoagulant |
| Uniphyllin Continus | theophylline | bronchospasm |
| Unisomnia | nitrazepam | hypnotic |
| Univer | verapamil | hypertension; angina |
| Uriben | nalidixic acid | urinary tract infections |

| Proprietary name | Approved name | Main action or indication |
| --- | --- | --- |
| Urispas | flavoxate | cystitis |
| Uromitexan | mesna | urotoxicity due to cyclophosphamide |
| Ursofalk | ursodeoxycholic acid | gall stones |
| Utinor | norfloxacin | urinary tract infections |
| Utovlan | ethisterone | progestogen |
| Uvistat | mexenone | sun screen |
| Valenac | diclofenac | arthritis |
| Valium | diazepam | anxiolytic; muscle relaxant |
| Vallergan | trimeprazine | sedative; pruritus |
| Valoid | cyclizine | antiemetic |
| Valtrex | valaciclovir | antiviral |
| Vancocin | vancomycin | antibiotic |
| Vascace | cilazapril | ACE inhibitor |
| Vasoxine | methoxamine | acute hypertension |
| Vectavir | penciclovir | antiviral |
| Velbe | vinblastine | cytotoxic |
| Velosef | cephradine | antibiotic |
| Ventolin | salbutamol | bronchospasm |
| Vepesid | etoposide | cytotoxic |
| Vermox | mebendazole | anthelmintic |
| Vesanoid | tretinoin | leukaemia |
| Vibramycin | doxycycline | antibiotic |
| Videx | didanosine | antiviral |
| Vidopen | ampicillin | antibiotic |
| Virazid | tribavirin | antiviral |

245

Approved and proprietary
names of drugs

| Proprietary name | Approved name | Main action or indication |
| --- | --- | --- |
| Virormone | testosterone | hypogonadism |
| Visclair | methylcysteine | mucolytic |
| Visken | pindolol | beta-blocker |
| Vistide | cidofovir | antiviral |
| Vivalan | viloxazine | antidepressant |
| Vividrin | sodium cromoglycate | allergic rhinitis |
| Volmax | salbutamol | bronchodilator |
| Volraman | diclofenac | arthritis |
| Voltarol | diclofenac | antirheumatic |
| Welldorm | chloral hydrate | hypnotic |
| Wellferon | interferon | leukaemia |
| Wellvone | atavaquone | antimalarial |
| Xalantan | latanoprost | glaucoma |
| Xanax | alprazolam | anxiolytic |
| Xatral | alfusozin | urinary retention |
| Xuret | metolazine | diuretic |
| Xylocaine | lignocaine | anaesthetic |
| Xylocard | lignocaine | cardiac arrhythmias |
| Yomesan | niclosamide | anthelmintic |
| Yutopar | ritodrine | premature labour |
| Zaditen | ketotifen | anti-asthmatic |
| Zadstat | metronidazole | trichomoniasis |
| Zamadol | tramadol | analgesic |
| Zanaflex | tizanidine | spasticity |
| Zantac | ranitidine | $H_2$-blocker |
| Zarontin | ethosuximide | anticonvulsant |

| Proprietary name | Approved name | Main action or indication |
|---|---|---|
| Zavedos | idarubicin | cytotoxic |
| Zerit | stavudine | antiviral |
| Zestril | lisinopril | ACE inhibitor |
| Zimovane | zopiclone | hypnotic |
| Zinacef | cefuroxime | antibiotic |
| Zinamide | pyrazinamide | tuberculosis |
| Zinga | nizatidine | peptic ulcer |
| Zinnat | cefuroxime | antibiotic |
| Zirtek | certirizine | antihistamine |
| Zispin | mirtazapine | antidepressant |
| Zithromax | azithromycin | antibiotic |
| Zocor | simvastatin | hyperlipidaemia |
| Zofran | ondansetron | antiemetic |
| Zoladex | goserlin | prostatic carcinoma |
| Zomacton | somatropin | growth hormone |
| Zomig | zolmitriptan | migraine |
| Zorac | tazarotene | psoriasis |
| Zoton | lanzoprazole | peptic ulcer |
| Zovirax | aciclovir | antiviral |
| Zydol | tramadol | analgesic |
| Zyloric | allopurinol | gout |
| Zyprexa | olanzapine | schizophrenia |

247

Approved and proprietary
names of drugs

| Orally active | Brand names | Daily dose range |
|---|---|---|
| cefaclor | Distaclor | 750 mg–4 g |
| cefadroxil | Baxan | 1–2 g |
| cefixime | Suprax | 200–400 mg |
| cefpodoxime | Orelox | 200–400 mg |
| ceftibuten | Cedax | 400 mg |
| cefuroxime | Zinnat | 500 mg–1 g |
| cephalexin | Ceporex, Keftex | 1–2 g |
| cephadrine | Velcef | 1–2 g |

| Cephalosporins given by IM or IV injection | | Daily dose range |
|---|---|---|
| cefodizime | Timecef | 2 g |
| cefotaxime | Claforan | 2–12 g |
| cefoxitin | Mefoxin | 3–12 g |
| cefpirome | Cefrom | 2–4 g |
| cefsulodin | Monospor | 1–4 g |
| ceftazidime | Fortum, Kefadim | 1–6 g |
| ceftizoxime | Cefizox | 2–8 g |
| ceftriaxone | Rocephin | 2–4 g |
| cefuroxime | Zinacef | 2–6 g |
| cephamandole | Kefadol | 2–12 g |
| cephazolin | Kefzol | 2–4 g |
| cephradine | Velosef | 2–8 g |

Table 34  Cephalosporins.

| Approved names | Brand names |
| --- | --- |
| chlortetracycline | Aureomycin |
| demeclocycline | Ledermycin |
| doxycycline | Nordox, Vibramycin |
| lymecycline | Tetralysal |
| minocycline | Minocin |
| oxytetracycline | Terramycin |

Table 35 Tetracyclines.

| Name | Dosage |
|---|---|
| cortisone | 25 mg |
| hydrocortisone | 20 mg |
| deflazacort | 6 mg |
| prednisone | 5 mg |
| prednisolone | 5 mg |
| methylprednisolone | 4 mg |
| triamcinolone | 4 mg |
| dexamethasone | 0.75 mg |
| betamethasone | 0.5 mg |

Table 36 Comparable doses of some corticosteroids.

| Name | Main action/target | Administration/injection |
|------|-------------------|--------------------------|
| amoxycillin | broad-spectrum | oral, i.m. |
| ampicillin | broad-spectrum | oral, i.m., i.v. |
| azlocillin | antipseudomonal | i.v. |
| benzylpenicillin | Gram-positive bacteria | i.m., i.v. |
| cloxacillin } <br> flucloxacillin } | penicillinase-producing <br> staphylococci | oral, i.m., i.v. |
| penicillin | see benzylpenicillin | |
| phenoxymethylpenicillin | as benzylpenicillin | oral |
| piperacillin | antipseudomonal | i.m., i.v. |
| pivampicillin | as ampicillin | oral |
| procaine-penicillin | long-acting penicillin | i.m. |
| temocillin | penicillinase-producing <br> Gram-negative bacteria | i.m., i.v. |
| ticarcillin | antipseudomonal | oral |

Table 37 Penicillins.

Penicillins

# Intravenous additives

The slow intravenous infusion of drugs has in some circumstances certain advantages over other injection methods, as a more even plasma level of the injected drug can be maintained over a longer period, and the disadvantages of a rapid bolus-type of injection are avoided. The method has its limitations as the addition of drugs to previously prepared i.v. fluids carries the risk of bacterial contamination, and strict aseptic precautions are essential during the preparation of any additive-containing i.v. fluid. In addition, incompatibility of the drug with the i.v. fluid may cause a loss of activity or an increase in toxicity, a risk that is increased if more than one drug is added to the infusion. Loss of activity may also occur because the stability of the drug is adversely influenced by dilution with the fluid, and in some cases the pH of the infusion may play an important part as far as the stability and activity of the drug are concerned.

The preparation of additive-containing fluids is best carried out in the hospital pharmacy. If nurses prepare any such solutions on the ward or at the bedside, they should be fully acquainted with the techniques required and be aware of the risks involved. In all cases, complete mixing or solution of the drug in the fluid is essential before i.v. infusion is commenced, and the giving set should not be used for more than 24 hours. Although the absence of any visual change in the appearance of the fluid is no guide to any loss of activity, any development or cloudiness in the solution, or a change of colour, is an indication that treatment should be stopped.

Intravenous additives are usually made to solutions of glucose 5%, or to sodium chloride solution 0.9%, although certain other fluids are also used, and any such extemporaneously prepared solution should be used as soon as possible, and only one bottle ought to be prepared at a time. Solutions containing sodium bicarbonate, mannitol, amino acids or blood products are not suitable vehicles for i.v. additives. The addition of drugs to i.v. fat emulsions is not recommended unless products specially formulated for the purpose are used. Such additions may break down the emulsion and cause embolism.

The i.v. infusion of drugs can be carried out by continuous or intermittent infusion. Some packs of continuous infusion fluids are designed to permit the addition of a drug in a way that reduces the risks of bacterial contamination, or the intermittent injection of a drug whilst the continuous infusion of the fluid is also taking place. With certain irritant cytotoxic drugs, the additive is not mixed with infusion fluid, but is injected via the tubing of a fast-running infusion fluid. Such a method permits the rapid dilution of the injected drug and so reduces the risks of vein irritation.

When a higher plasma level of a drug is required than can be obtained by continuous infusion, intermittent infusion is used, by which small volumes of about 100 ml of the drug solution are infused over 30–60 minutes. The method is used for drugs that are relatively unstable in dilute solution, such as amoxycillin and some other antibiotics, and for drugs that are unsuitable for administration by drip infusion.

In Table 38, the abbreviation G refers to glucose 5%, and S to sodium 0.9%, although some other standard solutions, such as Hartmann's Solution or Ringer's Solution, are used for additive-containing infusion fluids. In a few cases, Water for Injections (W) is preferred. CI refers to continuous i.v. infusion, I to intermittent infusion, and VDT to via drip tubing.

253

**Intravenous additives**

| Drug | Infusion fluid | Method of use |
|------|---------------|---------------|
| abciximab | G or S | CI |
| acetylcysteine | G | CI |
| aclarubicin | G or S | I (protect from light) |
| acyclovir | G or S | I |
| aldesleukin | G | CI |
| alfentanil | G or S | CI, I |
| alprostadil | G or S | CI |
| alteplase | S | CI, I |
| amikacin | G or S | I |
| aminophylline | G or S | CI |
| amiodarone | G | CI, I |
| amoxycillin | G or S | I |
| amphotericin | G | CI (protect from light) |
| ampicillin | G or S | I |
| amsacrine | G | I |
| atenolol | G or S | I |
| atracurium | G or S | CI |
| azathioprine | G or S | VDT |
| azlocillin | G or S | I |
| aztreonam | G or S | I |
| betamethasone | G or S | CI or VDT |
| bleomycin | S | I |
| bumetanide | G or S | I |

Table 38 Intravenous additives. Continued on pages 255–261.

| Drug | Infusion fluid | Method of use |
|------|----------------|---------------|
| calcium gluconate | G or S | CI (not with sodium bicarbonate) |
| carboplatin | G or S | CI |
| carmustine | G or S | I |
| cefodizime | G or S | I |
| cefotaxime | G or S | I |
| cefoxitin | G or S | I, VDT |
| cefsulodin | G or S | I, VDT |
| ceftazidime | G or S | I, VDT |
| ceftizoxime | G or S | I, VDT |
| ceftriaxone | G or S | CI, I |
| cefuroxime | G or S | I, VDT |
| cephamandole | G or S | I, VDT |
| cephazolin | G or S | I, VDT |
| cephradine | G or S | CI, I |
| chloramphenicol | G or S | I, VDT |
| chloroquine | S | CI |
| cimetidine | G or S | CI, I |
| cisatracurium | G or S | CI |
| cisplatin | S | CI |
| cladribine | S | CI |
| clarithromycin | G or S | I |
| clindamycin | G or S | CI, I |
| clomipramine | G or S | I |

Intravenous additives

| Drug | Infusion fluid | Method of use |
|------|----------------|---------------|
| clonazepam | G or S | I |
| cloxacillin | G or S | I, VDT |
| co-amoxiclav | S | I |
| co-fluampicil | G or S | I |
| colistin | G or S | CI, I |
| co-trimoxazole | G or S | I |
| cyclophosphamide | G or S | I, VDT |
| cyclosporin | G or S | CI |
| cytarabine | G or S | CI, I, VDT |
| dacarbazine | G or S | I |
| dactinomycin | G or S | I, VDT |
| daunorubicin | G | I |
| desferrioxamine | G or S | CI, I |
| dexamethasone | G or S | CI, I, VDT |
| diazepam | G or S | CI |
| diclofenac | G or S | CI, I |
| digoxin | G or S | CI |
| digoxin antibody | S | CI |
| dinoprost | G or S | CI |
| disodium etidronate | S | CI |
| disodium pamidronate | S | CI |
| disopyramide | G or S | CI, I |
| dobutamine | G or S | CI (not with sodium bicarbonate) |

| Drug | Infusion fluid | Method of use |
|------|----------------|---------------|
| docetaxel | G or S | CI |
| dopamine | G or S | CI |
| dopexamine | G or S | CI |
| doxorubicin | G or S | VDT |
| enoximone | S | CI, VDT |
| epirubicin | S | VDT |
| epoetin | S | I |
| epoprostenol | S | CI |
| erythromycin | G or S | CI, I |
| esmolol | G or S | CI, I |
| ethacrynic acid | G or S | VDT |
| etoposide | S | I |
| filgrastim | G | CI, I |
| flecainide | G or S | CI, I |
| flucloxacillin | G or S | I, VDT |
| fludarabine | S | I |
| flumazanil | G or S | CI |
| fluorouracil | G | CI, VDT |
| folinic acid | G or S | CI |
| foscarnet | G | CI |
| frusemide | S | CI |
| fusidic acid | G or S | CI |
| ganciclovir | G or S | I |
| gemcitabine | S | I |

257

**Intravenous additives**

| Drug | Infusion fluid | Method of use |
|------|----------------|---------------|
| gentamicin | G or S | I, VDT |
| glyceryl trinitrate | G or S | CI |
| granisetron | G or S | I |
| heparin | G or S | CI |
| hydralazine | S | CI |
| hydrocortisone | G or S | CI, I, VDT |
| idarubicin | S | VDT |
| ifosfamide | G or S | CI, I, VDT |
| imipenem | G or S | I |
| isoprenaline | G or S | CI (well diluted) |
| isosorbide dinitrate | G or S | CI |
| kanamycin | G or S | I |
| ketamine | G or S | CI |
| labetalol | G or S | I |
| lenograstim | S | I |
| lignocaine | G or S | CI (well diluted) |
| mecillinam | G or S | I |
| melphalan | S | CI, VDT |
| mesna | G or S | CI, VDT |
| metaraminol | G or S | CI, VDT |
| methocarbamol | G or S | I |
| methohexitone | G or S | I |
| methotrexate | G or S | I, VDT (well diluted) |
| methyldopa | G | I |

| Drug | Infusion fluid | Method of use |
|------|----------------|---------------|
| methylprednisolone | G or S | CI, I, VDT |
| metoclopramide | G or S | CI, I |
| mexiletine | G or S | CI |
| mezlocillin | G or S | CI |
| milrinone | G or S | CI |
| mitozantrone | G or S | VDT |
| mivacurium | G or S | CI |
| molgramostim | G or S | I |
| mustine | G or S | VDT |
| naloxone | G or S | CI |
| netilmicin | G or S | I, VDT |
| nimodipine | G or S | VDT |
| nizatidine | G or S | CI, I |
| noradrenaline | G or S | CI (well diluted) |
| ondansetron | G or S | CI, I |
| oxytocin | G | CI (well diluted) |
| paclitaxel | G or S | CI |
| pentamidine | G or S | I |
| pentostatin | G or S | I |
| phenoxybenzamine | S | I |
| phentolamine | G or S | I |
| phenylephrine | G or S | I |
| phenytoin | S | I |
| piperacillin | G or S | I |

259

Intravenous additives

| Drug | Infusion fluid | Method of use |
|------|----------------|---------------|
| polymyxin B | G | CI |
| potassium chloride | G or S | CI (well diluted) |
| propofol | G or S | VDT |
| quinine dihydrochloride | S | CI |
| ranitidine | G or S | I |
| rifampicin | G or S | I |
| ritodrine | G or S | CI (well diluted) |
| rocuronium | G or S | CI, VDT |
| salbutamol | G | CI |
| salcatonin | S | CI |
| sodium clodronate | S | CI |
| sodium nitroprusside | G | CI (well diluted; protect from light) |
| sodium valproate | G or S | CI, I |
| sotalol | G or S | CI, I |
| streptokinase | G or S | CI |
| sulphadiazine | S | CI |
| suxamethonium | G or S | CI |
| tacrolimus | G | CI |
| teicoplanin | G or S | I |
| temocillin | G or S | I |
| terbutaline | G | CI |
| tetracycline | G or S | CI |
| ticarcillin | G | I |

| Drug | Infusion fluid | Method of use |
|------|----------------|---------------|
| tobramycin | G or S | I, VDT |
| tramadol | G or S | CI, I |
| treosulfan | W | I |
| trimethoprim | G or S | VDT |
| tropisetron | G | I, VDT |
| urokinase | S | CI |
| vancomycin | G or S | I |
| vasopressin | G | I |
| vecuronium | G or S | I |
| vinblastine | S | VDT |
| vincristine | S | VDT |
| vindesine | G or S | VDT |
| zudovidine | G | I |

Intravenous additives

# Drugs and breast-feeding

Some drugs are known to be excreted to some extent in breast milk, and so should be avoided during breast-feeding, but in many cases information is scanty. Table 39 is only a general guide to the milk excretion of some standard drugs, and the omission of any drug does *not* imply that it is suitable for use during breast-feeding. Such use remains the responsibility of the prescriber. It might be wise to assume that if a drug of a certain class is listed, related drugs may have a similar pattern of excretion. If a drug is mentioned in more than one section, it may be that it is tolerated in low doses.

| Analgesics and anti-inflammatory drugs | Antimicrobial agents | Cardiovascular drugs; anticoagulants |
|---|---|---|
| **Drugs that are contraindicated** | | |
| gold compounds<br>phenylbutazone<br>penicillamine<br>indomethacin<br>colchicine<br>carisoprodol | chloramphenicol<br>tetracyclines<br>dapsone | amiodarone<br>ergotamine<br>phenindione |
| **Drugs for use under control** | | |
| salicylates | aminoglycosides<br>antimalarials<br>anthelmintics<br>ethambutol<br>isoniazid<br>metronidazole<br>nalidixic acid<br>sulphonamides | anti-arrhythmics<br>clonidine<br>nicoumalone |
| **Drugs usually considered safe in standard doses** | | |
| codeine<br>dextropropoxyphene<br>dihydrocodeine<br>ibuprofen<br>paracetamol<br>pentazocine<br>pethidine<br>salicylates | penicillins<br>cephalosporins<br>erythromycin<br>rifampicin<br>metronidazole<br>nitrofurantoin<br>antifungal agents<br>(except ketoconazole) | beta-blockers<br>digoxin<br>captopril<br>heparin<br>hydralazine<br>methyldopa<br>thiazide diuretics<br>warfarin |

**Table 39  Drugs and breast-feeding. Continued over.**

| CNS depressants: antidepressants; anticonvulsants | Drugs acting on the endocrine system; anticoagulants | Miscellaneous |
| --- | --- | --- |

### Drugs that are contraindicated

| | | |
| --- | --- | --- |
| doxepin<br>lithium salts | androgens<br>oestrogens<br>bromocriptine<br>cyproterone<br>carbimazole<br>corticosteroids<br>iodines | antineoplastics<br>atropine<br>calciferol<br>vitamin A |

### Drugs for use under control

| | | |
| --- | --- | --- |
| barbiturates<br>carbamazepine<br>benzodiazepines<br>phenothiazines<br>haloperidol<br>phenobarbitone<br>phenytoin<br>primidone<br>monoamine<br>  oxidase inhibitors | oestrogens<br>thyroxine<br>oral hypoglycaemics<br>corticosteroids<br>oral contraceptives | antihistamines<br>amantadine<br>aminophylline<br>anthraquinone laxatives<br>phenolphthalein<br>cimetidine<br>propantheline<br>ranitidine<br>sulphasalazine<br>theophylline |

### Drugs usually considered safe in standard doses

| | | |
| --- | --- | --- |
| benzodiazepines<br>phenothiazines<br>sodium valproate<br>tricyclic<br>  antidepressants | progestogens<br>ergometrine<br>insulin | oral bronchodilators<br>metoclopramide<br>sodium cromoglycate<br>vitamins<br>folic acid |

263

Drugs and breast-feeding

# Oral contraceptives

The prevention of conception by the oral use of oestrogen-progestogen hormone products is a highly effective method of fertility control, but it is not free from risks. Oral contraceptives are contraindicated when there is any history of thrombo-embolic disease, recurrent jaundice, liver disease, hyperlipidaemia, mammary and endometrial carcinoma and severe migraine. Side-effects include nausea, headache, weight gain, breast tenderness, depression, hypertension, benign hepatic tumours and reduced menstrual flow, which in some cases may amount to amenorrhoea. Care is necessary in hypertension, obesity, renal disease, varicose veins, asthma and epilepsy. Side-effects are considered to be more likely in women over the age of 35 and in cigarette smokers.

There is some evidence that the incidence of thrombo-embolic disease may be linked with the dose of oestrogen and, in general, those mixed products with a lower oestrogen content, yet which give adequate cycle control for the individual patient, should be used. On the other hand, those products with a higher dose of progestogen tend to reduce menstrual flow and increase weight gain.

Oral contraceptives fall into two groups, the oestrogen-progestogen group and the progestogen-only group. The former appear to act mainly by suppressing ovulation, but they may also influence the endometrium and hinder implantation. These are usually given in doses of one tablet from day 5–25 of the cycle, repeated after an interval of 7 days, but other dosage schemes are also in use. The so-called 'tri-phasic' products contain tablets of varying strengths of each constituent, and are designed to mimic the natural hormone cycle more closely than is possible with fixed dose products.

The progestogen-only products are considered to act by increasing the viscosity of cervical mucus, and so reduce sperm penetration. They are given in single daily doses, to be taken at the same time every day, and treatment must be continuous. Additional protection is necessary for the first 14 days, or if any dose is omitted. In general, they are considered less reliable than the mixed products, and they may cause menstrual irregularities.

Table 40 gives an indication of the range of products available.

| Brand name | Progestogen dose of product |
|---|---|
| **Mixed products containing 50 µg of mestranol** | |
| **Norinyl-1** | norethisterone 1 mg |
| **Ortho-Novin 1/50** | |
| **Mixed products containing 50 µg of ethinyloestradiol** | |
| **Ovran** | levonorgestrel 250 µg |
| **Mixed products containing 35 µg of ethinyloestradiol** | |
| **Brevinor** | norethisterone 500 µg |
| **Cylest** | desogestrel 250 µg |
| **Norimin** | norethisterone 1 mg |
| **Ovysmen** | norethisterone 500 µg |
| **Mixed products containing 30 µg of ethinyloestradiol** | |
| **Eugynon 30** | levonorgestrel 250 µg |
| **Loestrin 30** | norethisterone 1.5 mg |
| **Marvelon** | desogestrel 150 µg |
| **Microgynon 30** | levonorgestrel 150 µg |
| **Minulet** | gestodene 75 mg |
| **Ovran 30** | levonorgestrel 250 µg |
| **Ovranette** | levonorgestrel 150 µg |

Table 40  Oral contraceptives. Continued over.

265

Oral contraceptives

| Brand name | Progestogen dose of product |
|---|---|
| **Mixed products containing 20 μg of ethinyloestradiol** | |
| **Loestrin 20** | **norethisterone 1 mg** |
| **Mercilon** | **desogestrel 150 mg** |

Note: Logynon, Logynon ED, Binovum, Synaphase, Triadine, Triminulet, Trinordiol and TriNovum are mixed products containing tablets of different strengths of ethinyloestradiol and progestogen designed to give a phased hormonal effect.

| Progestogen-only products | |
|---|---|
| **Femulen** | **ethynodiol 500 μg** |
| **Micronor** | **norethisterone 350 μg** |
| **Microval** | **levonorgestrel 30 μg** |
| **Neogest** | **norgesterel 75 μg** |
| **Norgeston** | **levonorgestrel 30 μg** |
| **Noriday** | **norethisterone 350 μg** |

Note: Depo-Provera is an injectable product containing medroxyprogesterone. A dose of 150 mg by deep intra-muscular injection during the first 5 days of the cycle, repeated after 3 months, has also been used as a contraceptive. Similarly, norethisterone oenanthate 200 mg (Noristerat) may be given by deep intramuscular injection during the first 5 days of the cycle, and repeated once after 8 weeks.

Post-coital contraception has been obtained by the early administration of large doses of oestrogens, such as stilboestrol, in doses of 25 mg twice a day for 5 days. Mixed products containing levonorgestrel 250 μg and ethinyloestradiol 50 μg (Schering PC4; Ovran; Eugynon 50) are now preferred, and treatment should be commenced within 72 hrs, followed by a second dose 12 hrs later. The risk of vomiting can be reduced by giving an antiemetic such as prochlorperazine.

# Weights and measures

### Metric system

nanogram (ng) or 0.001 µg

microgram (mcg or µg) or 0.001 mg

milligram (mg) or 0.001 g

centigram (cg) or 0.01 g

decigram (dg) or 0.1 g

gram (g) = 1000 mg

(in prescriptions the abbreviation 'G' was formerly used, but is now obsolete.)

kilogram (kg) 1000 g

The metric measures of capacity which the nurse is likely to meet are the

millilitre (ml) which is approximately equal to the cubic centimetre (cc)

litre (l) = 1000 ml

# Abbreviations used in prescriptions

The use of Latin abbreviations in prescription-writing is no longer recommended; the directions for use should be written in English, and in full. The use of some time-hallowed abbreviations still persist, and the following list is a selection of those terms that may be met with occasionally.

*a.c. anti cibum*    before food
*aq. aqua*    water
*b.d. bis die*    twice a day
*c. cum*    with
*et*    and
*mitt. mitte*    send
*o.n. omni nocte*    every night
*p.c. post cibum*    after food
*p.r.n. pr re nata*    occasionally
*q.d. quater die*    4 times a day
*q.q.h. quarta quaque hora*    every 4 hours
*q.s. quantum sufficiat*    sufficient
*s.o.s. si opus sit*    when necessary
*stat. statim*    at once
*t.d.s. ter die sumendus*    to be taken 3 times a day
*t.i.d. ter in die*    3 times a day
*ung. unguentum*    ointment

**Notes:** The abbreviations s.c., i.m. and i.v. refer to subcutaneous, intramuscular and intravenous injections. It is usually made clear when a drug must be given by *slow* i.v. *infusion*.

The doses of a few drugs are based on the skin area of the body expressed as square metres, abbreviated to $m^2$.